Quality and Patient Safety in Medical Imaging

Jie Zhang
Editor

Quality and Patient Safety in Medical Imaging

A Modality-Based Approach

Springer

Editor
Jie Zhang
Department of Radiology
University of Kentucky
Lexington, KY, USA

ISBN 978-3-031-89006-2 ISBN 978-3-031-89007-9 (eBook)
https://doi.org/10.1007/978-3-031-89007-9

This Springer imprint is published by the registered company Springer Nature Switzerland AG
The registered company address is: Gewerbestrasse 11, 6330 Cham, Switzerland

Preface

Medical imaging technologies have become indispensable tools in the diagnosis and treatment of patients. Over the past few decades, the number of diagnostic imaging procedures has increased significantly, driven by continuous advancements in imaging technology. While these innovations have greatly enhanced diagnostic capabilities and patient outcomes, they have also underscored the critical need for maintaining high image quality and ensuring patient safety.

Given the broad scope of quality and patient safety in medical imaging, this book adopts a modality-based approach, focusing on imaging technologies commonly used in clinical practice. It covers radiography, fluoroscopy, computed tomography, dental imaging, bone densitometry, magnetic resonance imaging, ultrasound, breast imaging, and nuclear medicine.

This book is structured into nine chapters, authored by clinical medical physicists, radiologists, and/or radiology residents. Each provides a broad overview of fundamental principles, intrinsic safety considerations, quality control measures, and ongoing efforts to enhance imaging quality and safety. Comprehensive references are included to guide readers toward further resources on quality assurance and patient safety specific to each modality.

While this book does not aim to comprehensively cover every detail of these imaging modalities, it strives to address major topics and offer relevant references for further exploration. We hope this resource will serve as a concise yet essential guide to modality-specific quality and safety issues. However, broader quality and safety considerations—such as informatics and communication challenges that extend beyond imaging equipment—are not covered in this book.

This book is designed as a practical handbook for radiologists, medical physicists, radiologic technologists, healthcare professionals, researchers, and the public seeking to understand and implement best practices in medical imaging. Whether used as a reference for clinical practice, quality assurance programs, or academic study, this resource aims to contribute to the ongoing advancement of safe and high-quality imaging in healthcare.

We are grateful for the many valuable and constructive suggestions received during the preparation of this edition, but the opinions and conclusions expressed remain entirely those of the authors.

Lexington, KY, USA Jie Zhang

Contents

Contributors

Adrian Dawkins Department of Radiology, University of Kentucky, Lexington, KY, USA

Gary Ge Department of Radiology, University of Kentucky, Lexington, KY, USA

Nanditha George Department of Radiology, University of Kentucky, Lexington, KY, USA

Blaine T. Mischen Department of Radiology, University of Kentucky, Lexington, KY, USA

M. Elizabeth Oates Department of Radiology, University of Kentucky, Lexington, KY, USA

Brent Pressman Department of Radiology, University of Kentucky, Lexington, KY, USA

William F. Sensakovic Department of Radiology, Mayo Clinic, Phoenix, AZ, USA
Telerad Physics Teaching, LLC, Phoenix, AZ, USA

Margaret Szabunio Department of Radiology, University of Kentucky, Lexington, KY, USA

Xiaoqin Wang Department of Radiology, University of Kentucky, Lexington, KY, USA

Victor J. Weir Department of Veterans Affairs, Central Virginia VA Healthcare Systems (CVHCS), Richmond VA Medical Center, Richmond, VA, USA

Jie Zhang Department of Radiology, University of Kentucky, Lexington, KY, USA

Yifang Jimmy Zhou Department of Imaging, Cedars-Sinai Medical Center, Los Angeles, CA, USA

Radiography

1

Gary Ge, Victor J. Weir, and Jie Zhang

Introduction

Radiography was the first medical imaging technique developed following the discovery of x-rays on November 8, 1895 by the physicist Wilhelm Roentgen. By using the physical properties of x-rays, an image can be generated to display regions of varying density and composition.

Radiographic systems play a vital role in any radiology department due to their ease of use and availability in various configurations, including portable units [1–3]. While radiographic imaging may not provide the same level of detail as CT or MRI, its speed and simplicity make it indispensable across a wide range of medical imaging applications. These applications include, but not limited to, the evaluation of pulmonary diseases (e.g., edema, emphysema, and cancer), cardiovascular disorders, gastrointestinal disease, and musculoskeletal evaluations [4].

This chapter covers key aspects of patient safety and quality in radiography, including the fundamental principles of digital radiographic systems, common technologies and techniques for minimizing patient radiation exposure while maintaining diagnostic quality, quality control, relevant regulations, and ongoing efforts aimed at improving quality and patient safety in radiographic imaging.

Fundamental Principles of Radiography

Figure 1.1 shows a typical in-room radiography system and a mobile radiography unit. An x-ray tube generates x-rays by accelerating an electron beam at a tungsten target within x-ray tube, producing both Bremsstrahlung and characteristic x-rays. The x-rays are collimated into a beam that passes through the patient and is subsequently detected by an x-ray detector. As the x-ray beam interacts with the patient's anatomy, some portions of the beam are absorbed depending on tissue density and composition, creating the necessary contrast to visualize internal structures. This absorption process, while essential for producing diagnostic images, also exposes the patient to radiation. The final output is a 2D image representing internal ana-

G. Ge (✉) · J. Zhang
Department of Radiology, University of Kentucky, Lexington, KY, USA
e-mail: gyge222@uky.edu; jnzh222@uky.edu

V. J. Weir
Department of Veterans Affairs, Central Virginia VA Healthcare Systems (CVHCS), Richmond VA Medical Center, Richmond, VA, USA
e-mail: victor.weir@va.gov

J. Zhang (ed.), *Quality and Patient Safety in Medical Imaging*,
https://doi.org/10.1007/978-3-031-89007-9_1

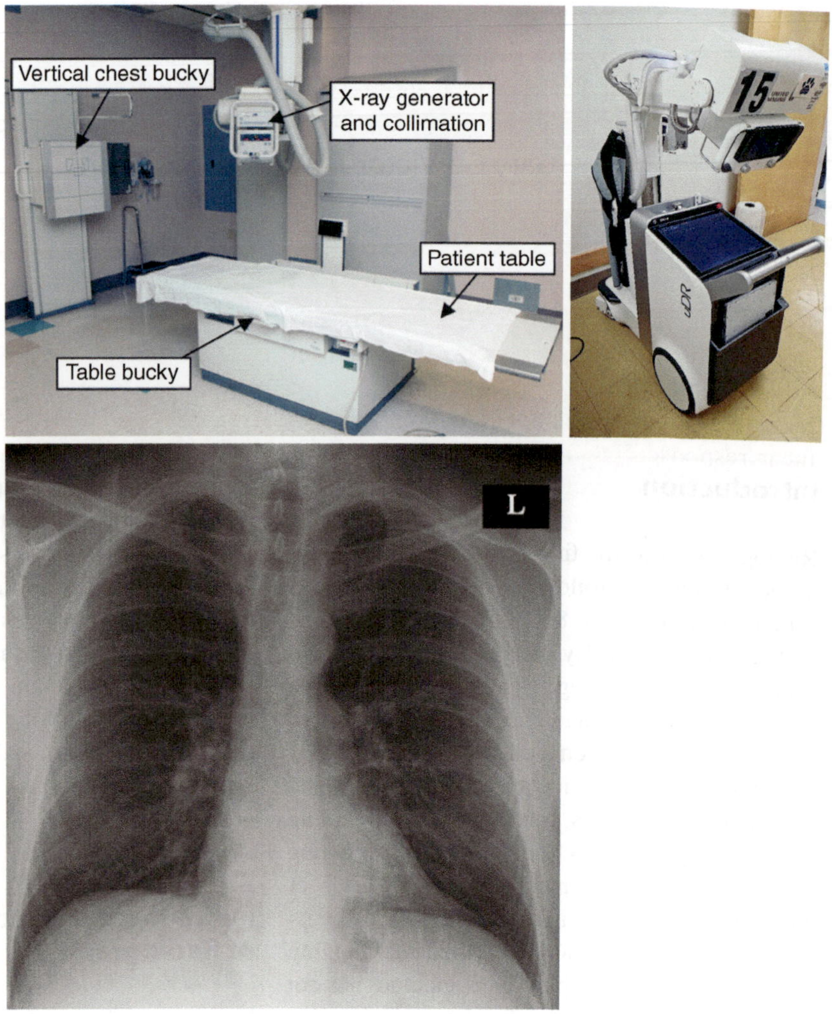

Fig. 1.1 A typical radiographic imaging system, mobile radiographic unit, and an example of anterior-posterior (AP) chest image

tomical structures superimposed on one another. Figure 1.2 provides a diagram illustrating this imaging process.

A primary distinguishing feature of radiographic units is the type of detector. Screen-film radiography, which relies on physical film to record x-ray images, was widely used in the past but has been replaced by modern digital detectors [5]. Digital detectors fall into two main categories, computed radiography (CR) and digital radiography (DR). CR uses a similar technique to screen-film radiography, except the photostimulable phosphor detec-

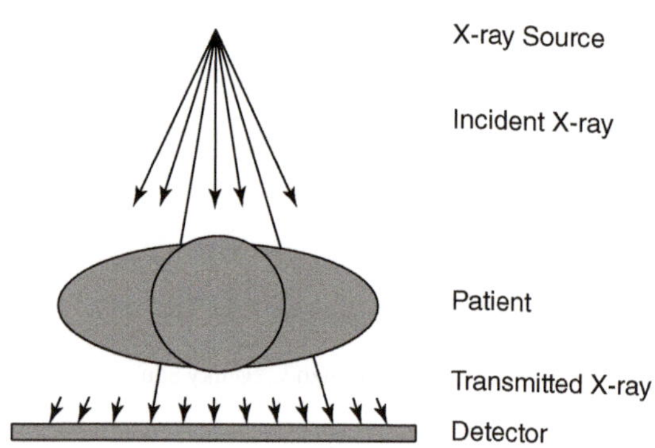

Fig. 1.2 A diagram showing how the x-rays travel from the x-ray source, through the patient, to the detector

tor that is used in CR is in a reusable cassette configuration [6]. DR is classified into indirect DR and direct DR. Indirect DR uses an amorphous silicon (a-Si) detector combined with a scintillator to convert x-rays to light photons, which are then transformed into electric charges and displayed visually. Direct DR employs an amorphous selenium (a-Se) flat panel detector to directly convert x-rays into electric charge, enabling immediate image display [7]. Analog detectors such as screen film and CR exhibit a sigmoidal response to radiation, while digital detectors (i.e., DR) exhibit a linear response. The linear response provides a much wider dynamic range, enabling better contrast resolution and reducing the impact of improper exposure factors [8]. DR's advantages include enhanced contrast resolution, expanded dynamic range, and minimized user errors due to automatic exposure correction. Post-processing techniques allow over- and underexposures to be adjusted to an acceptable quality level. Many digital detectors are also portable and able to be swapped and moved freely between different imaging equipment configurations from the same manufacturer, reducing the effect on clinic workflow in the case of detector failure.

Detectors often incorporate an additional component, the grid. The grid consists of a fine lattice of highly attenuating material, typically lead. This structure works to reduce scattered x-rays and improve image contrast. However, the grid also absorbs a portion of the primary x-ray beam which requires increased exposure to maintain image quality [9]. Improper grid alignment can result in reduced image contrast, making certain examination situations especially difficult to align properly, such as bedside portable examinations. Recent advances in post-processing algorithms have introduced techniques (e.g., Virtual Grid from Fujifilm) to achieve the noise reduction that grids provide, offering an alternative that sidesteps the disadvantages associated with physical grids [10]. These methods use model-based estimation of the scatter radiation and grid effect to improve image quality and reduce patient exposure.

Safety Concerns

Radiation Exposure

The inevitable issue associated with x-ray imaging techniques is radiation exposure. Compared to higher exposure imaging procedures, such as fluoroscopic interventional procedures and CT examinations, the radiation risk to patients during routine radiographic procedures is relatively low.

For various diagnostic radiography procedures, average effective doses for adults range from 0.001 mSv (e.g., extremities) to 6 mSv (e.g., barium enema). Two of the most common radiography examinations, an abdominal study and chest study will be 0.6 mSv and 0.1 mSv, respectively [2, 3]. As a point of comparison, the annual background radiation received by the general public from natural sources (not including medical or occupational exposure) is approximately 3 mSv [3].

Technique-Related Factors Impacting Patient Safety

Imaging technique plays a critical role in determining both the quality of radiographic images and the amount of radiation a patient receives during an examination. Key aspects of proper imaging technique include exposure control, beam quality, beam collimation, and patient positioning.

Exposure factor selection is particularly important in modern radiographic imaging due to the widespread adoption of digital detectors. This is primarily determined by the mAs setting used during image acquisition. In digital radiography, variations in exposure factor selection are automatically compensated by post-processing algorithms, ensuring a consistent image quality. However, this compensation can obscure inappropriately high or low exposures until the adjustment range is exceeded. This contrasts with conventional screen film imaging where underexposure results in a too-white film, and overexposure produces a too-black film, making exposure errors visually obvious. In digital radiography, underexposure creates noisy images, while both proper exposure and overexposure produce images with minimal noise, often preferred by radiologists. The brightness or darkness of digital images appear to depend mainly on post-processing parameters, not on actual acquisition technique. As a result, there is no direct visual indication of exposure level used, potentially leading to systematic overexpose, a phenomenon commonly referred to as "dose creep" [11, 12].

Dose creep can occur gradually if appropriate preventive measures are not in place. Many modern radiography machines provide an exposure indicator accessible to the technologist performing the examination. Dose area product (DAP), typically measured in units of uGy*m^2, is a common exposure metric displayed during planar x-ray examination, including radiography and fluoroscopy.

Automatic exposure control (AEC) is an effective tool for reducing patient radiation exposure and mitigating dose creep. AEC uses sensors in the radiograph detectors to measure incoming radiation levels and determine appropriate image exposure. Once the sensor detects a sufficient amount of radiation to produce a diagnostic quality image, the x-ray beam is automatically turned off. This process helps standardize the SNR between acquisitions of a given protocol, regardless of patient size, reducing reliance on technologists monitoring other exposure indications. However, AEC effectiveness depends on proper patient positioning and accurate alignment of the targeted anatomical region with the imaging detector. Incorrect alignment can result in increased radiation exposure compared to manual protocol, highlighting the importance of thorough training for technologists using AEC.

Proper patient setup is as crucial as selecting appropriate acquisition parameters such as kV and mAs. Correct patient positioning can significantly reduce radiation exposure to noncritical and/or radiosensitive organs. For example, positioning a female patient for a chest x-ray in a posterior-anterior (PA) orientation—facing away from the x-ray tube—can lower breast dose compared to the conventional anterior-posterior (AP) position. Incorrect patient positioning can lead to unusable images, often requiring repeat examinations and exposing the patient to additional, unnecessary radiation exposure. To prevent this, technologists should ensure accurate alignment of the targeted anatomy and remove any potential obstructions from the field of view (FOV).

Radiographic systems are equipped with collimators that adjust the size of the x-ray beam, allowing technologists to limit the beam to only the area of interest. Proper alignment of radiographic units is essential to minimize radiation exposure. During a patient preparation, the technologist should carefully adjust the collimator to cover only the necessary anatomical region. This practice reduces both patient radiation exposure and scatter radiation reaching the detector, thereby decreasing image noise. Although digital radiography offers post-processing tools such as cropping to remove unnecessary portions of an acquired image, this feature does not reduce patient radiation exposure. Proper collimation should always be performed during image acquisition. Poor-processing tools can help avoid repeat examinations in certain cases but should not be relied upon as a standard practice.

Manufacturers also implement various tools and technologies to reduce radiation exposure. One critical approach is the beam filter. Beam filters, typically made of aluminum or copper, are positioned at the x-ray output port. They absorb low-energy photons that would otherwise be absorbed by the patient without contributing meaningfully to the image [13]. By removing these low-energy photons, beam filters help lower the patient's radiation dose.

In addition, radiographic units report various metrics that provides information about patient radiation exposure. Dose area product (DAP), entrance skin exposure (ESE), and air kerma (AKR) are examples of metrics that provide an estimation of patient radiation exposure. There are other metrics, such as dose index (DI) and exposure index (EI), that do not measure patient exposure but instead serve as indicators

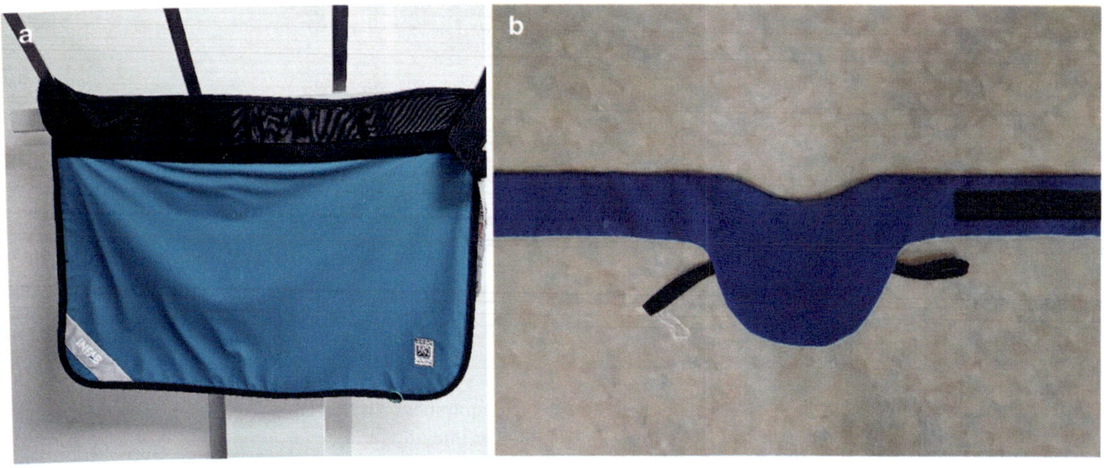

Fig. 1.3 A variety of personal shielding options including (**a**) a lead apron and (**b**) a lead thyroid shield

for whether the technique used to acquire the image was appropriate. Another valuable reference tool is the use of diagnostic reference levels (DRLs), which compile average dose data to establish baseline values for optimizing radiation safety [14].

Patient Shielding

In the past, patients had the option to wear leaded personal protective equipment, such as lead aprons, during image acquisition as a means to reduce radiation exposure [15]. Figure 1.3 shows a variety of personal shielding options. However, since 2019, industry and regulatory guidelines recommended against the use of routine gonadal shielding during abdominal or pelvic radiographic examinations [16–19]. There are several reasons for this, including:

- Risk of stochastic effects is lower than previously estimated.
- Modern imaging technology has significantly reduced patient radiation dose.
- Shielding equipment can interfere with AEC or obscure findings.
- External shielding does not mitigate patient dose resulting from internal scatter radiation.

Even in specific patient circumstances, such as pregnancy, best practices dictate tight collimation of the x-ray beam to limit the area of exposure to what is necessary.

Repeat Examinations

An important aspect of patient safety management deals with repeat examination analysis. Images can be retaken by technologists if the initial image was of insufficient diagnostic quality [20]. This ensures a higher-quality image for diagnostic interpretation but also increases the radiation the patient receives during their examination. There are many different reasons for a repeat examination [21].

- Artifacts
- Mispositioning
- Over-collimation
- Patient motion.
- Double exposure
- Inadequate inspiration
- Overexposed—*high exposure index*
- Underexposed—*low exposure index*
- Marker missing or wrong
- Wrong examination

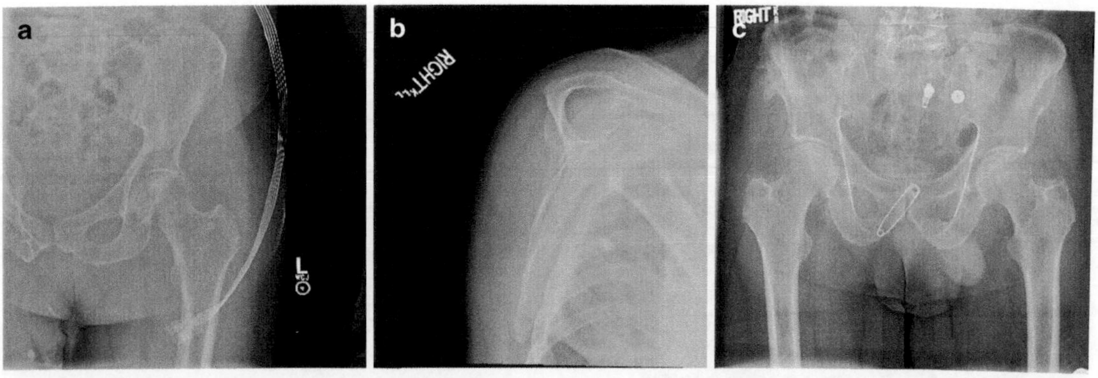

Fig. 1.4 Examples of rejected images that include (**a**) misplaced equipment (in this case a wire), (**b**) improper technique with too low of kVp, and (**c**) patient's clothing is present in the imaging field

- Wrong patient
- Lost image

With film-based radiography techniques, the primary cause of rejected images was due to improper exposure; however, with modern digital radiography, the primary reason for rejected images has become improper patient positioning [22]. Figure 1.4 shows some examples of rejected images. These situations often result in a repeat examination due to a loss of diagnostic information. From a safety standpoint, the priority is to reduce the number of repeat examinations to avoid exposing the patient to unnecessary radiation. Many modern digital radiography machines have the ability to keep track of repeat examinations; however, this requires active participation by the imaging technologist to provide accurate information. As such, technologists should be made aware of any features that allow repeat analysis during training and be encouraged to use them appropriately. When used properly, the repeat analysis data can be collected at regular intervals to determine what the most common reasons for repeat examinations are. This information can be useful in identifying potential areas of future training as well as providing insight into potential issues in the imaging workflow that may cause systemic errors [23, 24].

Radiation Monitoring

Many hospitals and healthcare systems have incorporated radiation monitoring systems. These software systems are integrated into the wider healthcare information infrastructure, typically interfacing with systems such as the picture archiving and communication system (PACS) and electronic health record (EHR) systems. They collect and catalogue many useful metrics about a healthcare system's practice, one of the most important being radiation dose information. Since the dose information is collected alongside all radiological acquisitions, radiation doses can be monitored at a system-wide level. This includes the monitoring of individual patients to ensure the prevention of potential radiation-induced injuries, the monitoring of imaging protocols to track usage and compliance with correct clinical technique, and identification of unnecessary examinations.

Quality Concerns

Quality Assurance Program

The quality assurance (QA) program is designed by the management to ensure the consistent quality of a product or service. It includes, but not limited to, customer feedback, employee empowerment, and quality control (QC). QC involves specific actions aimed at maintaining measurable aspects of a process within defined limits. These actions typically involve monitoring a process variable, comparing the measured value against a specific threshold, and taking corrective action if the threshold is exceeded [25–27].

The goal of an effective QC program is to ensure proper equipment performance to obtain high-quality images consistently while keeping patient radiation dose as low as reasonably achievable (ALARA). The periodic QC tests should be comprehensive and capable of detecting common system problems, while keeping them simple to implement and easy to maintain. An overambitious QC program, in terms of complexity or frequency of testing, may cease to be implemented at all.

Quality Control in Radiography

QC tests for radiographic systems require daily, weekly, monthly, quarterly, semiannual, and annual efforts [25, 28–32]. Since digital radiography eliminates the need for darkrooms, film, processing chemicals, and related waste management, QC efforts concentrate on the performance of imaging equipment and image processing systems. Essential QC tasks include:

- X-ray tube assessment.
- Collimation and beam alignment.
- Linearity of exposure.
- Spatial resolution (focal spot): Compared to a screen-film system, digital radiography has lower spatial resolution. Therefore, spatial resolution should be monitored more often than a screen-film system.

These QC measures are critical for maintaining high-quality diagnostic imaging while minimizing radiation exposure to patients and staff [33–36].

- X-ray tube assessment
- Collimation and beam alignment
- Linearity of exposure
- Spatial resolution (focal spot)

A typical annual survey of a digital radiography includes the following tests [37]:

1. Radiographic Unit Assembly Evaluation

   Radiographic unit assembly evaluation is performed to check if the unit is mechanically stable, and all moving parts move smoothly without obstruction to motion. All locks and detents (a mechanism that tends to stop a moving part in a specific location) should work properly. Image receptor holder assembly should be free from vibrations and held securely by assembly in any orientation. Image receptor should slide smoothly into holder assembly. Patient or operator should not be exposed to sharp or rough edges or other hazards. Operator technique control charts should be available in case the AEC fails. The operator should be protected during exposure by adequate radiation shielding. The exposure switch should be placed and secured in control booth to prevent the operator from taking exposures outside the control booth.
2. Collimation Assessment

   Collimation assessment is performed to check the source to image detector (SID) indicators. The consistency between indicated SID and actual SID should be verified. Deviation between x-ray field and light field as well as deviation between x-ray field and image receptor should also be verified. In general, numerical SID indicator should be accurate within 2% of measured SID. Deviation between x-ray field and light field and image receptor should be less than 2% of SID.
3. Radiographic Generator Assessment

   Radiographic generator assessment includes timer accuracy, radiation output with different kVp settings, radiation output reproducibility, x-ray beam quality (half-value layer), and exposure linearity. The accuracy and reproducibility of the timer stations on diagnostic x-ray equipment are important because they directly affect the mAs (milliampere-second) and hence the amount of radiation emitted. For a typical radiographic system, timer accuracy should be within 5%, x-ray output coefficient of variation should be less than 2%, exposure linearity should be less than 10%, and half-value layer should exceed the specified minimum values of Al filtration at different x-ray tube voltages.

4. kVp Accuracy and Reproducibility

   This test measures the peak electrical potential across the x-ray tube during operation. The accuracy of the x-ray tube kVp is critical since it affects both the intensity and quality of the x-rays reaching the image receptor. Inaccurate KV selections can have detrimental effects not only on image quality but on patient dose. The measured kVp should be within ±5% of the set value. The kVp coefficient of variation should be less than 2%.

5. Automatic Exposure Control (AEC) System Performance

   Automatic exposure control (phototiming and limiting circuits) terminates the exposure when a preset quantity of radiation has been detected. Part of AEC performance testing ensures the backup timer is properly set and functioning correctly. AEC is used to assure consistent radiographic images over a broad range of patient thicknesses. It tests if phototimer compensation for kVp and patient thickness is adequate.

6. Skin Entrance Exposure and Dose

   A table of skin entrance exposure limits is constructed and included in the annual physics report as a guide for the facility. These include regulatory limits and calculated entrance exposures, based on the machine parameters, for an average-sized adult patient. This table is checked every year to verify that the posted techniques result in patient entrance exposures that are in accordance with regulatory limits. This also can detect any dose creep in the facilities techniques.

7. Conventional Tomographic System Evaluation, if Applicable

   In radiography, a conventional tomographic function, if present, allows relative motions of the tube, patient, and detector to acquire an image that blurs all image planes of the object except the plane of interest. The evaluation of a conventional tomographic system ensures that slice thickness, positioning, and resolution are acceptable.

Radiographic Imaging Protocols

One of the main tools to maintain consistent image quality across an entire healthcare system is the implementation of standardized imaging protocols. These protocols establish baseline exposure settings for specific examination, ensuing consistent image quality and facilitating efficient examination indexing throughout the radiology department. Imaging protocols are typically configured when an imaging center is first established and are regularly reviewed and updated as new technologies, techniques, or recommendations emerge. National organizations, such as the American College of Radiology (ACR) and American Association of Physics in Medicine (AAPM), provide recommendations and best practice to guide healthcare systems in developing and maintaining standard radiographic protocols. In addition, manufacturer-provided default protocols along with radiographic can serve as a useful starting point for customization to meet specific clinical needs. The primary objectives of radiographic protocols are to ensure diagnostic image quality while minimizing patient dose. This requires optimization of exposure settings and collimation to ensure accurate and safe imaging.

An important exposure parameter to optimize for is kV. The kV setting determines the penetrating power of the x-ray beam and should be adjusted based on the anatomical region being imaged. Proper kV selection should be carefully considered before imaging to prevent suboptimal image quality and reduce the need for repeat examination [38]. Incorrect kV selection can negatively impact image contrast and diagnostic quality. For example, although higher-energy x-rays are more penetrating than low energy x-rays, using 100 kV instead of the typical 80 kV

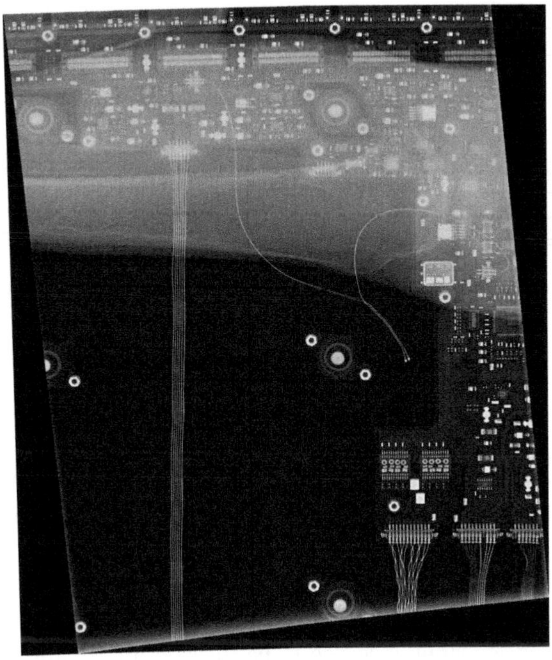

Fig. 1.5 A radiograph of a patient's leg that was improperly positioned over electronics embedded in the patient table

for an abdominal radiograph will result in reduced image contrast, making anatomical details harder to distinguish.

Another aspect of radiographic imaging that is important for image quality is x-ray beam alignment and collimation. Improper beam alignment can reduce the efficiency of the detector and produce nonuniform images if the beam is off-axis, decreasing diagnostic quality. Similarly, images that are tightly collimated to only what is necessary contain less noise from scatter, improving image quality. An improperly setup exposure, such as in Fig. 1.5, is detrimental to image quality and can lead to repeated imaging.

Basic Post-processing Techniques

Digital radiography provides significant flexibility through post-processing, enabling adjusting image quality after acquisition. Common techniques include image resizing, pixel intensity mapping, and spatial enhancement [39, 40].

Image resizing involves adjusting the image's dimensions or orientation. Techniques such as nearest-neighbor and bilinear interpolation are commonly used, while more advanced methods such as convolution-based cubic interpolation offer better scaling. Machine learning–based super resolution has emerged as a cutting-edge method, improving upscaling accuracy through trained models [41].

Pixel intensity mapping adjusts image brightness and contrast through a look-up table (LUT), modifying pixel intensity values. In clinical imaging, adjustments such as window level (WL) and window width (WW) are used for this purpose. S-shaped LUTs, designed to mimic film-based imaging, enhance a contrast with the volume of interest (VOI).

Spatial enhancement techniques improve spatial details through filters and algorithms. Common applications include noise reduction and edge enhancement, crucial for highlighting anatomical features while minimizing image artifacts.

These basic post-processing methods help optimize diagnostic quality while potentially reducing the need for retakes.

Advanced Post-processing Techniques

Advanced post-processing techniques enhance diagnostic accuracy by highlighting relevant visual information while minimizing superimposed structures. In digital radiography, challenges such as overlapping anatomical features, i.e., the ribcage in lung imaging, are addressed using techniques such as dual-energy subtraction.

Dual-energy subtraction exploits energy-dependent attenuation differences between bone and soft tissue [42]. Two x-ray acquisitions are taken at low (~60 kV) and high (~120 kV) energies. Since soft tissue attenuation changes less than that of bone, weighted scaling and subtraction isolate specific structures. While effective, this method requires two separate acquisitions or specialized "one-shot" systems to avoid motion artifacts [43].

Multifrequency processing (MFP) or multiscale processing enhance spatial and frequency features using Laplace segmentation, dividing images into spatial-frequency ranges for independent processing [9, 44]. Early implementations required manual adjustments, but modern version use automated algorithms, improving efficiency and clinic workflow. Machine learning–driven MFP is expected to further optimize task-specific imaging.

Computer-aided diagnosis (CAD) supports clinicians by identifying potential abnormalities [45, 46]. Some examples of techniques are temporal subtraction, image segmentation, and automated lesion detection.

Image Artifacts

Artifacts in radiography can significantly reduce diagnostic quality of images and impact patient safety when images require repeating. Image artifacts in radiography can be attributed to a variety of sources, including patient motion, detector errors, and device miscalibration [47–50]. Some common examples of artifacts are as follows:

- Patient motion
- Metal objects on patient (e.g., jewelry, clothing, medical devices)
- Detector ghosting/lag
- Dead pixels
- Backscatter
- Grid-line suppression failure

Because artifacts indicate improper patient preparation, positioning, and/or equipment malfunction, their appearance typically indicates that the patient must be reimaged, thus increasing their radiation dose.

Ongoing Efforts to Improve Quality and Patient Safety

Organizational Efforts

Professional organizations such as the AAPM, ACR, and the Radiological Society of North America (RSNA) all help provide up-to-date guidance on imaging technologies and best practices. In regard to radiographic imaging, AAPM has released multiple task group reports in the past that provide recommendations to ensure proper device functionality. The most recently published report specifically covering radiographic imaging is Task Group Report 151, which covers quality control in digital radiography [26]. Another relevant report is Task Group Report 305, which proposes a methodology to standardize reject analysis across different vendors [24]. The ACR has provided continued guidance on the appropriate usage of radiography in a clinical setting, having published many reports and practice parameters that are concerned with general radiography and the criteria for appropriate use in situations concerning at-risk populations, such as pregnant or pediatric patients. The RSNA serves as a major bridge between clinical settings and industry partners, helping to showcase new technologies and providing platforms for academic research to be discussed regarding these efforts.

The Image Gently campaign was launched in 2008 by the Alliance for Radiation Safety in Pediatric Imaging, with the ultimate goal to change practice by increasing awareness of the opportunities to promote radiation protection in the imaging of children [51]. The alliance represents a wide spectrum of health care providers whose roles relate to medical imaging, including four founding organizations, the Society for Pediatric Radiology (SPR), the American Society of Radiologic Technologists (ASRT), the ACR, and AAPM, as well as over 100 supporting groups representing equipment manufacturers, governmental agencies, and multiple international societies. These groups work together to improve pediatric patient care through medical imaging while controlling patient exposure to ionizing radiation. The Image Gently campaign includes all x-ray imaging modalities, such as CT, dental, DR, fluoroscopy, and interventional radiology, and provides essential information for radiologists, medical physicists, referring physicians, parents, and industry.

Similarly, the Image Wisely campaign concerns radiation safety in adult medical imaging [52]. It was created by the Joint Task Force on Adult

Radiation Protection, with the members consisting of the ACR, Radiological Society of North America (RSNA), AAPM, and ASRT. The Image Wisely campaign strives to lower the amount of radiation used in medically necessary imaging studies and to eliminate unnecessary procedures.

Industry Efforts

The technologies developed by industry are constantly evolving, incorporating new ideas and innovations to improve image quality. Current efforts by major industry vendors have increasingly focused on AI integration into the clinical workflow in a variety of different ways. Most commonly, it is introduced into post-processing procedures, leveraging advanced image processing techniques to extract more information from imaging than can be seen based on the initial image to improve diagnosis. Examples include temporal subtraction, image segmentation, and classification [43, 53]. AI-driven methods to improve image quality have also been developed. Super-resolution techniques upscale low-resolution images to high-resolution images, capable of providing additional detail without the need for additional imaging [54]. Deep learning–based denoising techniques remove image noise from radiographic images, which may allow low-dose images to achieve diagnostic quality [55, 56]. Machine learning has enabled virtual dual-energy subtraction, generating synthetic low-energy image from high-energy inputs, eliminating extra exposures [57]. AI integration does not only occur during image processing, it can also help improve clinical workflow. Ongoing research seeks to integrate AI models into preliminary screening workflows, supporting faster clinical decision-making [58].

Industry efforts do not solely focus on AI, as there have been advances made in the physical technologies as well. One such example is dynamic digital radiography (DDR), a technique that enables a radiographic unit to acquire images in rapid succession, similar to fluoroscopic units. This allows radiographic units to visualize the movement of patient anatomy, increasing the range of clinical applications that radiography can be used for. However, this technique has the potential to increase the exposure to patients and should be managed carefully [59].

Resources for Quality and Safety

Table 1.1 provides a summary of resources (e.g., QC recommendations, safety guidelines) for quality and safety specifically for radiographic imaging. The goal of this table is to facilitate quick access to those resources for readers.

Table 1.1 Resources for quality and patient safety

AAPM Report No. 4: Basic Quality Control in Diagnostic Radiology
AAPM Report No. 14: Performance Specifications and Acceptance Testing for X-Ray Generators and Automatic Exposure Control Devices
AAPM Report No. 15: Performance Evaluation and Quality Assurance in Digital Subtraction Angiography
AAPM Report No. 25: Protocols for the Radiation Safety Surveys of Diagnostic Radiological Equipment
AAPM Report No. 31: Standardized Methods for Measuring Diagnostic X-Ray Exposures
AAPM Report No. 58: Managing the Use of Fluoroscopy in Medical Institutions
AAPM Report No. 70: Cardiac Catheterization Equipment Performance
AAPM Report No. 93: Acceptance Testing and Quality Control of Photostimulable Storage Phosphor Imaging Systems
AAPM Report No. 116: An Exposure Indicator for Digital Radiography
AAPM Report No. 150: Acceptance Testing and Quality Control of Digital Radiographic Imaging Systems
AAPM Report No. 151: Ongoing Quality Control in Digital Radiography: Report of AAPM Imaging Physics Committee Task Group 151

(continued)

Table 1.1 (continued)

AAPM Report No. 232: Current State of Practice Regarding Digital Radiography Exposure Indicators and Deviation Indices: Report of AAPM Imaging Physics Committee Task Group 232
AAPM Report No. 305: Guidance for Standardization of Vendor-Neutral Reject Analysis in Radiography
ACR-SPR: Practice Parameter for General Radiography
ACR-SPR: Practice Parameter for the Performance of Abdominal Radiography
ACR-SPR: Practice Parameter for Imaging Pregnant or Potentially Pregnant Adolescents and Women With Ionizing Radiation
ACR-SPR-STR: Practice Parameter for the Performance of Chest Radiography
ACR-AAPM-SIIM-SPR: Practice Parameter for Digital Radiography
ACR-AAPM: Technical Standard for Diagnostic Medical Physics Performance Monitoring of Radiographic Equipment
CRCPD Publication 01–4: Quality Control Recommendations for Diagnostic Radiography, volume 3: Radiographic or Fluoroscopic Machines
CRCPD Publication No. E-10-2: Computed Radiography (CR) and Digital Radiography (DR) State X-Ray Inspection Protocol
EPA Federal Guidance Report No. 14: Radiation Protection Guidance for Diagnostic and Interventional X-Ray Procedures
FDA 21 CFR 1020: Code of Federal Regulations Title 21, Chapter I, Subchapter J: Radiological Health
NCRP Report No. 099: Quality Assurance for Diagnostic Imaging
NCRP Report No. 102: Medical X-Ray, Electron Beam and Gamma-Ray Protection for Energies Up to 50 MeV (Equipment Design, Performance and Use)
NCRP (2010). Report No. 168: Radiation Dose Management for Fluoroscopically-Guided Interventional Medical Procedures
NCRP Report No. 184: Medical Radiation Exposure of Patients in the United States
NCRP Statement No. 13: Recommendations for Ending Routine Gonadal Shielding During Abdominal and Pelvic Radiography
ICRP Publication 73: Radiological Protection and Safety in Medicine
NEMA: Test Standard for the Measurement of the Image Signal Uniformity of an X-Ray Image Intensifier (XRII) System
NEMA: Test Standard for the Determination of the Visible Entrance Field Size of an X-Ray Image Intensifier (XRII) System
NEMA: Characteristics of and Test Procedures for a Phantom to Benchmark Cardiac Fluoroscopic and Photographic Performance
NEMA: Test Standard for the Determination of the System Contrast Ratio (SCR) and the System Veiling Glare Index (SVGI) of an X-Ray Image Intensifier (XRII) System
NEMA: Test Standard for the Determination of the Radial Image Distortion of an X-Ray Image Intensifier (XRII) System
NEMA: Test Standard for the Determination of the Limiting Spatial Resolution of X-Ray Image Intensifier Systems
NEMA: Measurement of Dimensions and Properties of Focal Spots of Diagnostic X-Ray Tubes

AAPM American Association of Physicists in Medicine, *ACR* American College of Radiology, *CRCPD* Conference of Radiation Control Program Directors, *EPA* US Environmental Protection Agency, *FDA* US Food and Drug Administration, *ICRP* International Commission on Radiological Protection, *IEC* International Electrotechnical Commission, *NCRP* National Council on Radiation Protection and Measurements, *NEMA* National Electrical Manufacturers Association, *SIIM* Society for Imaging Informatics in Medicine, *SPR* Society for Pediatric Radiology

Chapter Summary

Radiographic imaging generally results in lower radiation exposure to patients compared to most other x-ray-based imaging techniques. However, it is still essential to take proper steps to minimize patient dose. Proper patient positioning and the use of appropriate imaging techniques are critical for ensuring both patient safety and high-quality diagnostic images. This approach reduces the likelihood of repeat examinations, further limiting radiation exposure. In addition, regular performance monitoring of radiographic imaging systems through a well-maintained QC program ensures optimal system functionality. Such programs contribute to patient safety, diagnostic accuracy, and the overall effectiveness of imaging procedures.

References

1. Bushberg JTS, Anthony J, Leidholdt EM Jr, Boone JM. The essential physics of medical imaging. 4th ed. Wolters Kluwer; 2020.
2. Mettler FA, et al. Patient exposure from radiologic and nuclear medicine procedures in the United States: procedure volume and effective dose for the period 2006–2016. Radiology. 2020;295(2):418–27.
3. Mettler FA Jr, et al. Report no. 184 – medical radiation exposure of patients in the United States. NCRP; 2019.
4. Busch HP. Digital radiography for clinical applications. Eur Radiol. 1997;7:S66–72.
5. Ritenour ER. Physics overview of screen-film radiography. Radiographics. 1996;16(4):903–16.
6. Sonoda M, et al. Computed radiography utilizing scanning laser stimulated luminescence. Radiology. 1983;148(3):833–8.
7. Chotas HG, Dobbins JT, Ravin CE. Principles of digital radiography with large-area, electronically readable detectors: a review of the basics. Radiology. 1999;210(3):595–9.
8. Ou X, et al. Recent development in X-ray imaging technology: future and challenges. Research (Wash D C). 2021;2021:9892152.
9. Lo WY, et al. Multiscale image processing and antiscatter grids in digital radiography. Vet Radiol Ultrasound. 2009;50(6):569–76.
10. Siddique AH, Ge G, Zhang J. Comparative evaluation of image quality between virtual grid and grid portable radiographic systems. Biomed Phys Eng Exp. 2024;10(5)
11. Schaefer-Prokop C, et al. Digital chest radiography: an update on modern technology, dose containment and control of image quality. Eur Radiol. 2008;18(9):1818–30.
12. Uffmann M, Schaefer-Prokop C. Digital radiography: the balance between image quality and required radiation dose. Eur J Radiol. 2009;72(2):202–8.
13. Jadva-Patel H. The use of thin metal filters to reduce dose to patients. Radiogr Today. 1991;57(651):18–22.
14. Mettler FA Jr, et al. Effective doses in radiology and diagnostic nuclear medicine: a Catalog. Radiology. 2008;248(1):254–63.
15. Daniels C, Furey E. The effectiveness of surface Lead shielding of gonads outside the primary X-ray beam. J Med Imaging Radiat Sci. 2008;39(4):189–91.
16. NCRP. Statement no. 13: recommendations for ending routine gonadal shielding during abdominal and pelvic radiography. National Council on Radiation Protection and Measurements; 2021.
17. AAPM. AAPM position statement on the use of patient gonadal and Fetal shielding. American Association of Physicists in Medicine; 2019.
18. Marsh RM, Silosky M. Patient shielding in diagnostic imaging: discontinuing a legacy practice. Am J Roentgenol. 2019;212(4):755–7.
19. Anaskevich L, et al. Reevaluating patient shielding: transitioning practices and perspectives in radiological protection. Radiol Phys Technol. 2024;
20. Nol J, Isouard G, Mirecki J. Digital repeat analysis; setup and operation. J Digit Imaging. 2006;19(2):159.
21. Waaler D, Hofmann B. Image rejects/retakes – radiographic challenges. Radiat Prot Dosim. 2010;139(1–3):375–9.
22. Peer S, et al. Comparative reject analysis in conventional film-screen and digital storage phosphor radiography. Radiat Prot Dosim. 2001;94(1–2):69–71.
23. Tzeng W-S, et al. Managing repeat digital radiography images – a systematic approach and improvement. J Med Syst. 2012;36(4):2697–704.
24. Little K, et al. AAPM task group report 305: guidance for standardization of vendor-neutral reject analysis in radiography. J Appl Clin Med Phys. 2023;24(5):e13938.
25. CRCPD, CRCPD Publication 01–4: Quality control recommendations for diagnostic radiography, volume 3: Radiographic or fluoroscopic machines 2001, Conference of radiation control program directors, Inc.
26. Jones AK, et al. Ongoing quality control in digital radiography: report of AAPM imaging physics committee task group 151. Med Phys. 2015;42(11):6658–70.
27. ACR-AAPM-SIIM-SPR. Practice parameter for digital radiography. American College of Radiology; 2022.
28. AAPM. Report no.4 BASIC QUALITY control in diagnostic radiology. American Association of Physicists in Medicine; 1977.
29. AAPM. Performance specifications and acceptance testing for x-ray generators and automatic exposure control devices. American Association of Physicists in Medicine; 1985.
30. AAPM. Report no. 31: standardized methods for measuring diagnostic x-ray exposures. American Association of Physicists in Medicine; 1990.
31. NCRP, Report no. 099: quality assurance for diagnostic imaging. 1998.
32. AAPM. Report no. 150: acceptance testing and quality control of digital radiographic imaging systems. American Association of Physicists in Medicine; 2024.
33. AAPM. AAPM report #15: performance evaluation and quality assurance in digital subtraction angiogra-

phy. American Association of Physicists in Medicine; 1985.
34. AAPM. AAPM report no. 25: protocols for the radiation safety surveys of diagnostic radiological equipment. American Association of Physicists in Medicine; 1988.
35. AAPM. AAPM report no. 116: an exposure indicator for digital radiography. American Association of Physicists in Medicine; 2009.
36. CRCPD. CRCPD publication no. E-10-2: computed radiography (CR) and digital radiography (DR) state x-ray inspection protocol. Conference of Radiation Control Program Directors; 2010.
37. Performance Standards for Ionizing Radiation Emitting Products, in 21 CFR 1020.31, FDA, Editor. 2005.
38. Bushong SC. Radiologic science for technologists : physics, biology, and protection. Elsevier Mosby: St. Louis; 2013.
39. Armato Iii SG, van Ginneken B. Anniversary paper: image processing and manipulation through the pages ofMedical physics. Med Phys. 2008;35(10):4488–500.
40. Prokop M, Neitzel U, Schaefer-Prokop C. Principles of image processing in digital chest radiography. J Thorac Imaging. 2003;18(3):148–64.
41. Siu WC, Hung KW. Review of image interpolation and super-resolution. In: Proceedings of The 2012 Asia Pacific signal and information processing association annual summit and conference. 2012.
42. Gupta A, et al. Dual energy imaging in cardiothoracic pathologies: a primer for radiologists and clinicians. Eur J Radiol Open. 2021:8.
43. MacMahon H, et al. Dual energy subtraction and temporal subtraction chest radiography. J Thorac Imaging. 2008;23(2):77–85.
44. Notohamiprodjo S, et al. Advances in multiscale image processing and its effects on image quality in skeletal radiography. Sci Rep. 2022;12(1):4726.
45. Doi K. Computer-aided diagnosis in medical imaging: historical review, current status and future potential. Comput Med Imaging Graph. 2007;31(4–5):198–211.
46. Abe H, et al. Computer-aided diagnosis in chest radiology. Semin Ultrasound CT MR. 2004;25(5):432–7.
47. Walz-Flannigan A, et al. Artifacts in digital radiography. Am J Roentgenol. 2012;198(1):156–61.
48. Shetty CM, et al. Computed radiography image artifacts revisited. Am J Roentgenol. 2011;196(1):W37–47.
49. Buckle CE, Udawatta V, Straus CM. Now you see it, now you don't: visual illusions in radiology. Radiographics. 2013;33(7):2087–102.
50. Walz-Flannigan AI, et al. Pictorial review of digital radiography artifacts. Radiographics. 2018;38(3):833–46.
51. The Alliance for Radiation Safety in Pediatric Imaging. ImageGently Web site: http://www.pedrad.org/associations/5364/ig/. [cited 2012 April 3rd].
52. The Image Wisely. http://www.imagewisely.org/. [cited 2012 04/03].
53. Agrawal T, Choudhary P. Segmentation and classification on chest radiography: a systematic survey. Vis Comput. 2023;39(3):875–913.
54. Huang Y, et al. Learn from orientation prior for radiograph super-resolution: orientation operator transformer. Comput Methods Prog Biomed. 2024;245:108000.
55. Sheikh BUH, Zafar A. Removing adversarial noise in X-ray images via total variation minimization and patch-based regularization for robust deep learning-based diagnosis. J Imaging Inform Med. 2024;37(6):3282–303.
56. Feghali JA, et al. New image quality and dose reduction technique for pediatric digital radiography. Diagn Interv Imaging. 2021;102(7–8):463–70.
57. Yamazaki A, et al. Development of artificial intelligence-based dual-energy subtraction for chest radiography. Appl Sci. 2023;13(12):7220.
58. Lee SM, et al. Deep learning applications in chest radiography and computed tomography: current state of the art. J Thorac Imaging. 2019;34(2):75–85.
59. Siddique A, et al. Assessment of radiation dose and shielding efficacy in DDR Versus mobile C-arm and portable X-ray systems. In: Annual meeting of the American Association of Physicists in Medicine. 2024: Los Angeles

Fluoroscopy and Interventional Radiology

2

Victor J. Weir and Gary Ge

Key Points

- Understand fundamental principles of fluoroscopy.
- Know relative risks associated with different fluoroscopy procedures.
- Recognize radiation dose to patients and exposure to staff.
- Quality control.
- Understand dose metrics in fluoroscopy.
- Patient radiation safety program.
- Current efforts to improve quality and patient safety.
- Use of Artificial Intelligence (AI) tools.
- Regulations/Guidelines regarding quality and patient safety.

Introduction

X-ray fluoroscopy is a valuable imaging modality for a wide range of diagnostic and therapeutic applications due to its real-time imaging capability and ease of patient access [1]. However, fluoroscopic procedures can result in significant radiation exposure to patients, making radiation safety a critical concern.

Fluoroscopy encompasses a broad range of procedures and uses various fluoroscopy unit configurations to meet diverse clinical needs. This chapter discusses different types of fluoroscopic procedures and their corresponding fluoroscopy machines, along with the risks associated with patient skin dose and techniques for dose reduction. Quality control measures for fluoroscopy machines, with emphasis on safety and image quality, will be discussed. Relevant regulations and regulatory bodies will be reviewed, with an assessment of their impact on patient dose. The use of AI is also introduced, particularly in interventional radiology (IR) and cardiac catheterization.

Fundamental Principles

Fluoroscopy is a dynamic radiographic imaging technique that acquires x-rays continuously or intermittently to produce images of the internal structures of a patient and is used to guide instruments in real-time during procedures. Similar to radiography, fluoroscopy is also a transmission-based projection imaging modality. A fluoroscopy imaging system consists of a specialized x-ray generator, an x-ray tube, a collimator, an

V. J. Weir
Department of Veterans Affairs, Central Virginia VA Healthcare Systems (CVHCS), Richmond VA Medical Center, Richmond, VA, USA
e-mail: victor.weir@va.gov

G. Ge (✉)
Department of Radiology, University of Kentucky, Lexington, KY, USA
e-mail: gyge222@uky.edu

J. Zhang (ed.), *Quality and Patient Safety in Medical Imaging*,
https://doi.org/10.1007/978-3-031-89007-9_2

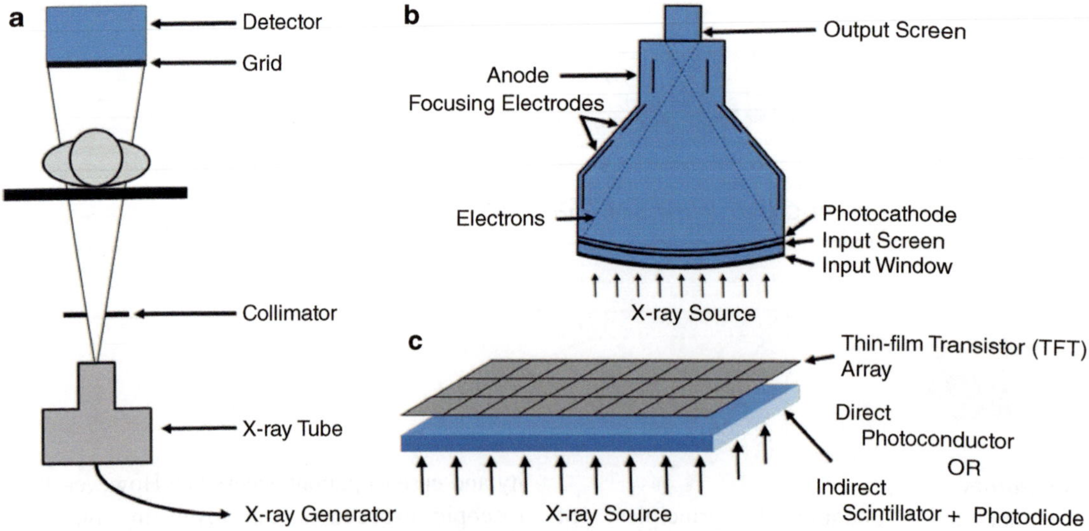

Fig. 2.1 (**a**) A diagram of the imaging chain for an under-table fluoroscopy unit. The detector of a fluoroscopy unit can be an image intensifier or a flat panel digital detector. (**b**) A diagram of an image intensifier. (**c**) A diagram of a flat panel digital detector

anti-scatter grid, and an x-ray detector. These devices are collectively referred to as the "imaging chain" and is shown in Fig. 2.1a. The x-ray detector is an image intensifier (II) on older fluoroscopy units. Flat panel digital detectors have replaced IIs in modern fluoroscopy devices, so the prevalence of II-based units has been decreasing over recent years.

An II consists of a photocathode screen (input screen) which converts x-rays into electrons. A diagram outlining an image intensifier is seen in Fig. 2.1b. Inside the II, electrons from the input screen are sped up by a high voltage and directed by special electrodes toward an anode that is also part of the output screen [2]. The image signal is boosted because the output screen is smaller than the input screen, so the electrons become more concentrated (i.e., minification gain). A second boost occurs when these electrons strike a fluorescent screen behind the anode, producing additional light photons (i.e., flux gain). To magnify the image, the machine adjusts the voltages on the focusing electrodes so that only a smaller region of the input window is used, effectively zooming in on the view. In magnification mode, the system automatically increases the x-ray output to keep the image bright, a process called automatic brightness control (ABC). Finally, a camera pointed at the output screen captures the images so they can be recorded and shown on a monitor [3, 4].

Flat panel detectors are digital detectors that convert x-ray photons into electrical signals (direct conversion systems), or into visible light, by a scintillating material, which is then converted into electrical signals (indirect conversion system). The electrical signals generated by the x-ray exposure are then collected by an array of thin-film transistors, which collect the signal and transfer it to be processed into images. Fig 2.1c shows the configuration for a digital detector. Flat panel detectors provide better stability, lower patient radiation doses, and wider dynamic ranges, compared to II fluoroscopy systems [4]. An example of a digital fluoroscopy unit is shown in Fig. 2.2.

Fluoroscopy units typically consist of an image receptor (detector) and an x-ray tube mounted on the same mechanical arm but can have different configurations of parts depending on the intended application. For instance, units designed for a gastrointestinal (GI) laboratory may have 15-inch detectors to allow a wider field of view (FOV) necessary for visualizing intesti-

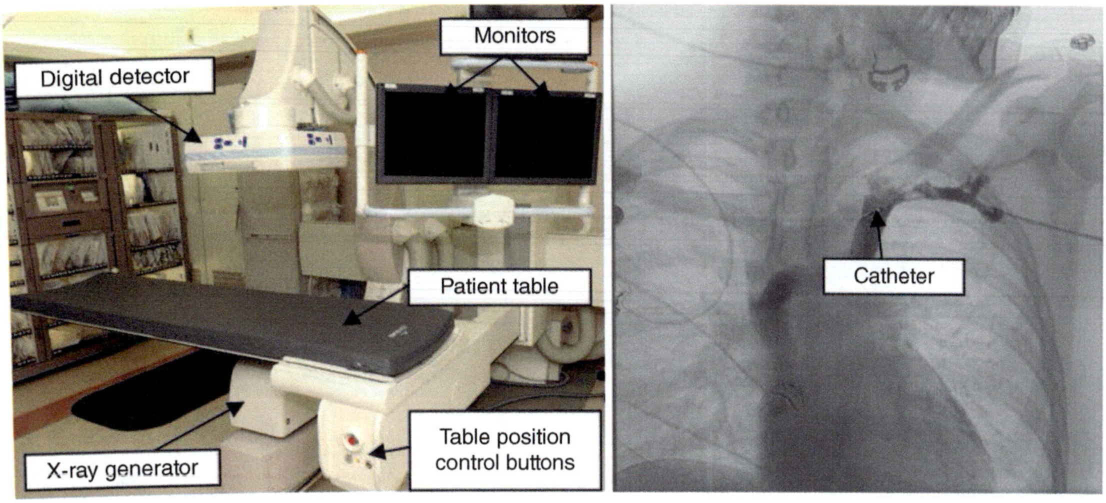

Fig. 2.2 A x-ray digital fluoroscopy system in a typical interventional radiology suite. The right image shows an example of thrombolysis procedure

nal tracts, while in the Cath lab, smaller detectors and narrower FOVs may be used, as the anatomy of interest is typically smaller, which reduces scatter noise in the images. Depending on the intended use, the x-ray tube may be mounted above or below the table, or on a free-rotating c-arm. Units that have a fixed x-ray tube position (i.e., above table or below table) provide appropriate visualization for simple procedures such as in GI labs. For more complex procedures that require precise positioning of medical devices or accurate visualization of complex patient anatomy, a c-arm mounted x-ray tube provides a wide degree of freedom, allowing the imaging plane to be oriented however necessary to visualize the treatment area.

Sources of Radiation Exposure in Interventional Fluoroscopy Applications

Fluoroscopy systems are configured differently to meet specific procedural requirements. For example, single-plane or biplane fixed c-arm systems are often used in interventional radiology and cardiac catheterization (Cath) labs for complex vascular and cardiac procedures, such as angioplasty, stent placement, and electrophysiology (EP) studies. Their fixed setup and dual-plane imaging capability (in the case of biplane systems) provide superior image quality and multiple angles for precise, real-time guidance (Fig. 2.3a, b).

In contrast, table-mounted fluoroscopy setups are commonly utilized in gastrointestinal and endourology suites. Having the x-ray tube and detector mounted on a specialized imaging table is beneficial for procedures like ureteroscopy, laser lithotripsy, and especially barium studies (e.g., barium swallow or enema), which may require the patient to be in a variety of positions, including standing. The table-mounted design ensures consistent patient positioning and uninterrupted imaging, which is vital for accurate diagnosis and therapy (Fig. 2.3c).

Finally, mobile c-arm units are frequently employed in operating rooms for orthopedic surgeries (e.g., fracture reductions, spinal instrumentation), vascular surgeries (e.g., endovascular repair), and other general surgical interventions. These mobile systems offer flexibility and ease of positioning around the sterile field. Mobile c-arms also play a key role in pain management, enabling accurate needle placement during epidural steroid injections, facet joint injections, or other spine-related procedures (Fig. 2.3d).

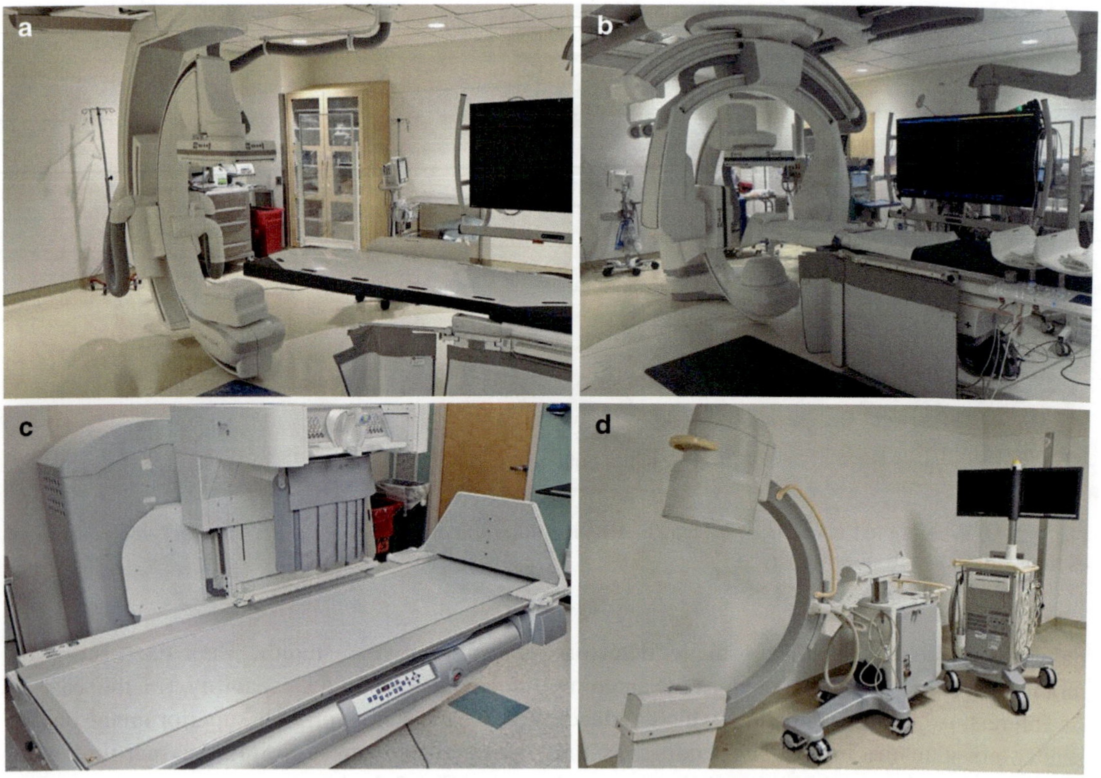

Fig. 2.3 (**a**) A typical fixed fluoroscopy unit for interventional procedures. (**b**) A typical biplane fluoroscopy unit for interventional procedures. (**c**) An under-table fluoroscopy unit used for non-interventional procedures. (**d**) A mobile c-arm unit

Safety Concerns in Fluoroscopy

Knowing Relative Risks Associated with Different Fluoroscopy Procedures

Patients are exposed to ionizing radiation during fluoroscopic procedures, presenting a risk for acute tissue reactions. These effects are localized to the area of exposure and can result from high doses during a single procedure. This is more likely to occur in patients undergoing procedures in the Cath labs, which typically last longer than other fluoroscopy procedures and frequently use high-dose rate recording (Cine) options. Dose rates may range from 1 mGy/min to several Gy/min if digital subtraction angiography (DSA), bolus chase or a Cine recording mode is used [5]. Although average times and displayed air kerma doses may often be less than 10 minutes and do not exceed the 2000 mGy (2Gy) threshold for skin effects, some cases may run longer than 90 minutes and exceed the 2000 mGy (2Gy) threshold.

EP labs are the next highest risk environment for potential patient skin effects. Most cases in the EP labs should fall below the 2 Gy [6, 7] threshold for early transient erythema, but that is not always the case; so special care should be taken to ensure doses remain low.

In the operating room (OR), the risk of high x-ray exposures to patients is relatively low due to the shorter fluoroscopy times required for fluoroscopy guidance. Only a few minutes of fluoroscopy may be required for an operation. Similarly, the pain clinic also requires short durations of fluoroscopy for needle guidance. Consequently, risks of tissue reactions for patients in the OR and pain clinic are low and often nonexistent [8].

In GI labs, radiation-related risks are relatively lower compared to Cath labs and EP lab cases. As in surgery, only a few minutes of fluoroscopy may be used. Also, in GI labs pulsed fluoroscopy is often used for observing contrast materials going through the digestive tract. Because of the low fluoroscopy times and lower doses employed, risks of acute skin effects are relatively low in GI cases compared to Cath lab cases. Due to the short times the x-ray beam is on under fluoroscopy guidance, there are usually little to no skin effects for these types of procedures [8].

Typical effective doses in fluoroscopy and interventional fluoroscopy are provided in reference [9]. In summary, for various interventional fluoroscopic procedures, adult effective doses range from 5 mSv (e.g., head/neck angiography) to 70 mSv (e.g., transjugular intrahepatic portosystemic shunt placement (TIPS)). Notably, patient doses for similar interventional fluoroscopic procedures can vary markedly, depending on the difficulty of the procedure as well as the skill of the operator.

Effects of Radiation Exposure

Biologic effects of radiation exposure are generally classified as either stochastic or tissue effects. For stochastic effects, there is no dose threshold, and the probability of occurrence increases with radiation exposure. Any radiation exposure could increase the risk of radiation-induced cancer or the probability of genetic effects. For tissue effects, the severity of effects increases with increased dose. However, there is a threshold dose below which no observable tissue effect occurs. According to the National Council on Radiation Protection & Measurements (NCRP) report No. 168 [10], there is no observable effect expected at any time if the single-site skin dose is less than 2 Gy. If the skin dose ranges from 2 to 5 Gy, prompt transient erythema may be observed, and early epilation may be expected, but hair loss can be recovered. For the dose range between 5 and 10 Gy, prompt erythema and early epilation may be observed. Patients may recover or expect permanent partial epilation or dermal atrophy induration. For a skin dose range from 10 to 15 Gy, in conjunction with prompt transient erythema and early epilation, possible dry or moist desquamation, permanent epilation, and telangiectasia may be expected. At higher doses greater than 15 Gy, in addition to all the abovementioned effects, dermal necrosis, deeper lesion, and late skin breakdown are expected, and surgical intervention may be required. It is very unlikely, but not impossible, to observe tissue reactions from diagnostic imaging procedures. Tissue reactions are more likely to occur because of interventional procedures.

Strategies to Reduce Patient Skin Dose

In fluoroscopic procedures, there are several best practices that help to limit patient exposure. Most important are the tools available on the fluoroscopy units themselves that help to reduce the amount of beam-on time required to complete exams. Last-image hold displays the most recent image on the monitor, allowing physicians to assess the patient without live exposure. Road mapping, often used during angiography, is an image processing technique that highlights vessels using pre- and post-contrast injection images for more efficient catheter placement. Low-dose and low-pulse rate modes can be selected to reduce x-ray output. The use of spacer cones in c-arms can help to ensure that the patient's skin surface does not come into close contact with the source of x-ray production. Additional tools like five-minute timers and displaying estimated dose information on monitors also help to remind operators to limit patient radiation exposure. Regulatory controls also limit the maximum exposure rate of any modern fluoroscopy unit to 10 R/min at 30 cm from the detector for normal fluoroscopy and 20 R/min for high-dose fluoroscopy.

In addition to the tools on the fluoroscopy units, there are techniques that operators can employ to reduce patient dose. Dose spreading is a technique where the x-ray tube is moved around so the x-ray beam enters different areas of the patient's surface during a procedure, thereby reducing the likelihood of any one area of skin receiving a high concentration of radiation. Positioning the patient as far from the x-ray tube as possible reduces the exposure to any portion of the patient's skin by taking advantage of the inverse square law. These practices can help reduce the incidence of skin injury. A review by Mahesh gives additional guidelines to reduce patient skin dose in fluoroscopy [11].

Quality Concerns

Quality Control in Fluoroscopy

Fluoroscopy requires daily, monthly, quarterly, and annual QC tests [12–18]. Annual evaluation of a fluoroscopic unit should include several QC tests as follows [19]:

1. Unit Assembly Evaluation

   Fluoroscopy unit assembly evaluation is performed to check if the unit is mechanically stable and all moving parts move smoothly without obstruction. There should be no mechanical failures in the motion control mechanisms of the various parts. All safety indicators (e.g., audible indicator sounds, fluoroscopy timer alarm, beam-on indicator) should be working correctly.
2. Collimation Assessment

   Collimation assessment is performed to ensure both the boundaries and centers of the x-ray field and image are consistent. Deviation between x-ray field and displayed image should be less than 2% of the source-to-image distance (SID).
3. kVp Accuracy and Reproducibility

   This test measures the peak electrical potential across the x-ray tube during operation. The accuracy of the x-ray tube kVp is critical since it affects both the intensity and quality of the x-rays reaching the image receptor. Inaccurate KV selections can have detrimental effects not only on image quality but also on patient dose. The measured kVp should be within ±5% of the set value. The kVp coefficient of variation should be less than 2%.
4. Air Kerma Evaluation

   This test measures the air kerma rate at the FDA determined distance from the x-ray tube focal spot. The value should not deviate more than 35% from the value displayed on the fluoroscopy unit. Maximum air kerma rate is also evaluated to ensure regulatory compliance with the FDA limits of 10R/min and 20R/min for normal and mA boost mode, respectively.
5. Half-Value Layer Evaluation

   Measurement of the half-value layer (HVL) of the x-ray beam ensures sufficient filtration according to FDA regulations. Filtration is necessary to remove low-energy x-rays that contribute to patient dose but not to image quality.
6. Image Quality Evaluation

   Evaluation of high- and low-contrast resolution annually helps to identify degradation in image quality over the lifetime of a fluoroscopy unit. This can be performed with a variety of specialized phantoms and should be conducted in a consistent manner to ensure accurate measurements.

The evaluations are required by the Joint Commission (JC) as part of their guidelines. Also, several states require annual equipment performance evaluations (EPE) of fluoroscopy equipment not to exceed 14 months. Any deviations from these tests should be corrected by a qualified service engineer within 30 days of reporting. Because some test failures fall under different timelines for repair, it is important for physicists and service technicians to consult the rules and regulations in their state.

Image Artifacts

Artifacts in fluoroscopy can significantly affect patient safety and image quality. They are associated with a variety of mechanical and electrical sources, primarily concerning the detector [4, 20]. Some artifacts, such as S-distortion in II systems and dead pixels or ghosting in flat panel digital systems, can severely degrade the image quality of a fluoroscopic unit, making diagnostic assessments more difficult. This degradation often results in prolonged examination time, potentially increasing patient radiation exposure beyond the necessary levels.

Ongoing Efforts to Improve Quality and Patient Safety

Patient safety and quality require a long-term, continuous effort that involves every practical aspect and commitment to education programs. Various organizations/associations, e.g., the NCRP and the American College of Radiology (ACR), have made numerous recommendations/guidelines concerning patient safety and quality programs. In the following, we discuss some recent efforts by organizations, clinical practice, and industry.

Federal/Organizational Efforts

Professional organizations such as the ACR, the American Association of Physics in Medicine (AAPM), and the Radiological Society of North America (RSNA) all help to provide up-to-date guidance on imaging technologies and best practices. Regarding fluoroscopy, AAPM has released multiple task group reports in the past that provide recommendations to ensure proper device functionality. The most recently published report specifically covering fluoroscopy is Task Group Report 272, which covers acceptance testing and evaluation of fluoroscopy units [19].

The Image Gently and Image Wisely campaigns are large-scale efforts to ensure safe, effective imaging of pediatric and adult populations, respectively. Both organizations are composed of a coalition of many professional and governmental organizations committed to the core tenets of safety in diagnostic imaging. These organizations have been covered in more detail in the previous chapter, and more information can be found at their respective websites [21, 22].

Clinical Efforts

Safety and quality improvement should be the goal of every radiologic imaging facility. While x-ray imaging and its associated radiation risks are inevitable, questions should be continually asked, e.g., Is the procedure necessary? Have all providers of imaging services that use radiation optimized their protocols? Do we have additional ways to further reduce radiation exposure? Are there alternative modalities available to provide the diagnostic information needed?

General techniques to reduce radiation exposure while preserving image quality include protocol optimization and collimation to the region of interest. Protocol optimization plays a key role in dose reduction of x-ray imaging. Initiatives of the Image Gently-Step Lightly and Image Wisely campaigns are primarily focused on protocol optimization. In the following, we discuss some efforts in practice to reduce radiation dose besides protocol optimization [23].

Industry Efforts

Vendors commonly provide a handbook of recommended quality control activities and, if under contract, also carry out routine preventative maintenance. While field engineers can keep the scanner running smoothly, they are generally not trained in assessing image quality and dealing with radiation safety issues. Several manufacturers of fluoroscopy equipment have taken steps to reduce patient dose by providing specialized dose sparing protocols that incorporate the use of copper filters and adjustable pulse rates. The use of different thicknesses of copper filtration reduces dose by filtering out low energy photons that otherwise get absorbed in the patient. Copper filters may range from 0.1 mm to 0.3 mm in some settings. Reducing the pulse rate during procedures also reduces dose. The use of software enhancements can improve image quality while keeping doses low. Automatic exposure control (AEC) reduces patient dose by adjusting x-ray exposure based on patient thickness and density. Technological advances and improvements in x-ray detector technology like flat panel detectors can also reduce patient dose as improved detector response and detection efficiency means less radiation is required to generate images. Furthermore, real-time dose monitoring is a feature present on modern fluoroscopes that provide real-time feedback on patient radiation dose, allowing the radiologists to adjust techniques during the procedure. Currently, several manufacturers also provide dose tracking software to log patient radiation doses across multiple imaging modalities and procedures, helping to prevent cumulative dose buildup that could result in radiation-induced injury. All these features have made IR procedures safer for patients.

Image processing techniques developed and introduced by vendors can provide additional dose reductions beyond advancements in physical technologies. Lessray® (NuVasive, Inc.) is a technology that uses proprietary software algorithms and hardware. It takes advantage of the largely static nature of spine fluoroscopy procedures by combining an initial traditional fluoroscopy image with subsequent ultralow dose images. The low-dose images are used to update the position of an advancing tool, while the high-detail traditional fluoroscopy image provides visualization of the surrounding anatomy. The result is far lower radiation exposure during procedures that can benefit from this technique [24]. Additional image processing efforts include virtual augmentation of fluoroscopic images with overlays of 3D models of tools or implants and 3D multi-planar reconstructions of fluoroscopic images on advanced c-arm units [24]. All these techniques are designed to improve accuracy and efficiency within a procedure, helping to improve both clinical outcomes and reduce patient radiation exposure.

Advances in Artificial Intelligence (AI) in Fluoroscopy

AI has gained wide acceptance and use in diagnostic radiology compared to interventional radiology primarily due to challenges associated with the complex and dynamic nature of procedures. Several reviews of the use of AI in IR have highlighted the difficulties and challenges of implementing AI in the field. According to a recent review, there are many barriers that limit the use of AI applications in the dynamic procedures of interventional radiology [25]. The authors explore the evolving applications of AI in preprocedural, intraprocedural, and post-procedural settings to improve patient selection, treatment planning and execution, procedural training, intraprocedural augmentation, and treatment follow-up. It was acknowledged that the complexities of the various techniques have presented several challenges and ethical dilemmas that have limited AI integration into IR cases. Another review also examined challenges contributing to scarcity of AI in IR [26]. The authors point out that the IR workflow is an amalgam of multiple intertwined and often simultaneous processes that include diagnostic imaging and other procedures that cannot adequately be addressed by the typical AI agents currently available. They call for a broader generalized solution that they acknowledge is currently unattainable. In specific and focused applications, AI has been used to reduce radiation exposure in fluoroscopically guided endoscopy procedures [27]. Dose reduction was achieved by using AI-controlled secondary collimator shutter blades that reduce patient dose by reducing radiation passing through the primary collimator.

Resources for Quality and Patient Safety

Table 2.1 provides a summary of resources (e.g., QC recommendations, safety guidelines) for quality and patient safety in fluoroscopy. We include a selection of relevant references from major organizations. The goal of this table is to facilitate readers for quick access to those resources.

It needs to be pointed out that most organizations do not function as enforcement agencies. Agencies that enforce the implementation of the recommendations/guidelines include the FDA, Nuclear Regulatory Commission (NRC),

Table 2.1 Resources for quality and safety of diagnostic imaging modalities

AAPM Report No. 4: Basic Quality Control in Diagnostic Radiology
AAPM Report No. 14: Performance Specifications and Acceptance Testing for X-Ray Generators and Automatic Exposure Control Devices
AAPM Report No. 15: Performance Evaluation and Quality Assurance in Digital Subtraction Angiography
AAPM Report No. 25: Protocols for the Radiation Safety Surveys of Diagnostic Radiological Equipment
AAPM Report No. 31: Standardized Methods for Measuring Diagnostic X-Ray Exposures
AAPM Report No. 58: Managing the Use of Fluoroscopy in Medical Institutions
AAPM Report No. 70: Cardiac Catheterization Equipment Performance
AAPM Report No. 93: Acceptance Testing and Quality Control of Photostimulable Storage Phosphor Imaging Systems
AAPM Report No. 116: An Exposure Indicator for Digital Radiography
AAPM Report No. 125: Functionality and Operation of Fluoroscopic Automatic Brightness Control/Automatic Dose Rate Control Logic in Modern Cardiovascular and Interventional Angiography Systems
AAPM Report No. 251: Survey of Pediatric Fluoroscopic Air Kerma Rate Values and Recommended Application of Results
AAPM Report No. 272: Comprehensive Acceptance Testing and Evaluation of Fluoroscopy Imaging Systems
AAPM Report No. 357: Estimation of Patient Skin Dose in Fluoroscopy: Summary of a Joint Report by AAPM TG357 and EFOMP
AAPM Medical Physics Practice Guideline 12.a: Fluoroscopy Dose Management
ACR–AAPM Technical Standard for Management of the Use of Radiation in Fluoroscopic Procedures
ACR–AAPM Technical Standard for Diagnostic Medical Physics Performance Monitoring of Fluoroscopic Equipment
ACR–AAPM–SPR Practice Parameter for Diagnostic Reference Levels and Achievable Doses in Medical X-Ray Imaging
ACR–SPR Practice Parameter for Imaging Pregnant or Potentially Pregnant Patients with Ionizing Radiation
CRCPD Publication 01–4: Quality control recommendations for diagnostic radiography, volume 3: Radiographic or Fluoroscopic Machines
CRCPD Publication No. E-10-2: Computed Radiography (CR) and Digital Radiography (DR) State X-Ray Inspection Protocol
EPA Federal Guidance Report No. 14: Radiation Protection Guidance for Diagnostic and Interventional X-Ray Procedures
FDA 21 CFR 1020: Code of Federal Regulations Title 21, Chapter I, Subchapter J: Radiological Health
ICRP Publication 73: Radiological Protection and Safety in Medicine
ICRP Publication 117: Radiological Protection in Fluoroscopically Guided Procedures Performed Outside the Imaging Department
ICRP Publication 139: Occupational Radiological Protection in Interventional Procedures
NCRP Report No. 099: Quality Assurance for Diagnostic Imaging
NCRP Report No. 102: Medical X-Ray, Electron Beam and Gamma-Ray Protection for Energies Up to 50 MeV (Equipment Design, Performance and Use)
NCRP (2010). Report No. 168: Radiation Dose Management for Fluoroscopically-Guided Interventional Medical Procedures
NCRP Statement 11: Outline of Administrative Policies for Quality Assurance and Peer Review of Tissue Reactions Associated with Fluoroscopically-Guided Interventions
NEMA: Test Standard for the Measurement of the Image Signal Uniformity of an X-Ray Image Intensifier (XRII) System
NEMA: Test Standard for the Determination of the Visible Entrance Field Size of an X-Ray Image Intensifier (XRII) System
NEMA: Characteristics of and Test Procedures for a Phantom to Benchmark Cardiac Fluoroscopic and Photographic Performance
NEMA: Test Standard for the Determination of the System Contrast Ratio (SCR) and the System Veiling Glare Index (SVGI) of an X-Ray Image Intensifier (XRII) System

(continued)

Table 2.1 (continued)

NEMA: Test Standard for the Determination of the Radial Image Distortion of an X-Ray Image Intensifier (XRII) System
NEMA: Test Standard for the Determination of the Limiting Spatial Resolution of X-Ray Image Intensifier Systems
NEMA: Measurement of Dimensions and Properties of Focal Spots of Diagnostic X-Ray Tubes

AAPM American Association of Physicists in Medicine, *ACR* American College of Radiology, *CRCPD* Conference of Radiation Control Program Directors, *FDA* US Food and Drug Administration, *ICRP* International Commission on Radiological Protection, *IEC International Electrotechnical Commission, NCRP* National Council on Radiation Protection and Measurements, *NEMA* National Electrical Manufacturers Association

Environment Protection Agency (EPA), Occupational Safety and Health Administration (OSHA), and agreement States.

Summary

This chapter reviews the use of fluoroscopy for imaging guidance under various imaging and interventional radiology applications. Different types of fluoroscopy devices and their key features are briefly described. Methods for reducing patient dose while maintaining image quality are discussed, along with efforts from both industry and healthcare institutions to enhance patient safety. The importance of a QA program is emphasized. A list of resources is provided at the end of the chapter to guide readers to further information.

References

1. Saeed M, et al. MR fluoroscopy in vascular and cardiac interventions. Int J Cardiovasc Imaging. 2012;28(1):117–37.
2. Hendee WR, Ritenour ER, Hoffmann KR. Medical imaging physics. Med Phys. 2003;30(4):730.
3. Maher KP, Malone JF. Digital fluoroscopy: a new development in medical imaging. Contemp Phys. 1986;27(6):533–52.
4. Nickoloff EL. AAPM/RSNA physics tutorial for residents: physics of flat-panel fluoroscopy systems. Radiographics. 2011;31(2):591–602.
5. Balter S, et al. Fluoroscopically guided interventional procedures: a review of radiation effects on patients' skin and hair. Radiology. 2010;254(2):326–41.
6. Geleijns J, Wondergem J. X-ray imaging and the skin: radiation biology, patient dosimetry and observed effects. Radiat Prot Dosim. 2005; 114(1–3):121–5.
7. Koenig TR, et al. Skin injuries from fluoroscopically guided procedures: part 1, characteristics of radiation injury. Am J Roentgenol. 2001;177(1):3–11.
8. YiLi Zhou M, et al. Fluoroscopy radiation safety for spine interventional pain procedures in university teaching hospitals. Pain Physician. 2005;8(1)
9. Mettler FA, et al. Effective doses in radiology and diagnostic nuclear medicine: a Catalog1. Radiology. 2008;248(1):254–63.
10. NCRP. Report no. 168 –radiation dose Management for Fluoroscopically-Guided Interventional Medical Procedures (2010). National Council on Radiation Protection; 2010.
11. Mahesh M. Fluoroscopy: patient radiation exposure issues. Radiographics. 2001;21(4):1033–45.
12. AAPM. AAPM report #15: performance evaluation and quality assurance in digital subtraction angiography. American Association of Physicists in Medicine; 1985.
13. AAPM. AAPM report no. 58: managing the use of fluoroscopy in medical institutions. American Association of Physicists in Medicine; 1998.
14. AAPM. AAPM report no. 64: cardiac catheterization equipment performance. American Association of Physicist in Medicine; 2001.
15. AAPM. AAPM report no. 93: acceptance testing and quality control of photostimulable storage phosphor imaging systems 2006. American Association of Physicists in Medicine.
16. AAPM. AAPM report no. 116: an exposure indicator for digital radiography. American Association of Physicists in Medicine; 2009.
17. CRCPD, CRCPD publication 01–4: quality control recommendations for diagnostic radiography, volume 3: radiographic or fluoroscopic machines 2001, Conference of Radiation Control Program Directors.
18. NCRP, Report No. 168: Radiation dose management for fluoroscopically-guided interventional medical procedures. 2010.
19. Lin P-JP, et al. AAPM Task Group Report 272: comprehensive acceptance testing and evaluation of fluoroscopy imaging systems. Med Phys. 2022;49(4):e1–e49.
20. Keating TC, Bohl DD, Hamid KS. A review of fluoroscopic image-intensifier Artifacts and the next generation of Isocentric C-arm imaging. JBJS Reviews. 2018;6(12):e4.

21. Image Wisely. www.imagewisely.org.
22. Image Gently. www.imagegently.org.
23. Wilting J, et al. A rational approach to dose reduction in CT: individualized scan protocols. Eur Radiol. 2001;11(12):2627–32.
24. Keil H, Trapp O. Fluoroscopic imaging: new advances. Injury. 2022;53:S8–S15.
25. von Ende E, et al. Artificial intelligence, augmented reality, and virtual reality advances and applications in interventional radiology. Diagnostics. 2023;13(5):892.
26. Mazaheri S, et al. Challenges of implementing artificial intelligence in interventional radiology. In: Seminars in interventional radiology. Thieme Medical; 2021.
27. Bang JY, et al. Use of artificial intelligence to reduce radiation exposure at fluoroscopy-guided endoscopic procedures. Am J Gastroenterol. 2020;115(4):555–61.

Computed Tomography

3

Yifang Jimmy Zhou

Key Points

- CT dose optimization depends on the diagnosis task.
- CT dose should be adjusted according to the protocol and patient size. Dedicated pediatric protocols should be used for pediatric patients.
- The low kV imaging should be used in studies with iodine contrast agents.
- Suggestions are given for CT dose and protocol management.

Introduction

Applications of multi-detector computed tomography (MDCT) have been expanded tremendously since its introduction in 1998 [1–3]. In the meantime, concerns have been raised about the patient dose in the public communities [4–6]. Whereas the radiation risk is debatable at the diagnostic x-ray energy range [7–12], it is the consensus among many that it is a prudent approach to assume the risk to be proportional to the dose. The approach suggests a smaller risk at a lower dose without any threshold. However, excessive dose reduction may compromise the diagnosis accuracy. In fact, the image quality demand is diagnosis task specific. For instance, the image quality requirement is different for routine brain CT studies as compared to hydrocephalous CT studies. Therefore, the goal of dose reduction effort should be pursued to meet the task-specific diagnosis requirement.

In order to optimize dose using the aforementioned approach, a good understanding of the factors impacting the image quality and dose is essential. The factors can be categorized into two domains: those determined by the design of the CT system and those determined by the operators. In the following sections, we will first discuss the basic design of the multi-detector CT system and then introduce the CT dose concept and address image quality. The CT protocol and dose management are discussed in detail thereafter. A summary of the chapter is given at the end.

Basic Design of Multi-detector CT System

Hardware Design

All current multi-detector CT systems use a rotation-rotation design. With this design, the x-ray tube and the detector rotate together (Fig. 3.1) with a high speed (the rotation time can be as short as 0.23 s for modern scanners). The x-ray beam is collimated to a relatively thin beam so the x-ray use efficiency is very low. Therefore,

Y. J. Zhou (✉)
Department of Imaging, Cedars-Sinai Medical Center, Los Angeles, CA, USA
e-mail: Jimmy.Zhou@cshs.org

J. Zhang (ed.), *Quality and Patient Safety in Medical Imaging*,
https://doi.org/10.1007/978-3-031-89007-9_3

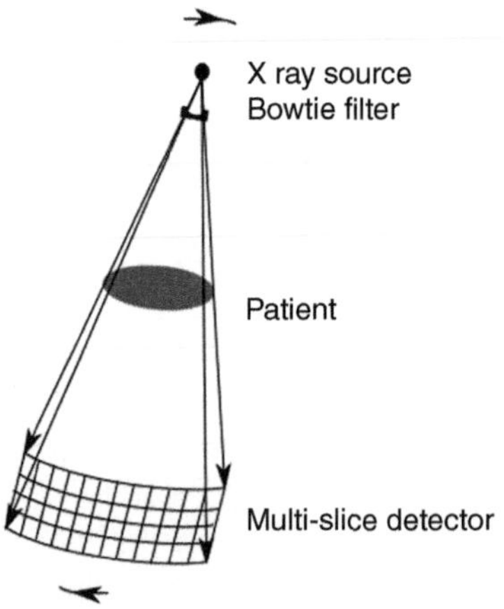

Fig. 3.1 Major components of the CT scan system

the tube design to dissipate the heat rapidly (mega heat units per minute) is vital. Because of the lower kV use in contrast imaging or in dual energy CT, the higher mA rating (1000 mA or more) is implemented on the state-of-the-art systems to compensate the signal loss. The beam coverage at the CT iso-center ranges from several centimeters to 16 cm. In order to make the intensity and spectrum more uniform across the detector, bowtie-shaped filters are installed in the x-ray tube to compensate different attenuations across the body contour. The filter absorbs the least x-rays along the beam path to the center of the body and the most x-rays along the path to the peripheries. Typically, various bowtie filters are implemented depending on the body parts. The spectrum uniformity is important to reduce the beam-hardening effects such as dark bands formed between the highly attenuated objects. The bowtie filter also makes the post-patient scatter more uniform, so the scatter correction is more effective. It impacts the low-contrast detectability as well, which will be elaborated on in the later sections.

The detector system consists of multiple rows along the longitudinal direction, from 4 rows in the 1990s to 320 rows in the state-of-the-art design. Each detector row consists of several hundreds of detector elements. The detector material (CdWO4, Gd_2O_2S, other vendor proprietary) is critical in that not only is it necessary to produce high light output, but also the light needs to decay rapidly (in microseconds) to avoid the signal lag [13]. For CT systems using scintillator-based detectors, the detector elements are usually structured, and reflective coating is used. Their size and thickness impact the image resolution and dose efficiency. The x-ray photons, after passing through the patient and interacting with the detector elements, are converted into light photons. The light photons are then converted to electric signals in the photodiodes via the photo-electric effect. The signal is amplified and digitized for each element. The signal readout speed needs to be fast enough to keep up with the data flow rate. To appreciate the technical challenge, we can take a 256-row scanner as an example: if the number of detector elements is 900 per row and number of projections is 1000 per rotation, and if 16 bits are used for each data point, the total bits required in each rotation are $256 \times 900 \times 1000 \times 16 = 3.686$ GBits. If the rotation time is 0.28 s, the data rate is about 13 Gbits per second.

The scatter generated from the patient is significant. Not only does it degrade the contrast-to-noise ratio, but also it generates artifacts such as streaks and dark bands. To reduce the scatter, the anti-scatter grid (ASG) is implemented in front of the detector. Since the detector rotates together with the x-ray source for modern MDCT, the configuration of the ASG can be such that it focuses toward the x-ray source. For 64-slice or of narrower beam CT scanners, one-dimensional (1D) ASG rejecting the in-plane scatter is typically effective enough [14, 15]. For CT systems of wider beam, the scatter rejection between detector rows needs to be considered as well, so 2D or 3D AGD has been utilized [16].

For multi-detector detector CT systems, there are two radiation phenomena worth further discussions. The first is called overranging: the radiation caused by additional rotations at the start and the end of the helical scan is shown in Fig. 3.2. The additional rotations are necessary in order to interpolate the data in the intended clinical range for image reconstruction. With the increase of detector rows, the radiation from overranging becomes a concern [17]. To alleviate

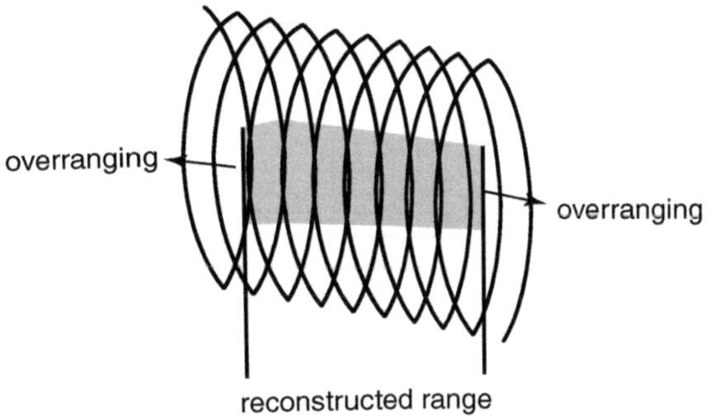

Fig. 3.2 Overranging in helical scans

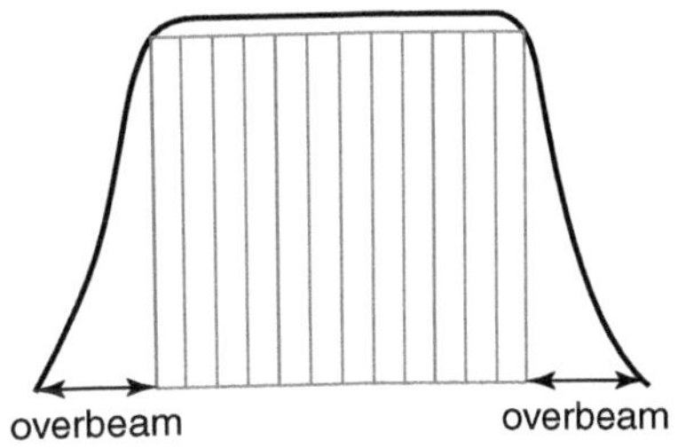

Fig. 3.3 Overbeaming due to penumbra

the problem, dynamically adjusted collimation (smart or active collimation) has been implemented to cut off the part of the radiation that is not required by the interpolation algorithm [18]. The second radiation phenomenon is called overbeaming: the penumbra goes beyond the detector array in the longitudinal direction as shown in Fig. 3.3. It is a necessity in order to make the radiation on the detectors uniform. Overbeaming is a bigger concern for four-slice scanners because the penumbra occupies a significant portion of the total radiation range. For the scanners with more detector rows, the penumbra portion takes a less percentage, so it is less of a concern for modern scanners.

Software Design

Software design includes CT reconstruction, scatter correction, beam hardening correction, photon starving correction, and others. We will elaborate more on CT reconstruction. Until recently, filtered backprojection (FBP) algorithms had been the standard practice for CT reconstruction. Filtered backprojection is a process of backprojecting the filtered projection data (sinogram), where the filter (kernel) compensates the projection caused nonuniform spatial sampling from the center to the periphery of the object. The shape of the kernel determines the sharpness of the image, be it named bone, lung, or soft tissue. The advantage of FBP is the fast speed owing to the analytical solutions and the utilization of fast Fourier transform (FFT) [19]. However, the FBP algorithm does not model the photon statistics or imaging hardware, so the noise inherently associated with the signal in the reconstruction process is manifested in the resulted image after the fact [20, 21]. The noise is strongly coupled with the dose, so the lower dose leads to the higher noise. Another limitation of the FBP reconstruction is that it assumes a certain degree of continuity about the attenuation coefficient in the object. When a highly attenuated foreign object such as a metallic implant is in the patient, significant streak artifacts are observed.

The limitations of the FBP reconstruction are alleviated using iterative reconstructions (IR) [22–24]. The concept of IR is not new, but it has been revitalized for clinical use owing to the ever increased computing power. The basic idea of IR is to take the photon statistics and/or imaging optics into consideration. The initial image data can be a set of constant attenuation coefficients or FBP image. The image data are forward projected with the photon statistics and/or imaging optics considered. The results are compared with the measured sinogram. Depending on the tolerance to the difference and the corresponding regularization term, the data are updated following an iteration equation. For instance, one way to perform iteration is to find the image data with the most likelihood to generate the sonogram by assuming that the photons observe Poisson statistics. Attributing the photon fluctuation to noise and using iterations to extract the best possible image data make the resulted image significantly less dependent on the dose. Therefore, iterative reconstructions have enabled lower dose imaging. In practice, the application of IR is usually constrained due to the compromise of image quality especially of noise texture and spatial resolution. This issue will be revisited in the following section.

CT Dose and Image Quality

CT Dose Index, Dose-Length Product, and Effective Dose

Unlike two-dimensional projection imaging where the dose is exponentially reduced as the x-ray beam passes through the body, the CT dose inside the body is more uniformly distributed due to the nature of its tomographic imaging. The general CT dose computation is to obtain the average dose across the axial slab of a certain thickness. Because the slab area varies from patient to patient, the dose is patient size specific. This dose estimate is defined as the size-specific dose estimate (SSDE) by the American Association of Physicists in Medicine (AAPM) [25].

However, the widely used volume CT dose index ($CTDI_{vol}$) is not a metric of the patient dose. It is rather a measure of the machine's output. To better explain the $CTDI_{vol}$, it is necessary to introduce another quantity called CT dose index (CTDI) [26]. For a contiguous axial scan on a phantom, one would like to find the dose to a cross section at the longitudinal center. The average dose to the section is equal to the contributions from the primary beam as well as from the scatter from all other scans at the other longitudinal parts, normalized by the section thickness. In practice, the integral (summation) only goes as far as ±50 mm about the section of interest, assuming that the scatter contribution beyond this range is negligible. The corresponding CTDI is called $CTDI_{100}$. As for the scatter material, irrelevant to the patient size, only two fixed cylindrical acrylic phantoms are defined, both at the length of 15 cm, with diameters of 16 cm and 32 cm, simulating the head and the body, respectively [27].

With the standard phantoms, the average dose across the section can be calculated using the weighted summation of the results near the surface and at the center as follows, according to the Monte Carlo simulation:

$$CTDI_w = \frac{1}{3} CTDI_{center} + \frac{2}{3} CTDI_{surface}, \quad (3.1)$$

The resulted quantity $CTDI_w$ is called weighted CTDI. $CTDI_{center}$ and $CTDI_{surface}$ can be measured by placing a 100 mm ion chamber at the center and near the surface, respectively.

All the aforementioned CTDIs are defined for contiguous axial scans only. For helical scans, one needs to take the beam sparseness into consideration, as shown in Fig. 3.4, where the pitch is the table movement per rotation divided by the total beam width at the iso-center. Obviously, the CTDI increases as the beam is denser. This leads to the concept of volume CT dose index ($CTDI_{vol}$):

$$CTDI_{vol} = CTDI_w / \text{pitch}. \quad (3.2)$$

According to the regulatory requirements in Europe and in the United States, the $CTDI_{vol}$ is always reported on the scanner. Because it is readily available, it can be mistakenly treated as the patient dose. In fact, the patient dose deviates from the $CTDI_{vol}$ depending on the patient size. For instance, for an abdomen scan, if the patient size is smaller than 32 cm, the patient dose is larger than the $CTDI_{vol}$ (32 cm). The opposite is true for a bigger patient. The size-specific dose estimate (SSDE) can be obtained from the $CTDI_{vol}$ using conversion tables given by the AAPM Task Group 204 [25]. For any given set of radiation parameters, the smaller patient receives higher dose. This fact along with the higher radiation sensitivity of children justifies the need of

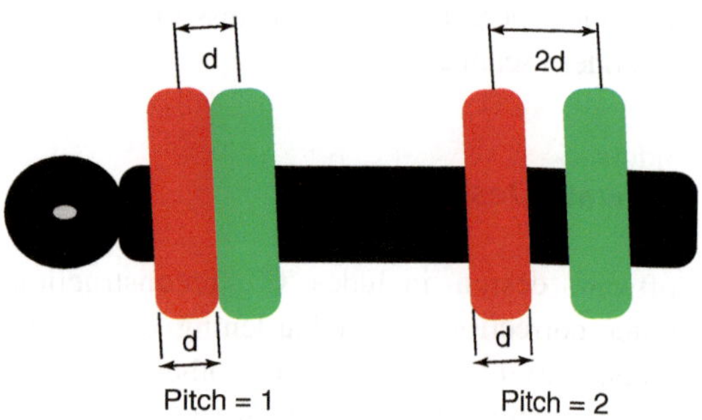

Fig. 3.4 Helical scans with different pitches. d is the total beam width

imaging gently for pediatric patients. This subject will be discussed again when the image quality aspect is addressed.

Although Eq. (3.2) considers the beam sparseness in the helical scan, there are certain non-helical scans where the scatter from neighbor rotations is either not in existence or substantially sparse. For instance, in the cine perfusion scan, the table does not move. In the step-and-shoot high-resolution chest CT, the typical table increment is significantly bigger than the beam width (10 mm movement with 1 mm collimation). In either of these cases, the reported $CTDI_{vol}$ may overestimate the CT dose if appropriate correction is not taken.

In addition to $CTDI_{vol}$, another frequently used dose metric is called dose-length product (DLP). DLP is the product of $CTDI_{vol}$ and scan length. The typical unit for DLP is mGy● cm. Whereas the $CTDI_{vol}$ represents a local average dose to a slab of the defined phantom, the DLP is related to the total radiation energy imparted on the phantom. Therefore, $CTDI_{vol}$ is only additive for the overlapped region from multiple series in a study, but the DLP is additive from all these series.

Effective dose is defined as the whole body equivalent dose from the radiation of limited body regions. Effective dose is typically in the unit of mSv. As DLP is related to the total imparted energy, the effective dose can be obtained from the DLP. The conversion factor, called *k* factor in units of mSv● mGy^{-1}● cm^{-1}, is defined to convert the DLP to the effective dose. The *k* factor is radiation sensitivity dependent; therefore, it depends on the patient organ and age. For example, it is 0.0031 mSv● mGy^{-1}● cm^{-1} for adult's head and neck, but 0.013 mSv● mGy^{-1}● cm^{-1} for a 1-year old. The readers are suggested to refer to the ICRP report 102 for further details [28].

Effective dose is a good metric for radiation management in practice, but it should not be used for patient radiation risk assessment. The risk assessment is very complex. Even the latest report for Biologic Effects of Ionizing Radiation (BEIR 7) [29] from US National Academy of Sciences has met critiques [30, 31].

Image Quality

As mentioned in the introduction, dose reduction cannot be conducted without considering image quality. One may assume that better image quality is always associated with more dose, but the image quality response to dose is not proportional. In fact, the quality improvement is less significant or even saturated with increased dose after the dose reaches a certain point. The details will be addressed later. With regard to image quality for routine CT studies, the most concerned aspects include low-contrast detectability and spatial resolution.

Low-Contrast Detectability

Low-contrast detectability (LCD) is vital for CT. It is the capability of the CT system to resolve the lesions with different low-contrast scales from the surroundings. This can be qualitatively characterized by evaluating an array of structures with various contrast and sizes in a phantom, such as Catphan, QRM, or the phantom from American College of Radiology [32–34]. However, this approach cannot be used to establish the quantitative relationship between the LCD and patient dose.

For a well-designed CT system, the LCD is determined by the quantum noise of the CT image, which varies at different spatial scales. To quantify the LCD, a concept called statistically defined low-contrast detectability (SD-LCD) was proposed [35, 36]. The concept can be understood in such a manner: assume that if the same image acquisition is repeated, the CT number in the reconstructed image will not remain the same but fluctuates following a certain statistical distribution. The amplitude of the fluctuation changes as the interested area changes, reflecting the noise dependence on the spatial scale. To make the quantification easier, one does not have to repeat the acquisition many times. Rather, as shown in Fig. 3.5a, one can choose any specified area matching the lesion size to segment the uniform background (such as water) into an array of such areas. The average CT number in each area will fluctuate. For any lesion with the size of the area, the background fluctuation must be small enough

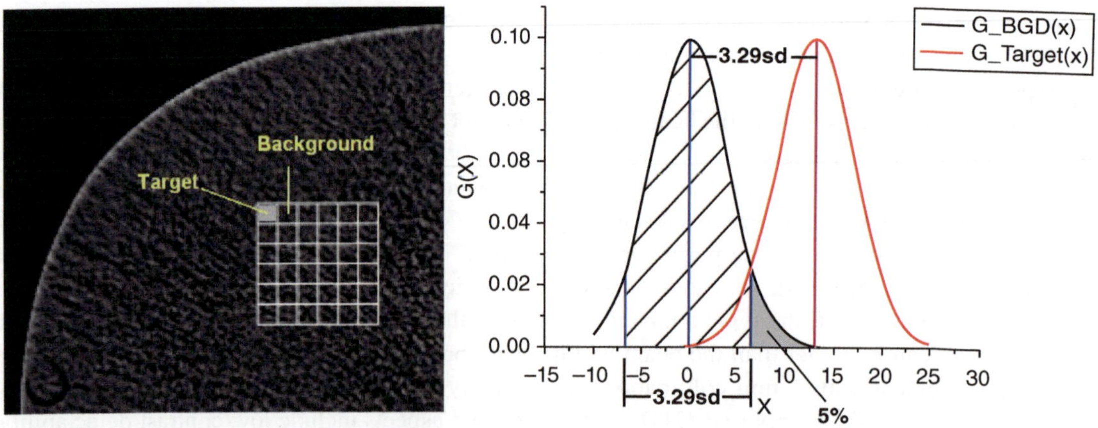

Fig. 3.5 A matrix formed by repeating the squared element in the uniform region (**a**. left). Separation of two Gaussian distributions with 5% overlap (**b**. right)

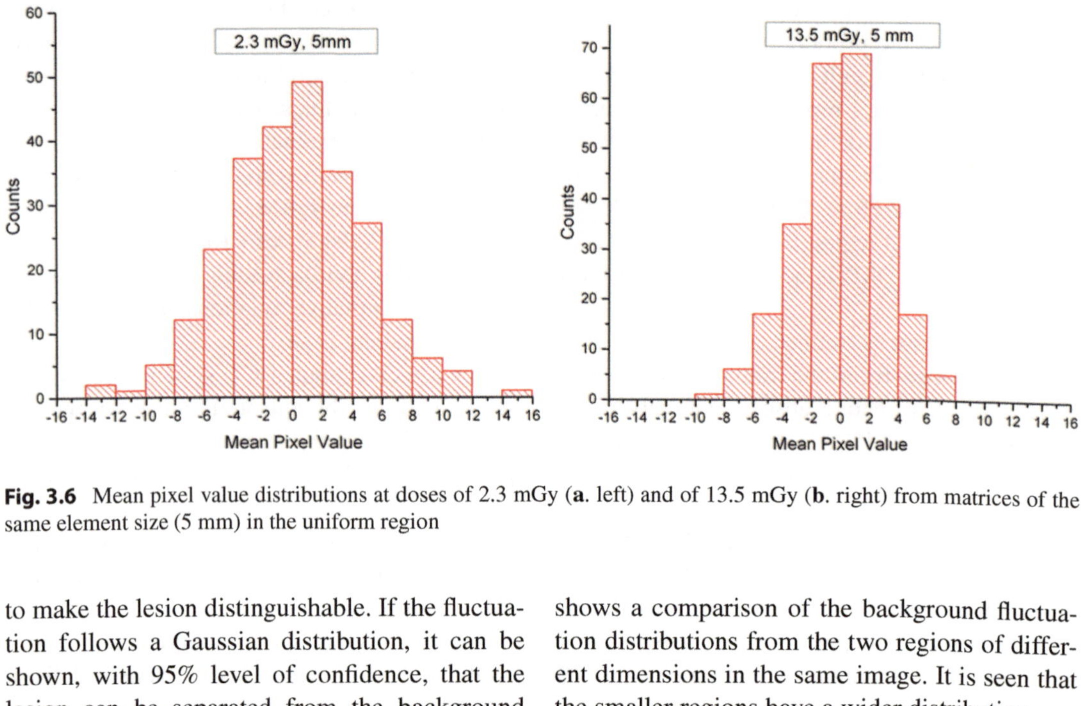

Fig. 3.6 Mean pixel value distributions at doses of 2.3 mGy (**a**. left) and of 13.5 mGy (**b**. right) from matrices of the same element size (5 mm) in the uniform region

to make the lesion distinguishable. If the fluctuation follows a Gaussian distribution, it can be shown, with 95% level of confidence, that the lesion can be separated from the background when the contrast is 3.29 times the standard deviation of the distribution (Fig. 3.5b) [35, 36]. This threshold can serve as the minimum detectable contrast (MDC). The lower the MDC, the better the low-contrast detectability. Figure 3.6 shows a comparison of the background fluctuation distributions from two images with different doses (thus different noises). As demonstrated, for the regions of the same dimension, the noisier image shows a wider distribution. Figure 3.7 shows a comparison of the background fluctuation distributions from the two regions of different dimensions in the same image. It is seen that the smaller regions have a wider distribution.

Zhou et al. used a simplified model to show that, for FBP reconstructed images, the MDC for a lesion depends on the following factors [37, 38]:

Lesion size—the MDC is inversely proportional to the size.

Dose—the MDC is inversely proportional to the square root of the dose.

Patient size—the larger the patient size, the higher the MDC (i.e., lower detectability).

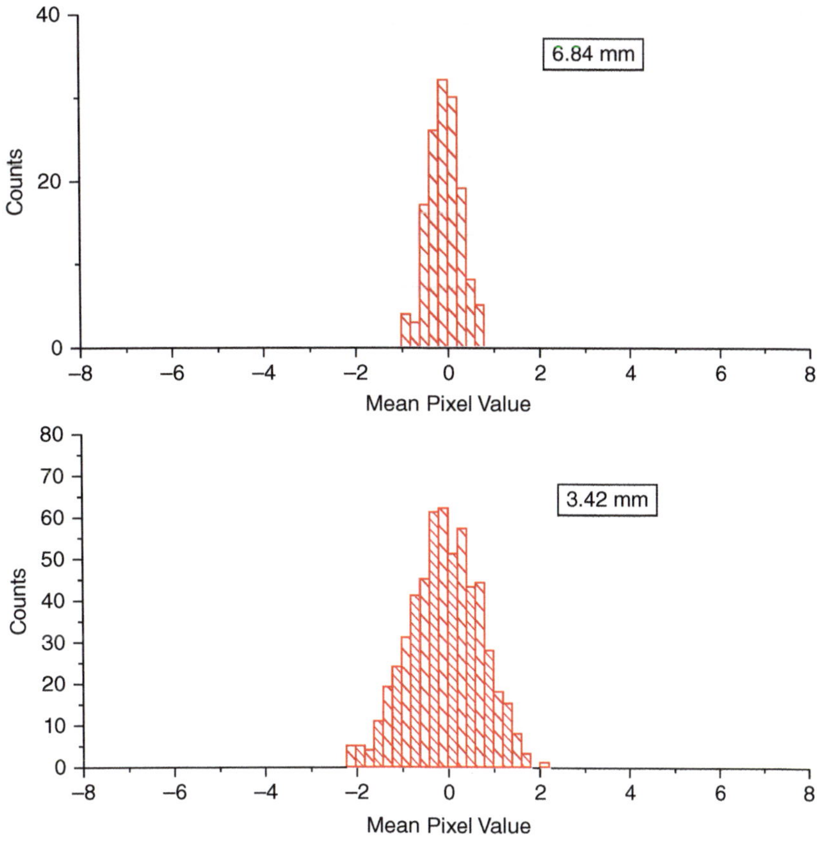

Fig. 3.7 Mean pixel value distribution at the same dose from matrices of element sizes of 6.84 mm and 3.42 mm in the uniform region

The relationship is not linear and strongly depends on the bowtie filter design.

Slice width—the MDC is inversely proportional to the square root of the slice width.

Other design factors—especially the detector efficiency, the detector element size, the reconstruction kernel, and the energy spectrum of the incident photons at the detector after passing through the bowtie filter and the patient.

For the end users, the adjustable factors include the kVp, mA, rotation time, slide width, and the reconstruction method. The dose is proportional to the milliampere rotation time product (mAs) and to the x-ray tube voltage (kVp) to a certain power (typically bigger than 2). The patient size is important as smaller patients need much lower dose than larger patients to reach the same low-contrast detectability. The slice width needs to be reasonably chosen to meet the task requirement with certain constraints. First, if the small structure is to be assessed, the partial volume effect is a concern for thicker images. Second, for some scanners, the primary reconstructed images need to be thin enough in order to reformat the orthogonal images with good quality.

The task-specific diagnosis is an important consideration when the above factors are altered. The intrinsic contrast of the lesion can be relatively high for some diagnoses such as virtual colonoscopy, hydrocephalus, kidney stone, coronary artery calcium, and lung screening. These tasks can therefore tolerate higher noise or lower patient dose. For examinations using the iodine contrast, the contrast enhancement may cope with noisier images depending on whether the focus is on angiography or/and on lesion assessment in the soft tissue. Further details will be discussed in the later section.

Iterative reconstructions (IR) has gained popularity as they suppress the noise for potentially better low-contrast detection and lower patient dose [39–41]. However, caution should be used for the application of IR. First, not all IR algorithms are the same. The popular algorithms may only consider the photon statistics along the projections, the x-ray optics details, such as the focal spot size, voxel size, and detector element size, are not included. The simplification enables faster reconstruction but smears out the edges as dissimilar pixels in adjacency are penalized in the iteration process. Second, the radiologist may not feel confident with the appearance of the image texture obtained entirely from IR. Therefore, a certain blending between the IR and filtered backprojection reconstructed images is utilized in practice. The degree of the blending depends on the radiologist's satisfaction. Last, the model-based iterative reconstruction (MBIR) considering the x-ray optics appears to be promising [42], but the current computing time (about 30 min per scan) is too long to be implemented in practice [43]. To ease the problem, an intermediate approach using a blending of FBP and MBIR has been implemented.

Although model-based iterative reconstructions are supposed to deliver very good image quality in principle, the convergence control from iterations remains to be a significant challenge due to many parameters to be tuned. Deep learning image reconstructions (DLIR) have gained more attention recently [44]. The details of DLIR are beyond the scope of this chapter, but the basic idea is to train the low-dose images toward the high-dose target images reconstructed with FBP. The deep learning network updates a very large set of parameters during the training process. The final images are expected to be of similar noise texture in the high-dose FBP images.

Spatial Resolution

Spatial resolution can be referred to the closest distance between the two adjacent structures that the system is able to resolve. Typically, a high-contrast bar pattern consisting of various line pair densities is used to characterize the spatial resolution in practice. The utilization of "line pair" reflects that there are always two adjacent structures to be resolved. For three-dimensional imaging such as CT, spatial resolution can be separately characterized in the scan plane (x-y) and in the longitudinal direction (z). Spatial resolution intrinsically depends on the focal spot size, the reconstruction algorithm, the detector element size, the data sampling density, and other design factors. To improve the spatial resolution in the longitudinal direction, a straightforward approach is to use lower pitch in the helical scan. From the design perspective, various techniques to oversample the projection data have been implemented by the manufacturers such as focal spot deflection (Siemens and GE) and double-slice technology (Canon) [45–47]. The focal spot deflection deflects the electron beam inside the x-ray tube so that the x-ray beam shifts back and forth either in the scan plane or in the longitudinal direction. For scans using the wide (cone) beam, the double-slice technology takes advantage of the cone beam volume data contributed to each voxel at different detectors. The approach realizes fine reconstruction intervals for high-resolution applications.

One may often confuse the spatial resolution with the pixel size or voxel size. They are different concepts. Spatial resolution depends on the focal spot size, reconstruction algorithm, detector element size, data sampling density, and other design factors, whereas the pixel or voxel size only depends on the displayed field of view and the image matrix size. For instance, the lung filter typically is of a high frequency pass, and the spatial resolution in the axial plane is about nine line pairs per centimeter. For the same pixel size, if the standard tissue filter is used, the spatial resolution is only seven line pairs per centimeter. Figure 3.8 demonstrates the difference using the American College of Radiology (ACR) CT phantom.

The spatial resolution in the final image depends not only on the system design but also on the choice of the slice thickness and reconstruction field of view (displayed field of view). For lesions smaller than the slice thickness in the same direction, they are averaged across the thickness so the intensity profile is reduced. This effect is called partial volume effect. If the inferior resolution in the scan plane is due to the

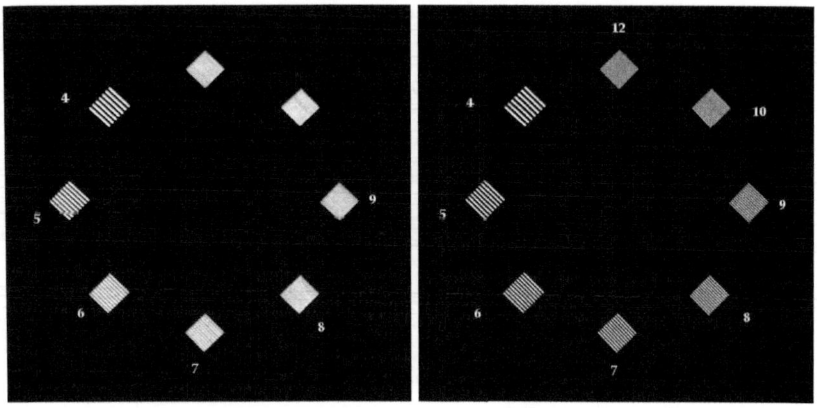

Fig. 3.8 Resolution pattern in the ACR phantom for an abdomen scan (**a**. left) and a high-resolution chest scan (**b**. right). The standard tissue filter was used in the abdomen scan, and the lung filter was used. 1.25 mm slice width was reconstructed for both images for comparison

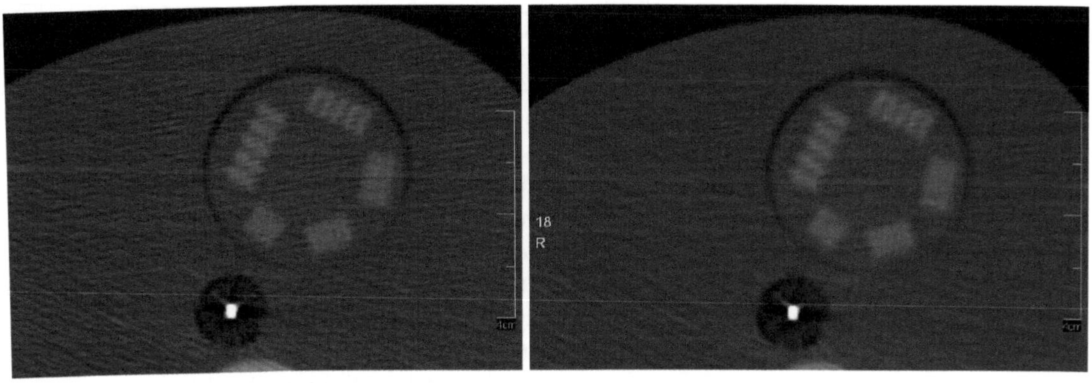

Fig. 3.9 High-contrast line pattern difference at different IR settings (left: GE ASIR = 0. Right: GE ASIR = 100%) for a small phantom mimicking the elbow at the lateral side of the adult anthropomorphic phantom

choice of bigger pixel, the displayed field of view and the slice width can be made smaller. For instance, for assessment of the lesions in abdomen CT, the field of view is typically 36 cm. The corresponding pixel size is about 0.7 mm. Resolution equal to or better than 0.7 mm is easier to realize in practice (~ 7 line pairs per cm) on most modern MDCT. However, for cardiac CT imaging, the displayed view of 16 cm for the heart coverage gives the pixel size of 0.315 mm. A resolution matching this size is very challenging. In reality, this resolution is necessary for coronary stent imaging and coronary calcification assessment. In the former case, the small stent diameter can be 2–3 mm [48]. This fact along with the blooming effect (from beam hardening and partial volume effect) makes the in-stent lumen assessment a challenge. A sub-millimeter resolution is needed. In the latter case, the calcification size can be in submillimeter. If the in-plane resolution is worse than the pixel size, then a 1 mm calcified lesion only occupies less than 3 pixels, making it difficult to be discerned.

We shall briefly discuss the impact of iterative reconstructions (IR) to spatial resolution. As mentioned in 4.1, the spatial resolution is compromised at higher degree of iterative reconstructions. Figure 3.9 shows the high-contrast line pattern difference at different IR settings (GE ASIR 0 and 100%) for a small phantom mimicking the elbow at the lateral side of the adult anthropomorphic phantom.

For low-contrast structures, the edge is also smeared by the use of IR. Figure 3.10 demonstrates the edge profile difference for a 7 mm low-contrast insert (2% contrast). It is clear that the low-contrast edge is more blurred by the

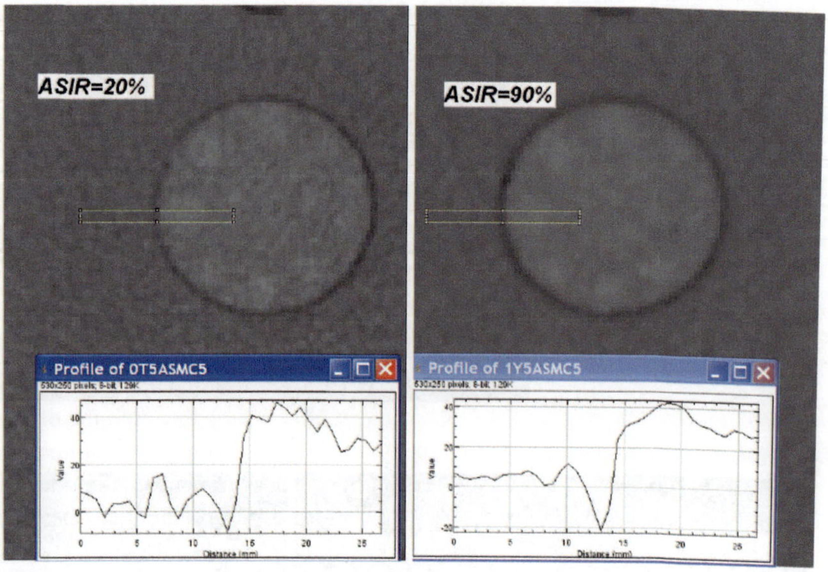

Fig. 3.10 Edge profile difference for a 7 mm low-contrast insert

higher percentage of IR. In fact, due to the nonlinearity of IR, it was found that the spatial resolution is low-contrast dependent for IR-formed images [49]. This is true even for images using deep learning image reconstructions. The detail of this topic is beyond the scope of this chapter.

CT Image Artifacts

CT artifacts [50–53] are the visually discernable discrepancies of the reconstructed CT numbers from those representing the true attenuation of the object in study. The causes of artifacts can originate from various factors, such as patient movement, metal implant in the body, polychromatic spectrum nature of the CT beam, detector module fault, CT x-ray tube arching, foreign object in the CT tube housing or on the mylar window of the CT gantry, and others. The article of Barrett and Keat can be referred for a good review of CT artifacts.

Among the frequently encountered artifacts, **motion artifacts** cause image misregistration streaks and blurring. They can be mitigated by using breath-holding and immobilization aids. **Beam hardening artifacts** are presented as dark bands between the high-attenuation objects such as bony structures. They are due to the lower-attenuation coefficients from the contribution of higher-energy photons after passing through the high-attenuation objects. Beam hardening can be mitigated with specialized filters or software adjustments. **Partial volume effect** is caused by large slice thicknesses, where multiple tissue types are averaged within a single voxel. This averaging can blur details or create streaks, particularly when different densities are present in one voxel. An example of this artifact presentation is blooming artifact in calcified coronary arteries. The calcifications appear bigger than the true size. Using thinner slices helps minimize this effect by capturing more detailed structures. **Metal artifacts** are seen as bright streaks or starbursts around metal implants or other dense objects in the scan field, due to the strong x-ray attenuation by metals that goes beyond the normal range of attenuation of the human organs. Techniques such as patient repositioning, higher kV, virtual monochromatic imaging with dual energy, or single energy metal artifact reduction software can reduce these artifacts. **Truncation artifacts** occur when part of the scanned anatomy extends beyond the scanner's field of view, often in patients with broad anatomy or in cases where positioning is suboptimal. This causes bright or dark shading at the edges of the scan, as the CT reconstruction algorithm misinterprets missing data, sometimes creating streaks or distortion near the boundary. Avoiding truncation artifacts involves adjusting the field of view to capture the entire area of interest or repositioning the patient to fit fully within the scan range. Some scanners offer software-based solutions to estimate and correct the missing information, though careful positioning remains a reliable method to prevent these artifacts. Addressing these artifacts often requires a combination of protocol optimization, hardware adjustments, and patient preparation to maintain the highest possible imaging quality.

CT Dose Reduction: Practical Considerations

As CT radiation becomes a public concern, it is necessary to reduce the dose in general. However, the task cannot be carried out without meeting the diagnosis needs. To find the acquisition techniques corresponding to the minimum dose for the diagnosis requirement is a dose optimization process. Since the diagnosis is task specific, there is no simple and universal procedure to follow for the optimization.

It is often a misconception that better image quality is always realized with increased dose. For the low-contrast lesion detection, the quality-dose relationship is rather nonlinear, meaning that the detectability improvement with higher doses is negligible after the dose reaches a certain point. Figure 3.11 shows the minimum detectable contrast (MDC) as a function of the dose for the low-contrast targets of two sizes (7.0 mm and 3.5 mm) for a medium size abdomen phantom. As demonstrated, the MDC curve flattens after certain dose values (15 mGy and 23 mGy, for 7 mm and 3.5 mm, respectively). These values can serve as the optimal doses for the assessment of the corresponding lesions.

As far as the radiation output is concerned, one can adjust either the x-ray tube voltage (kVp) or current (mA). The effects of the two adjustments differ. The kVp adjustment changes the x-ray spectrum in addition to the photon flux, whereas mA adjustment only impacts the number of photons. Higher kVp means less beam hardening and better penetration through the patient. Therefore, it is recommended for the exams with severe photon-starving or with metal hardware. Lower kVp

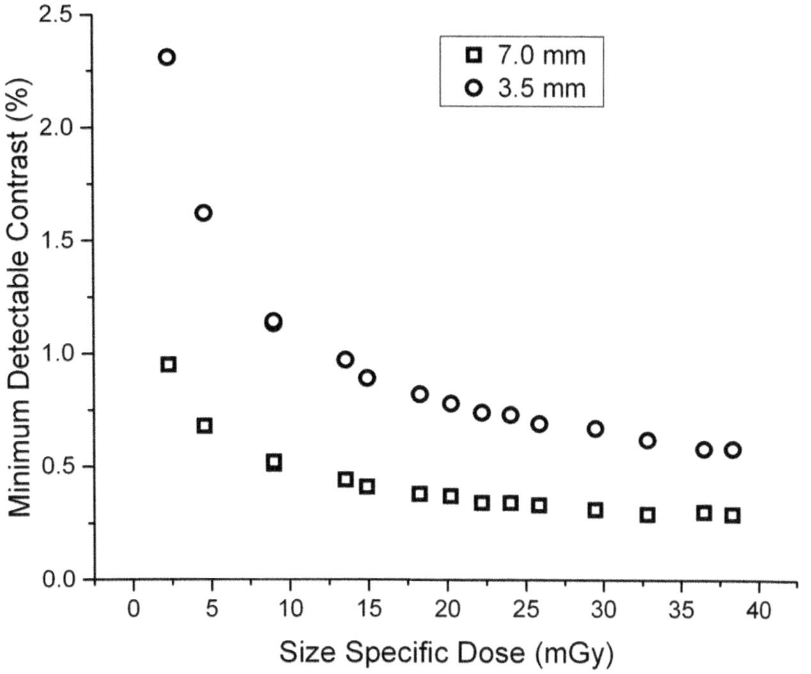

Fig. 3.11 Minimum detectable contrast (MDC) as a function of the dose for the low-contrast targets of different sizes (7.0 mm and 3.5 mm) for a medium abdomen phantom. The images were reconstructed using the filtered backprojection

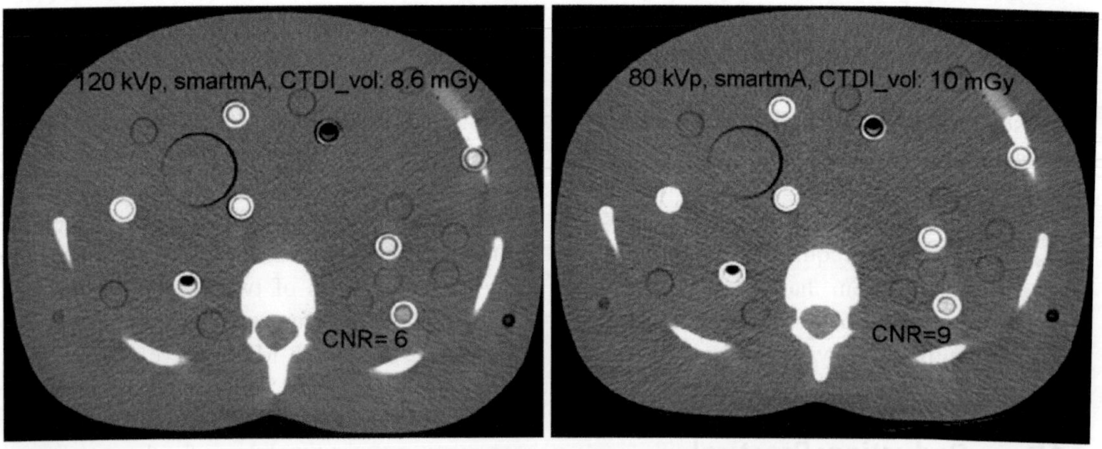

Fig. 3.12 Results of keeping the same noise at 120 kVp and 80 kVp for the ATOM phantom (CIRS, VA, USA) scanned with a GE VCT scanner by using GE's smartmA. The small circular regions were filled with various iodine concentrations

can significantly enhance the iodine contrast, which can be used to tolerate noisier surroundings; so a dose reduction is practical. The details of lower kVp imaging will be further discussed in the following subsection. For mA adjustment, there are situations where the reduction of mA, hence the dose, is obviously achievable, when the higher intrinsic contrast presents as the diagnosis target, such as kidney stone, hydrocephalous, colonoscopy, angiography, calcium scoring, and the like. In other situations, where the lesion is subtle such as tumors in the liver, the tolerance to the noise is limited. The mA reduction is accordingly limited. Therefore, the mA selection is highly task dependent. For the same task, to reach consistent noise from different organs of the scan or from different patients, the mA needs to be altered in a more systematic manner. The most popular approach performing this function is called automatic tube current modulation (ATCM), which will be addressed later.

kVp Adjustment for Iodine Contrast Enhancement

In studies using iodine contrast, the contrast can be enhanced using lower kVps. As the kVp decreases, the iodine contrast increases as the effective energy is closer to the iodine's k-edge, although the enhancement is less appreciated for bigger patients due to the beam hardening effect [54]. However, if the milliampere (mA) is kept the same when the kVp is lower, the noise will increase more significantly. At different kVps, one may have different choices to address the target image quality: keep the same noise, keep the same contrast-to-noise ratio, or find a solution in between, for the concerned region. Figure 3.12 shows the results of keeping the same noise at 120 kVp and at 80 kVp for the ATOM phantom (CIRS-Sun Nuclear, VA, USA) scanned with a GE VCT scanner by using GE's smartmA. It is seen that the dose increases with this choice. Figure 3.13 shows the results using the second choice by targeting the same iodine contrast-to-noise ratio. This choice leads to dose reduction and is the most appropriate for CT angiography. If the primary task is not only angiography but also toward nearby soft tissue, the mA needs to be adjusted higher to be between the first two aforementioned choices. The details of the mA/kVp for different tasks are beyond the scope of this chapter [55]. To make this process easier for the user, CT manufacturers have implemented the semiautomatic kV/mA adjustment on the newer scanners using different commercial terms, such as Care kV, kV assist, sure KV, and so on. The adjustment is first made by the user's selection of the task (see Fig. 3.14), be it angiography,

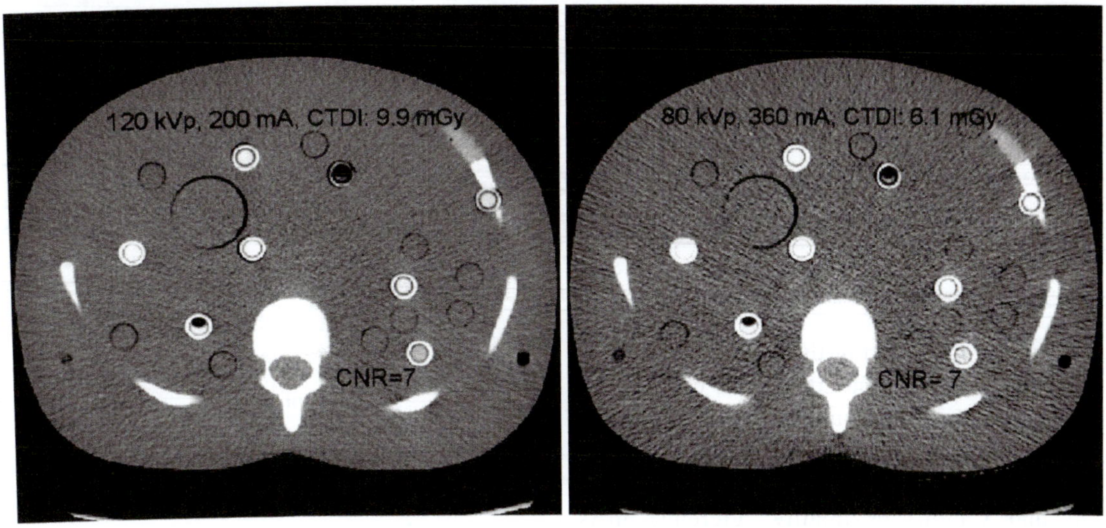

Fig. 3.13 Results by targeting the same iodine contrast-to-noise ratio. The small circular regions were filled with various iodine concentrations

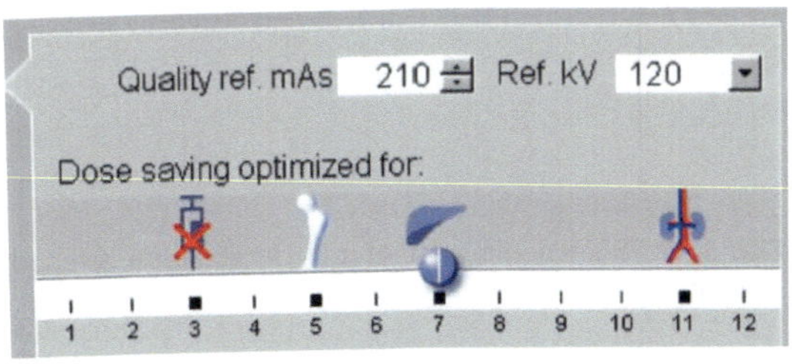

Fig. 3.14 Graphical user interfaces of Care kV (left, Siemens) and kV Assist (right, GE)

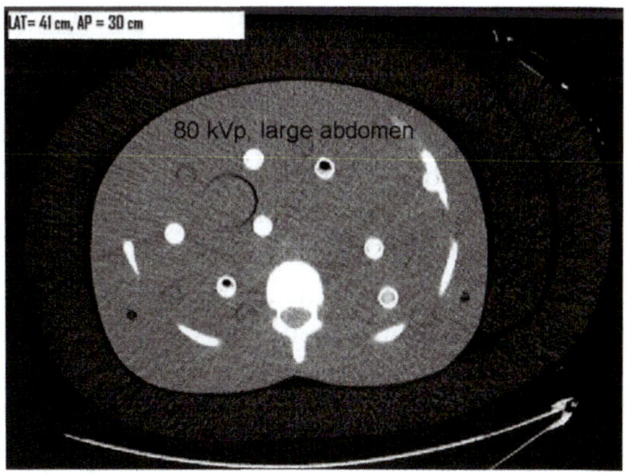

Fig. 3.15 Artifacts at 80 kVp for a large phantom due to photon starving and beam hardening

contrast-enhanced studies, bone imaging or soft tissue only, and then by the automatic selection of the kV and mA for the task. Figure 3.14 shows a graphical user interface of Siemens' Care KV.

Finally, it should be pointed out that the benefits gained by the iodine contrast enhancement at lower kV may be significantly compromised by the severe artifacts if the patient is large. As seen in Fig. 3.15, the artifacts at 80 kVp for a large phantom make the low kVp selection inappropriate.

Automatic Tube Current Modulation (ATCM)

For the same patient, the penetration of the x-ray is different for different body parts in the beam. For instance, the penetration through the anterior-posterior (AP) dimension is easier than that through the lateral dimension. The corresponding mA should be adjusted smaller as shown in the left figure in Fig. 3.16. Similarly, the penetration through the chest is significantly easier than that through the abdomen. To reach the similar image quality, the required mA for the chest should be significantly smaller as seen in the right figure in Fig. 3.16.

To take all the above factors into the design is the task of automatic tube current modulation (ATCM). The key is to choose an acceptable

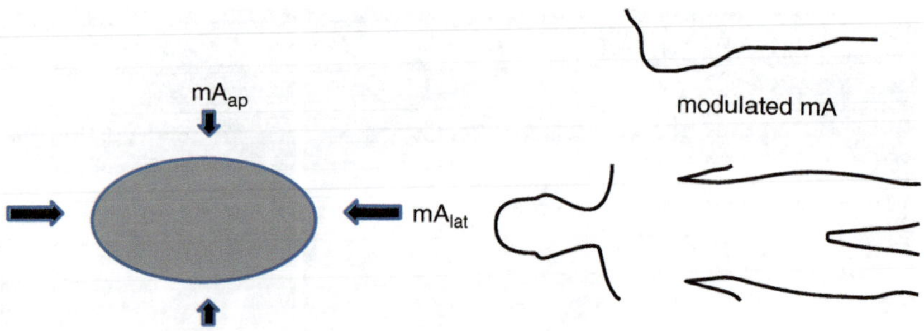

Fig. 3.16 mA modulation at different rotation angles and along the longitudinal dimension

quality surrogate during the scan planning and assure that the surrogate drives the correct mA during the scan. The quality surrogate can be the noise in a water equivalent phantom (noise index or standard deviation as implemented by GE and Canon) or quality reference mAs matching a predefined reference patient (implemented by Siemens and similarly by Philips) [56–58]. The patient size can be estimated from the scan projection radiographs (SPR) (scout views). If the noise index is prescribed, its relationship to the mA can be directly obtained through a look-up-table for the estimated patient size. To prevent the patient from over or under exposure, the user can define the upper and lower bounds of the mA. The latest development of the ATCM using noise index contains a feature called profile prescription where the "size-adjustable noise index (SANI)" is used. This allows the user to choose the patient size based noise index for fine-tuning of the dose. If the reference mAs is used, such as in Siemens Care Dose 4D, the mA during the scan is derived from a predefined curve that mandates adequate diagnosis quality at different patient sizes [57, 59]. In this modulation scheme, adequate diagnosis quality does not correspond to a constant noise. Rather, the noise increases with the patient size [53]. This means that more noise can be tolerated for larger patients due to the increased visceral fat (thus better contrast) and radiation concern, whereas the opposite is true for slim and pediatric patients. The deviation of the curve from the constant noise is related to the "modulation strength" (less deviation corresponds to strong modulation, as seen in Fig. 3.17), which can be selected by the user. A further mA fine-tuning is automatically made during the scan to account for the attenuation change due to contrast or patient organ motion.

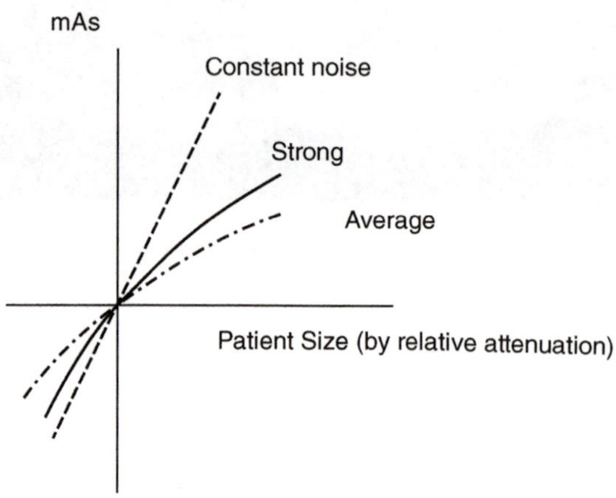

Fig. 3.17 Sketch diagram of mA modulation strength control with Care Dose

In order to address the task-specific diagnosis, adequate choice of the noise index or quality reference mAs is important. This is currently done empirically. For example, for the assessment of kidney stones, a noise index of 17 or higher may be appropriate for the slice thickness of 5 mm, whereas a noise index of 11.4 may be needed for the liver lesion diagnosis (see Fig. 3.18 for comparison). It is desired to derive these noise indices or quality reference mAs from the required contrast percentage and lesion size for the known patient size. Certain research effort has been made toward this goal [60].

In either of the aforementioned ATCM implementations, the $CTDI_{vol}$ can be estimated post the scan projection radiograph but prior to the actual scan. This estimate is displayed on the acquisition console. The feature is useful for the user to judge the dose before the scan.

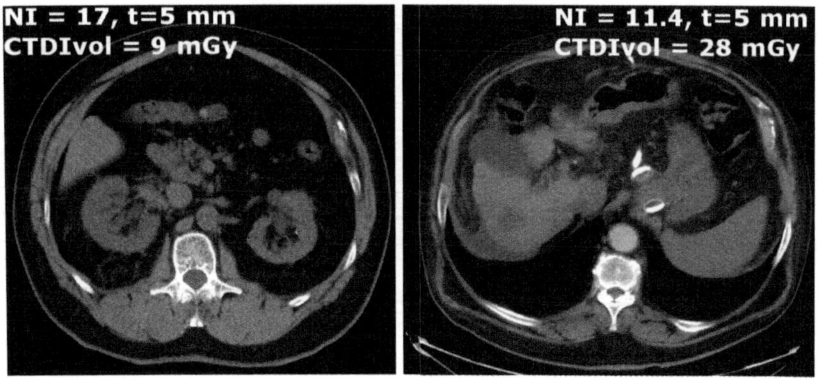

Fig. 3.18 Noise index comparison for different tasks. (Left: kidney stone. Right: liver lesion. The right patient is also bigger)

Pitfalls of CT Dose Optimization

When the attempt is made to optimize the patient dose in CT, especially when ATCM is utilized, several important caveats have to be addressed. Unexpected results may occur if cautions are not used.

ATCM, Primary Reconstruction Thickness, and IR Strength

For some scanners, the prescribed quality surrogate with ATCM is directly associated with the slice thickness of the primary (or the first) reconstruction. For a given quality surrogate, the dose consequences are substantially different at different primary reconstruction thicknesses. As far as the slice thickness selection is concerned, it is the total photon flux per unit volume that determines the dose, as shown in Fig. 3.19. If the same noise index (thus the same photon flux) is prescribed for half of the primary reconstruction thickness, the same photon flux has to be packed into the thinner slices from the original thickness. The total photon flux to the same anatomical range is doubled. The radiation dose therefore increases by a factor of 2. In order to achieve the same dose for the thinner slice prescription, the photon flux to the thinner slices needs to be half of that delivered to the thicker slices. The expected noise accordingly increases by a factor of $\sqrt{2}$. This reasoning is critical when a new noise index is specified with a new primary slice thickness. For the systems using the quality reference mAs in the ATCM, the similar principle applies. Thinner slices lead to noisier images for the same quality reference mAs, or a bigger quality reference mAs is required for the same noise.

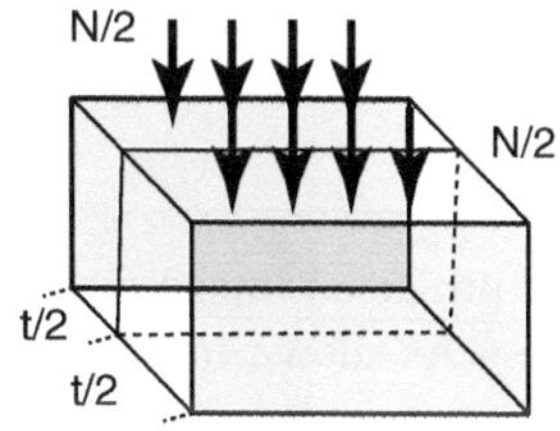

Fig. 3.19 Photon flux per unit volume determines the dose at different slice thicknesses

The dose determination from the above primary thickness and quality surrogate get even more complicated for some newer scanner models when the third-generation IR reconstruction is prospectively involved in the dose prescription. This was found in GE revolution scanners. A previous study has analyzed the data and found a quantitative relationship among the dose, patient size, primary thickness, and the IR strength [61].

The situation varies depending on the manufacturers. For example, the Canon CT separately specifies the surrogate quality index (standard deviation) and the thickness that is independent of the clinical reconstruction thickness.

ATCM and Patient Positioning

Another factor that may not receive enough attention from the user is the patient positioning. The importance can be illustrated in Fig. 3.21. When the ATCM is used, the mA modulation is determined by the scan projection radiograph. Specifically, the patient size estimate is directly

Fig. 3.20 Consequences of different patient positions

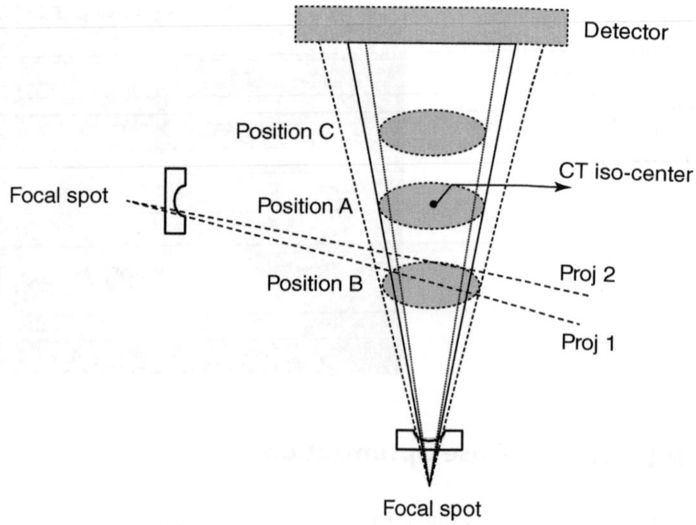

related to the projected image that is table position dependent. As shown in the figure, position A places the patient to the CT's iso-center, whereas positions B and C result in bigger and smaller projected images, respectively. Therefore, position B modulates the mA to higher values and delivers more patient dose. The opposite is true for position C. Another major concern of mispositioning the patient originates from the misalignment of the patient with respect to the bowtie filter. As mentioned in Section "Basic design of multi-detector CT system", the bowtie filter is designed to attenuate the least x-ray at the center and the most x-ray at the periphery so that the photon intensity and spectrum are more equalized after passing through the patient. This is no longer true if the patient is not positioned at the CT's iso-center. For instance, for patient position B in Fig. 3.20, projection 1 travels through the thicker paths of both the bowtie and the patient, resulting in poor photon flux to the detector. In the meantime, projection 2 travels through the thinner path of the bowtie to the surface of the patient, leading to the overdose to the region.

Other Considerations

In addition to the pitfalls aforementioned, it is worthwhile to discuss the other issues that may be misunderstood or hidden in practice.

The first consideration is about the implementation of Image Gently. It is well recognized that the reduced dose should be applied to younger patients. However, how to adjust the dose to the same detectability need for different patient sizes is challenging. Due to the limitation of $CTDI_{vol}$ defined only on either of the two phantoms of diameters of 16 am and 32 cm, $CTDI_{vol}$ does not vary with the patient size for the fixed radiation technique. The AAPM proposed that size-specific dose estimate (SSDE) adequately reflects the impact of the patient size [25], so that the SSDE is bigger for smaller patients for the given radiation technique. Accordingly, there may be suggestions to use the same SSDE for different patients to achieve the dose reduction goal for younger patients. However, if the objective is to obtain the same low-contrast detectability for smaller patients, further dose reduction should be considered [38]. This point is demonstrated in a phantom study in Fig. 3.21, where the low-contrast detectability is substantially better for the phantom mimicking the 1-year old patient with the same SSDE. Of course, one needs to consider the lack of visceral fat for pediatric patients so the intrinsic contrast may be lower. The required dose may need to be adjusted slightly higher than mandated by the consistent low-contrast detectability from the adult patient.

The next pitfall is the selection of the rotation time. Shorter rotation time can be used to reduce the motion artifacts. However, the selection should be made carefully when the ATCM is used.

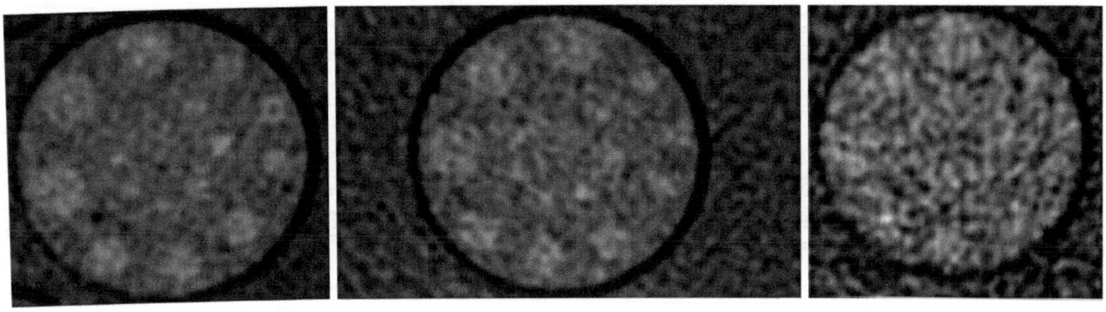

Fig. 3.21 Low-contrast inserts in the abdomen phantoms for (left to right) 1-year-old, 5-year–old, and adult. SSDE = 8.9 mGy for all

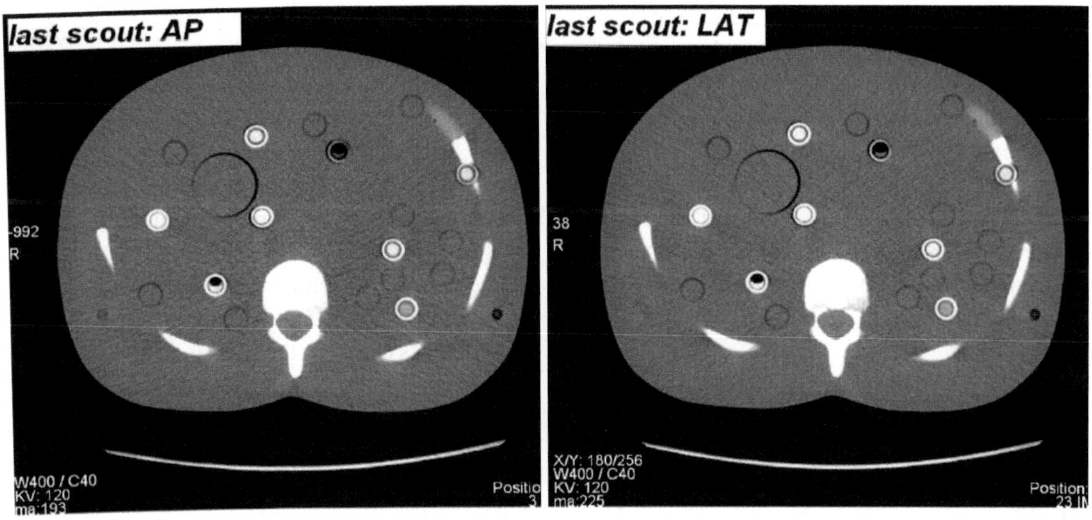

Fig. 3.22 mA was modulated differently depending on the lastly acquired scout on the GE VCT scanner

The reason is that it is the effective milliampere-second (mAs) that determines whether the prescribed quality factor is met. If the rotation time is too short, it drives the mA to a higher value that may exceed the upper bound of the mA range. This results in a flat rather than a modulated mA for the scan and suboptimal image quality. As one of the schemes to mitigate the problem, some machines automatically choose a lower pitch so the required mA can be smaller. However, this feature is not available for many scanners.

The third consideration is about the use of the automatic kV feature. As pointed out earlier, the choice of lower kV may not be optimal for very large patients if the artifacts of the photon starving and beam hardening severely overshadow the iodine contrast enhancement. For a similar reason, caution should be used for patients with significant metal implants. Furthermore, cardiac CT angiography should not be acquired at the low kV if one of the following situations occurs: the calcium distribution is dense or the calcium score is high from the calcium score scan, or the patient has stents. The blooming artifacts are significant at lower kVp, and the automatic kV software typically does not detect these subtleties adequately.

The fourth consideration is the order of the scan projection radiographs (SPR) for some machines. The ATCM on some scanner models uses the most recent SPR to determine the mA modulation. On these scanners, the dose consequence may be different depending on whether the AP or lateral view is lastly acquired. Figure 3.22 shows the mA difference on GE VCT scanner.

CT Dose Management

Standards and Rules

The US National Electrical Manufacturers Association (NEMA) published a standard agreed among CT manufacturers specifying four attributes that help perform optimization or management of ionizing radiation while still enabling the system to deliver the image quality needed by the physician [62]. The standard, called NEMA XR-29, consists of the following items:

1. DICOM-compliant structure dose report.
2. Dose check features. This includes defining notification values (NV) for different scans and alert value (AV) per scanner across different exams.
3. Automatic exposure control: Dose should be modulated for different patient sizes.
4. Reference adult and pediatric protocols. Dedicated pediatric protocols should be established

The US Center for Medicare and Medicaid Services (CMS) require the adherence to the NEMA XR-29 for full reimbursement starting January 2016 [63]. If the scanner is NEMA XR-29 compliant [62], it allows the user to define various dose notification values (NV) for different scans. A warning dialog appears if the $CTDI_{vol}$ exceeds the NV, and the user is required to give a reason if the scan is proceeded without revision (see Fig. 3.23 for GE's implementation). XR-29 also defines an alert value (AV) that is valid at the exam level for all CT exams. The default value is typically 1000 mGy but can be adjusted tighter at the user's discretion. If the exam is about to exceed the AV, a more restrictive control dialog appears that mandates not only the reason but also the user's logon name and password.

More recently, the CMS has published the final rules about implementing new electronic clinical quality measures (eCQM 1074, 1206, and 1056) called "excessive radiation dose or inadequate imaging quality for diagnostic CT in adults." The rules address both CT radiation and image quality by defining upper bound values for patient-size adjusted dose-length product (DLP) and global noise from 18 CT exams [64–66]. A viable implementation of the new eCQM is to include the metrics in the electronic medical record (EMR) of the patient. It requires a seamless integration of CT dose tracking system with the EMR.

The Joint Commission in the United States further established the diagnostic imaging standards that requires, among others, annual performance evaluations of CT by a medical physicist, CT radiation dose tracking, CT protocol review, and annual education on Image Wisely and Image Gently using CT [67].

The American College of Radiology (ACR) has long established the CT accreditation standards. The accreditation includes different modules, head and neck, chest, abdomen, and cardiac. The site is required to send clinical and phantom images for the selected modules. There are defined dose and contrast-to-noise thresholds for the phantom images matching the clinical images. This process can help the imaging site to tune the corresponding protocols to be compliant, although the scope only applies to the chosen modules for the accreditation application. To obtain further dose information from a national database, the site can participate the national CT radiation dose registry (NRDR) implemented by ACR. The dose information from the protocols with good statistical data can serve as a good reference for the site.

Image Gently for Pediatric Patients

The NEMA XR-29 requires dedicated protocols for pediatric studies. Furthermore, the Alliance of Image Gently is founded by Society for Pediatric Radiology, American College of Radiology, American Society for Radiologic Technologists, and the American Association of Physicists in Medicine. CT modality is one of the important modalities in the mission. The effort is vital because pediatric patients are more sensitive to radiation. It is suggested that the parents receive

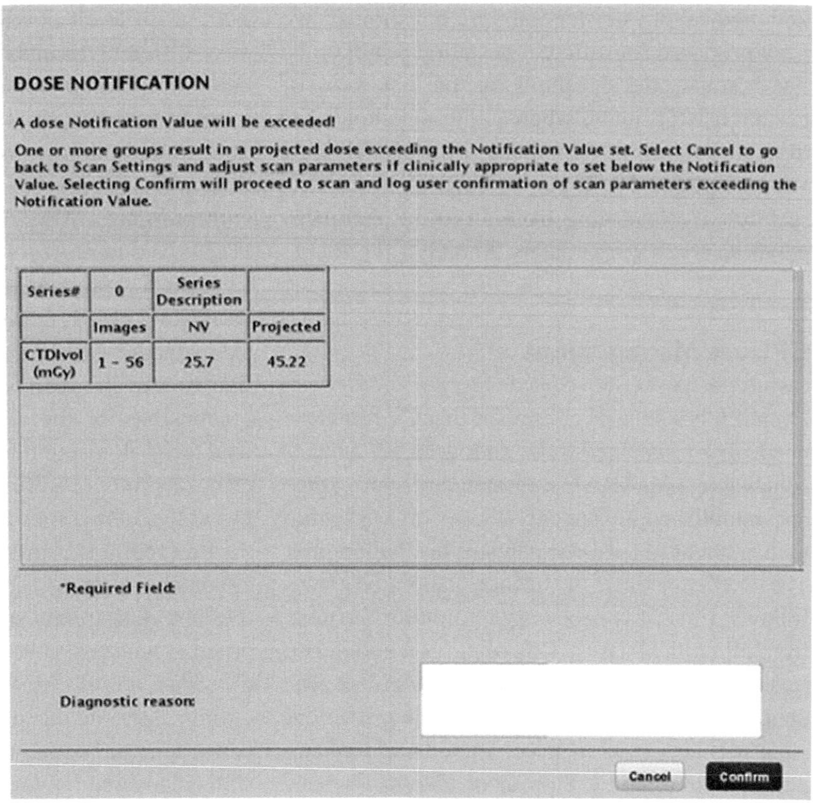

Fig. 3.23 Example of the NV warning dialog

the necessary information about the options for alternative non-radiation examinations by discussing with the referring physicians. If the CT exam is medically justified, it is a consensus to deliver radiation as low as reasonably achievable (ALARA). Therefore, it is prudent to apply age- and size-dependent dose thresholds in pediatric protocols. The success can be achieved by using automatic dose modulation with possible lower kV selections for the body habitus or by using age-tuned manual techniques for the head studies. To find reference doses, one can refer to the US national benchmarks published by Kanal et al. for the top ten pediatric CT examinations [68]. The data were gathered from the US national dose registry for the patients 18 years old or younger. The work classified the age to four groups (0–1, 1–2, 2–6, and 6–18). In practice, the site may choose more age group granularities to practice ALARA.

CT for Pregnant Patients

Non-radiation imaging modalities should be the first choice for pregnant patients if the imaged area is on or near the fetus. However, CT imaging may be still necessary for some patients. Hence, special caution should be used when imaging these patients. If the primary beam is far from the fetus, such as in head exams, there should not be concerns about the dose to the fetus. If the fetus is to be exposed to the primary beam, the diagnosis task should be discussed with the radiologist to determine if the scan length can be further limited. In addition, the technique itself should be adjusted to be patient size dependent for the task. The use of lead apron is not recommended in this situation because significant artifacts can occur to compromise the diagnosis. For the cases where the fetus is exposed to the primary beam, it is suggested to perform a fetal dose estimate by a qualified medical physicist. Fetal dose thresholds have been proposed for different gestation time points. For example, the threshold for the first week of gestation is 50 mGy, whereas the thresholds for the other fetus development time are at least 100 mGy [69, 70]. To put information in the perspective, the fetal dose from a typical abdomen-pelvis scan is approximately 20 mGy [71].

CT Dose Management

Even if it is a general consensus that CT radiation needs to be managed to be as low as reasonably achievable (ALARA), and standards and rules are established to support the effort, systemic management of CT dose can still be challenging. The challenges can be further elaborated on as follows: First, it is necessary to monitor the dose from all clinical cases. This requires a good dose tracking tool. Since the dose is protocol dependent, and protocol names vary among different sites, it is important to select a good tool that can perform automatic CT protocol mapping whenever a scanner or a protocol is added. The systems requiring a manual protocol mapping will be hard to maintain. Another challenge is to define reasonable dose alert levels that trigger notifications to the medical physicists or lead technologists. The thresholds need to be protocol specific and patient size dependent. It is noted that the ACR published the national benchmarks for the top ten CT protocols: the dose reference level (DRL) and achievable dose (AD), corresponding to the 75th and 50th percentiles, respectively. An imaging site can use its own 50th percentile data to compare to the DRL [72]. However, there are hundreds of CT protocols used for many large imaging sites. It is necessary to carefully define their own ALARA-based alert levels for many protocols. One may start using the 90th or 95th percentile for each protocol and each patient size group and gradually reduce the alert level by diligently checking the image quality and revising the CT protocols. The CT protocol review and revision thus come into play naturally. It also introduces an additional challenge: many sites handle a large number of scanners of different makes and models that contain very different formats of protocols. It is practically important to obtain a unified format for protocol review [73]. It is even more desirable to be able to compare protocols at any two specified time points using the formatted protocols. One can configure a Website on the intranet to host the HTML-based protocols.

For CT dose management, the recommended workflow is to (1) define the protocol and patient-size-specific dose alert levels, (2) track the cases that exceed the alert levels and find the reasons responsible for the alerts, (3) interact with the lead technologist to find if the alert is from human error or protocol setting, (4) coach the technologist if the alert comes from the operator or revise the protocol if it is justified, (5) update the protocol database, and (6) adjust the alert thresholds as the new data trends suggest [73]. This iteration process will make continuous improvement of the dose optimization effort. Furthermore, the outlier cases in the process can serve as good educational material for annual education sessions mandated by the Joint Commission.

Ongoing Efforts to Improve Quality and Safety

Efforts to improve quality and patient safety in CT by organizations, clinical practice, and industry are discussed in the following [68, 72, 74]:

Federal/Organizational Efforts

The Image Gently and Image Wisely campaigns improve patient safety by promoting radiation dose reduction in CT scans, which minimizes the potential risks associated with radiation exposure, particularly in children and patients requiring frequent imaging. While dose reduction can lead to increased image noise, potentially affecting diagnostic quality, these campaigns emphasize using advanced techniques, i.e., iterative reconstruction and age- or size-specific protocols, to preserve image quality at lower doses. By balancing safety and diagnostic accuracy, these initiatives support high-quality imaging practices that protect patients while still providing reliable diagnostic information.

The ACR is another organization that promotes quality and patient safety. Besides ACR CT accreditation, the ACR CT Dose Index Registry (DIR) is an important tool that enhances patient safety and imaging quality by allowing facilities to monitor, compare, and optimize radiation doses in CT scans. By contributing to and accessing national benchmarks for CT dose indices, facilities can evaluate their radiation usage against established standards, identifying opportunities to reduce exposure while maintaining image quality. This benchmarking process helps facilities track dose trends, address potential outliers, and implement dose reduction strategies tailored to specific patient demographics, clinical indications, and scan protocols. The DIR promotes transparency and encourages continuous improvement in CT practices, ultimately supporting safer imaging by reducing unnecessary radiation exposure and ensuring consistent, high-quality diagnostic outcomes across institutions.

The recent CMS rules about the new electronic clinical quality measures about excessive CT radiation and inadequate image quality are expected to further CT dose optimization. This aspect was briefly discussed in Section "CT dose management". Further details can be found in Section "Resources for quality and safety".

Resources for Quality and Safety

Table 3.1 provides a summary of resources (e.g., QC recommendations, safety guidelines) for quality and safety of diagnostic imaging modalities, including those related to mammography for completeness. We include a selection of relevant references from the major organizations. The goal of this table is to facilitate readers for a quick access to those resources.

It needs to be pointed out that most organizations do not function as enforcement agencies. Regulatory agencies that enforce the implementation of the recommendations/guidelines include the FDA, Nuclear Regulatory Commission (NRC), Environment Protection Agency (EPA), Occupational Safety and Health Administration (OSHA), and agreement States.

Table 3.1 Resources for quality and safety of diagnostic imaging modalities

CT imaging
AAPM Report No. 96: The Measurement, Reporting and Management of Radiation Dose in CT
AAPM Report No. 111: Comprehensive Methodology for the Evaluation of Radiation Dose in X-Ray Computed Tomography
AAPM Report No. 204: Size-Specific Dose Estimates (SSDE) in Pediatric and Adult Body CT Examinations
IEC (2010) 60601–60602: Medical Electrical Equipment. Part 2–44: Particular Requirements for the Basic Safety and Essential Performance of X-Ray Equipment for Computed Tomography
ICRP 102 (2007): Managing Patient Dose in Multi-detector Computed Tomography (MDCT)
NCRP 184 (2019): Medical Radiation Exposure of Patients in the United States
NEMA XR 29: Standard Attributes on CT Equipment Related to Dose Optimization and Management
CMS: 2024 Hospital Inpatient Quality Reporting (IQR) Program Final Rule
CMS: 2024 Hospital Outpatient Quality Reporting (OQR) Program Final Rule
CMS: 2024 Medicare Physician Fee Schedule (PFS) Final Rule
National Research Council: Health Risks from Exposure to Low Levels of Ionizing Radiation. BEIR VII Phase 2
ACR (2023): ACR–AAPM–SPR Practice Parameter for Diagnostic Reference Levels and Achievable Doses in Medical X-Ray Imaging
Image Gently Alliance: http://imagegently.org

AAPM American Association of Physicists in Medicine, *ACR* American College of Radiology, *FDA* US Food and Drug Administration, *ICRP* International Commission on Radiological Protection, *NCRP* National Council on Radiation Protection, *IEC* International Electrotechnical Commission, *CMS* US Centers for Medicare & Medicaid Services

Summary

In this chapter, several important aspects related to dose and image quality in CT have been discussed. The summary is listed as follows:

- CTDI is a radiation output measurement instead of a patient dose metric.
- CT dose optimization depends on the diagnosis task.
- CT dose should be adjusted according to the patient size and age. This effort aligns with Image Wisely and Gently.
- Due to its nonlinear response to dose, the image quality may not improve appreciably with dose increase if the dose exceeds a certain value for the task.
- Low kVp imaging enhances the iodine contrast, so more noise may be tolerated if high-contrast lesion is the concern. This helps dose reduction.
- Automatic tube current modulation eases the user from manual parameter tuning for consistent image quality, but its use calls for careful attention for several pitfalls, such as patient position, scout acquisition order, and others.
- A sustainable program for CT dose and protocol management calls for a system support including dose tracking with size- or age-specific thresholds, protocol extraction, protocol review, revision, and approval.

Glossary

MDCT Multi-detector computed tomography
CTDI Computed tomography dose index
$CTDI_{free\text{-}in\text{-}air}$ Computed tomography dose index measured free-in-air
$CTDI_w$ Weighted computed tomography dose index
$CTDI_{vol}$ Volume computed tomography dose index
SSDE Size-specific dose estimate
FBP Filtered backprojection
IR Iterative reconstruction
ASIR Adaptive statistical iterative reconstruction
MBIR Model-based iterative reconstruction
DLIR Deep learning image reconstruction
AP Anterior-posterior
LAT Lateral
ATCM Automatic tube current modulation
AEC Automatic exposure control
LCD Low-contrast detectability
MCD Minimum detectable contrast
AAPM Assocation of American Physicists in Medicine
NEMA National Electrical Manufacturers Association
IEC International Electrotechnical Commission

References

1. Hu H. Multi-slice helical CT: scan and reconstruction. Med Phys. 1999;26:5–18. https://doi.org/10.1118/1.598470.
2. Klingenbeck-Regn K, Schaller S, Flohr T, et al. Subsecond multi-slice computed tomography: basics and applications. Eur J Radiol. 1999;31:110–24.
3. McCollough CH, Zink FE. Performance evaluation of a multi-slice CT system. Med Phys. 1999;26:2223–30. https://doi.org/10.1118/1.598777.
4. Smith-Bindman R, Lipson J, Marcus R, et al. Radiation dose associated with common computed tomography examinations and the associated lifetime attributable risk of cancer. Arch Intern Med. 2009;169:2078–86. https://doi.org/10.1001/archinternmed.2009.427.
5. Lewis MA, Edyvean S. Patient dose reduction in CT. Br J Radiol. 2005;78:880–3. https://doi.org/10.1259/bjr/75960844.
6. Shrimpton PC, Hillier MC, Lewis MA, Dunn M. National survey of doses from CT in the UK: 2003. Br J Radiol. 2006;79:968–80. https://doi.org/10.1259/bjr/93277434.
7. National Research Council. Health risks from exposure to low levels of ionizing radiation. BEIR VII phase 2. Washington, DC: National Academies Press; 2006.
8. Pierce DA, Preston DL. Radiation-related cancer risks at low doses among atomic bomb survivors. Radiat Res. 2000;154:178–86.
9. Preston DL, Ron E, Tokuoka S, et al. Solid cancer incidence in atomic bomb survivors: 1958-1998. Radiat Res. 2007;168:1–64. https://doi.org/10.1667/rr0763.1.
10. Cardis E, Vrijheid M, Blettner M, et al. The 15-country collaborative study of cancer risk among radiation workers in the nuclear industry: estimates of radiation-related cancer risks. Radiat Res. 2007;167:396–416. https://doi.org/10.1667/rr0553.1.
11. Tubiana M. Dose-effect relationship and estimation of the carcinogenic effects of low doses of ionizing radi-

ation: the joint report of the Academie des Sciences (Paris) and of the Academie Nationale de Medecine. Int J Radiat Oncol Biol Phys. 2005;63:317–9. https://doi.org/10.1016/j.ijrobp.2005.06.013.
12. Tubiana M, Feinendegen LE, Yang C, Kaminski JM. The linear no-threshold relationship is inconsistent with radiation biologic and experimental data. Radiology. 2009;251:13–22. https://doi.org/10.1148/radiol.2511080671.
13. Ronda CR. Scintillators. In: Ronda CR, editor. Luminescence: from theory to applications. Wiley; 2007.
14. Engel KJ, Herrmann C, Zeitler G. X-ray scattering in single- and dual-source CT. Med Phys. 2008;35:318–32. https://doi.org/10.1118/1.2820901.
15. Glover GH. Compton scatter effects in CT reconstructions. Med Phys. 1982;9:860–7. https://doi.org/10.1118/1.595197.
16. Vogtmeier G, Engel KJ, et al. Two-dimensional anti-scatter-grids for computed tomography detectors. In: SPIE Proc6913, Med. Imaging 2008, p. 6913
17. van der Molen AJ, Geleijns J. Overranging in multisection CT: quantification and relative contribution to dose--comparison of four 16-section CT scanners. Radiology. 2007;242:208–16. https://doi.org/10.1148/radiol.2421051350.
18. Christner JA, Zavaletta VA, Eusemann CD, et al. Dose reduction in helical CT: dynamically adjustable z-axis X-ray beam collimation. AJR Am J Roentgenol. 2010;194:W49–55. https://doi.org/10.2214/ajr.09.2878.
19. Kak AC, Slaney M. Principles of computerized tomographic imaging. Philadelphia: Society for Industrial and Applied Mathematics; 2001.
20. Geyer LL, Schoepf UJ, Meinel FG, et al. State of the art: iterative CT reconstruction techniques1. Radiology. 2015;276:339–57. https://doi.org/10.1148/radiol.2015132766.
21. Deak Z, Grimm JM, Treitl M, et al. Filtered back projection, adaptive statistical iterative reconstruction, and a model-based iterative reconstruction in abdominal CT: an experimental clinical study. Radiology. 2013;266:197–206. https://doi.org/10.1148/radiol.12112707.
22. Buzug T. SpringerLink (Online service), 2008. Computed tomography from photon statistics to modern cone-beam CT.
23. Neroladaki A, Botsikas D, Boudabbous S, et al. Computed tomography of the chest with model-based iterative reconstruction using a radiation exposure similar to chest X-ray examination: preliminary observations. Eur Radiol. 2013;23:360–6. https://doi.org/10.1007/s00330-012-2627-7.
24. Hou Y, Xu S, Guo W, et al. The optimal dose reduction level using iterative reconstruction with prospective ECG-triggered coronary CTA using 256-slice MDCT. Eur J Radiol. 2012;81:3905–11. https://doi.org/10.1016/j.ejrad.2012.06.022.
25. AAPM. Size-specific dose estimates (SSDE) in pediatric and adult body CT examinations. College Park: American Asociation of Physicists in Medicine; 2011.
26. Shope TB, Gagne RM, Johnson GC. A method for describing the doses delivered by transmission x-ray computed tomography. Med Phys. 1981;8:488–95. https://doi.org/10.1118/1.594995.
27. AAPM. The measurement, reporting and management of radiation dose in CT. College Park: American Association of Physicisits in Medicine; 2008.
28. Valentin J. Managing patient dose in multi-detector computed tomography(MDCT). ICRP Publication 102. Ann ICRP. 2007. https://doi.org/10.1016/j.icrp.2007.09.001
29. (2006) Health risks from exposure to low levels of ionizing radiation: BEIR VII Phase 2.
30. Siegel JA, Greenspan BS, Maurer AH, et al. The BEIR VII estimates of low-dose radiation health risks are based on faulty assumptions and data analyses: a call for reassessment. J Nucl Med. 2018; https://doi.org/10.2967/jnumed.117.206219.
31. O'Connor MK. Risk of low-dose radiation and the BEIR VII report: a critical review of what it does and doesn't say. Phys Med. 2017;
32. Hernandez-Giron I, Calzado A, Geleijns J, et al. Low contrast detectability performance of model observers based on CT phantom images: kVp influence. Phys Med. 2015;31:798–807. https://doi.org/10.1016/j.ejmp.2015.04.012.
33. Racine D, Ba AH, Ott JG, et al. Objective assessment of low contrast detectability in computed tomography with channelized Hotelling observer. Phys Med. 2016;32:76–83. https://doi.org/10.1016/j.ejmp.2015.09.011.
34. Saiprasad G, Filliben J, Peskin A, et al. Evaluation of low-contrast detectability of iterative reconstruction across multiple institutions, ct scanner manufacturers, and radiation exposure levels. Radiology. 2015;277:124–33. https://doi.org/10.1148/radiol.2015141260.
35. Chao EH, Toth TL, Bromberg NB, et al. A statistical method of defining low contrast detectability. Radiology. 2000;217:162.
36. Hsieh J. Computed tomography : principles, design, artifacts, and recent advances. Bellingham: SPIE Press; 2003.
37. Zhou Y, Scott A, Allahverdian J, et al. On the relationship of minimum detectable contrast to dose and lesion size in abdominal CT. Phys Med Biol. 2015;60:7671–94. https://doi.org/10.1088/0031-9155/60/19/7671.
38. Zhou Y, Nute J, Scott A, Lee C. Consistent low-contrast detectability for variable patient sizes and corresponding dose in abdominal CT. Med Phys. 2017;44:861–72. https://doi.org/10.1002/mp.12085.
39. Singh S, Kalra MK, Hsieh J, et al. Abdominal CT: comparison of adaptive statistical iterative and filtered back projection reconstruction techniques. Radiology. 2010;257:373–83. https://doi.org/10.1148/radiol.10092212.

40. Solomon J, Mileto A, Ramirez-Giraldo JC, Samei E. Diagnostic performance of an advanced Modeled iterative reconstruction algorithm for low-contrast detectability with a third-generation dual-source multidetector CT scanner: potential for radiation dose reduction in a multireader study. Radiology. 2015;275:735–45. https://doi.org/10.1148/radiol.15142005.
41. Raman SP, Johnson PT, Deshmukh S, et al. CT dose reduction applications: available tools on the latest generation of CT scanners. J Am Coll Radiol. 2013;10:37–41. https://doi.org/10.1016/j.jacr.2012.06.025.
42. Katsura M, Matsuda I, Akahane M, et al. Model-based iterative reconstruction technique for ultralow-dose chest CT: comparison of pulmonary nodule detectability with the adaptive statistical iterative reconstruction technique. Investig Radiol. 2013;48:206–12. https://doi.org/10.1097/RLI.0b013e31827efc3a.
43. Sun JH, Yu T, Liu JR, et al. Image quality improvement using model-based iterative reconstruction in low dose chest CT for children with necrotizing pneumonia. BMC Med Imaging. 2017;17. https://doi.org/ARTN2410.1186/s12880-017-0177-9
44. Koetzier LR, Mastrodicasa D, Szczykutowicz TP, et al. Deep learning image reconstruction for CT: technical principles and clinical prospects. Radiology. 2023;
45. Heismann B, Schmidt B, Flohr T. Spectral computed tomography. SPIE. 2012
46. Rubert N, Szczykutowicz T, Ranallo F. Improvement in CT image resolution due to the use of focal spot deflection and increased sampling. J Appl Clin Med Phys. 2016;17:452–66.
47. Zamyatin AA, Nakanishi S. Extension of the reconstruction field of view and truncation correction using sinogram decomposition. Med Phys. 2007;34:1593–604. https://doi.org/10.1118/1.2721656.
48. Geyer LL, Glenn GR, De Cecco CN, et al. CT evaluation of small-diameter coronary artery stents: effect of an integrated circuit detector with iterative reconstruction. Radiology. 2015;276:706–14. https://doi.org/10.1148/radiol.15140427.
49. Yu L, Vrieze TJ, Leng S, et al. Technical note: measuring contrast- and noise-dependent spatial resolution of an iterative reconstruction method in CT using ensemble averaging. Med Phys. 2015;42:2261–7. https://doi.org/10.1118/1.4916802.
50. Barrett JF, Keat N. Artifacts in CT: recognition and avoidance. Radiographics. 2004;
51. Boas FE, Fleischmann D. CT artifacts: Causes and reduction techniques. Imaging Med. 2012;
52. Selles M, van Osch J, Maas M, et al. Advances in metal artifact reduction in CT images: a review of traditional and novel metal artifact reduction techniques. Eur J Radiol. 2024;
53. Pack JD, Xu M, Wang G, et al. Cardiac CT blooming artifacts: clinical significance, root causes and potential solutions. Vis Comput Ind Biomed Art. 2022;
54. Boone JM, Geraghty EM, Seibert JA, Wootton-Gorges SL. Dose reduction in pediatric CT: a rational approach. Radiology. 2003;228:352–60. https://doi.org/10.1148/radiol.2282020471.
55. Yu L, Li H, Fletcher JG, McCollough CH. Automatic selection of tube potential for radiation dose reduction in CT: a general strategy. Med Phys. 2010;37:234–43. https://doi.org/10.1118/1.3264614.
56. Kalra MK, Maher MM, Kamath RS, et al. Sixteen-detector row CT of abdomen and pelvis: study for optimization of Z-axis modulation technique performed in 153 patients. Radiology. 2004;233:241–9. https://doi.org/10.1148/radiol.2331031505.
57. Solomon JB, Li X, Samei E. Relating noise to image quality indicators in CT examinations with tube current modulation. AJR Am J Roentgenol. 2013;200:592–600. https://doi.org/10.2214/AJR.12.8580.
58. McCollough CH, Bruesewitz MR, Kofler JM Jr. CT dose reduction and dose management tools: overview of available options. Radiographics. 2006;26:503–12. https://doi.org/10.1148/rg.262055138.
59. Papadakis AE, Perisinakis K, Damilakis J. Automatic exposure control in CT: the effect of patient size, anatomical region and prescribed modulation strength on tube current and image quality. Eur Radiol. 2014;24:2520–31. https://doi.org/10.1007/s00330-014-3309-4.
60. Nute J, Zhou Y, Scott A, Lee C. Relationship between pixel noise and task-specific low contrast detectability for various patient sizes in abdomen CT. Med Phys. 2016;43 https://doi.org/10.1118/1.4958214.
61. Scott AW, Alancherry ASP, Lee C, et al. Computed tomography dose index determination in dose modulation prospectively involving the third-generation iterative reconstruction and noise index. J Appl Clin Med Phys. 2024; https://doi.org/10.1002/acm2.14167.
62. NEMA. Standard attributes on CT equipment related to dose optimization and management. Rosslyn: National Electrical Manufacturers Association; 2013.
63. (2015) Medicare Program; Revisions to Payment Policies Under the Physician Fee Schedule and Other Revisions to Part B for CY 2016. Final rule with comment period. Fed Regist.
64. Smith-Bindman R, Yu S, Wang Y, et al. An image quality-informed framework for CT characterization. Radiology. 2022; https://doi.org/10.1148/radiol.2021210591.
65. Christianson O, Winslow J, Frush DP, Samei E. Automated technique to measure noise in clinical CT examinations. Am J Roentgenol. 2015; https://doi.org/10.2214/AJR.14.13613.
66. Malkus A, Szczykutowicz TP. A method to extract image noise level from patient images in CT. Med Phys. 2017; https://doi.org/10.1002/mp.12240.
67. Standards changes for organizations providing diagnostic imaging services. Jt Comm Perspect. 2014;34:5–19.
68. Kanal KM, Butler PF, Chatfield MB, et al. U.S. diagnostic reference levels and achievable doses for 10

pediatric CT examinations. Radiology. 2022; https://doi.org/10.1148/radiol.2021211241.
69. Wagner LK, Lester RGSL. Exposure of the pregnant patient to diagnostic radiations: a guide to medical management. Madison: Medical Physics; 1997.
70. Streffer C, Shore R, Konermann G, et al. Biological effects after prenatal irradiation (embryo and fetus). A report of the International Commission on Radiological Protection. Ann ICRP. 2003
71. Sensakovic WF, Royall I, Hough M, et al. Fetal dosimetry at CT: a primer. Radiographics. 2020; https://doi.org/10.1148/rg.2020190166.
72. Kanal KM, Butler PF, Sengupta D, et al. U.S. diagnostic reference levels and achievable doses for 10 adult CT examinations. Radiology. 2017; https://doi.org/10.1148/radiol.2017161911.
73. Eastman E, Pressman BD, Roy L, Zhou Y. A holistic approach to CT protocol and dose management. J Am Coll Radiol. 2024; https://doi.org/10.1016/j.jacr.2024.01.008.
74. Little BP, Duong PA, Knighton J, et al. A comprehensive CT dose reduction program using the ACR dose index registry. J Am Coll Radiol. 2015; https://doi.org/10.1016/j.jacr.2015.07.020.

Dental Imaging

4

Victor J. Weir

Key Points

1. Modalities for dental imaging
2. Quality concerns
3. Risks and safety concerns
4. Quality assurance and quality control
5. Regulations and guidelines for dental imaging
6. Efforts to improve safety and quality

Introduction

Dental radiography in various forms has been aided by major innovations in the field of dental imaging [1–3]. The transition from radiographic films to digital imaging plates now enables immediate readout after imaging. In dental radiography, an image receptor is inserted into the mouth, a single x-ray exposure is acquired, and the image receptor processed or read out to produce an image. Although additional exposures can be captured by repositioning the receptor, this method only supports limited intraoral and oblique lateral projections of a patient's teeth and jaw health.

A more advanced approach uses sequential exposures with a narrow x-ray beam and reciprocal movement of the source and detector along an arced trajectory, creating a panoramic image of the teeth and jaws. Panoramic dental imaging provides a broader view of a patient's dental health [4]. In some areas, panoramic imaging has been supplanted by dental maxillofacials using computed tomography (CT) imaging or cone beam CT (CBCT). Dental maxillofacial imaging is fast, straightforward, and allows for multiple views of a patient's jaw health [5–10]. CT maxillofacials may be ordered in case of facial trauma or for orthodontic treatment planning. Specialized CBCT devices tailored for dental maxillofacials are now available and marketed for use in dental offices [11]. These CBCT devices allow low-dose images to be taken of multiple areas of the jaw [8, 10], an advantage when compared to higher-dose maxillofacial imaging performed on conventional CT scanners [7]. The use of CBCT devices specially designed for dental imaging competes with CT maxillofacials performed on conventional CT scanners.

Another aspect of dental imaging that is becoming more common is the use of handheld radiographic devices [12–17]. These portable, battery-powered devices are ideal for imaging patients with limited mobility, those in remote areas, military applications on the battlefield, forensic orthodontics, and crime scenes.

Patient safety is a cornerstone of modern dental imaging practice. As technologies advance, minimizing radiation exposure while ensuring

V. J. Weir (✉)
Department of Veterans Affairs, Central Virginia VA Healthcare Systems (CVHCS), Richmond VA Medical Center, Richmond, VA, USA
e-mail: victor.weir@va.gov

J. Zhang (ed.), *Quality and Patient Safety in Medical Imaging*,
https://doi.org/10.1007/978-3-031-89007-9_4

diagnostic accuracy remains a critical challenge. The goal of this chapter is to discuss the value of various dental imaging technologies used in the diagnosis and management of diseases associated with the teeth and jaws, as well as evaluate image quality and radiation dose from the point of view of safety and efficacy. Principles of patient safety in dental imaging, the risks associated with various imaging modalities, and strategies for mitigating these risks are explored. Methods for dose reduction and image quality enhancement are reviewed, along with emerging technologies such as artificial intelligence (AI) applications for diagnosis, decision-making, and treatment prognosis prediction. Regulations pertaining to dental imaging are also discussed.

Dental Imaging Modalities

There are several types of dental radiographic images, all requiring exposure to ionizing radiation to create a diagnostic-quality image. Intraoral radiographs involve placing the image receptor inside the patient's mouth, while extraorals position the image receptor outside the mouth. Intraorals are further classified into periapical, bitewing, or occlusal radiographs, based on the positioning device used and the receptor size.

Intraoral bitewing radiographs are one of the most common types done. During the procedure, the image receptor (also called x-ray detector) is positioned inside the mouth adjacent to the teeth, and x-ray images are captured using a dental x-ray machine (Fig. 4.1a). The typical tube potential for dental intraoral imaging is at least 60kVp, with some tubes also offering 70KVp. These x-rays provide the dentist with detailed views of specific areas in the mouth, aiding in the diagnosis of dental conditions. Figure 4.1b shows a typical intraoral image of the teeth.

As part of a routine dental examination, comprehensive dental radiographs are performed annually to assess bone health beneath the gum line, detect bone loss, evaluate gum disease, identify the presence of plaque, and check cavities. Historically, intraoral bitewings were conducted exclusively using conventional screen-film image receptors. These analog x-ray detectors consist of phosphor screens that detect x-rays and photographic films that record the images. The film must be chemically processed and developed before the dentist can review the results.

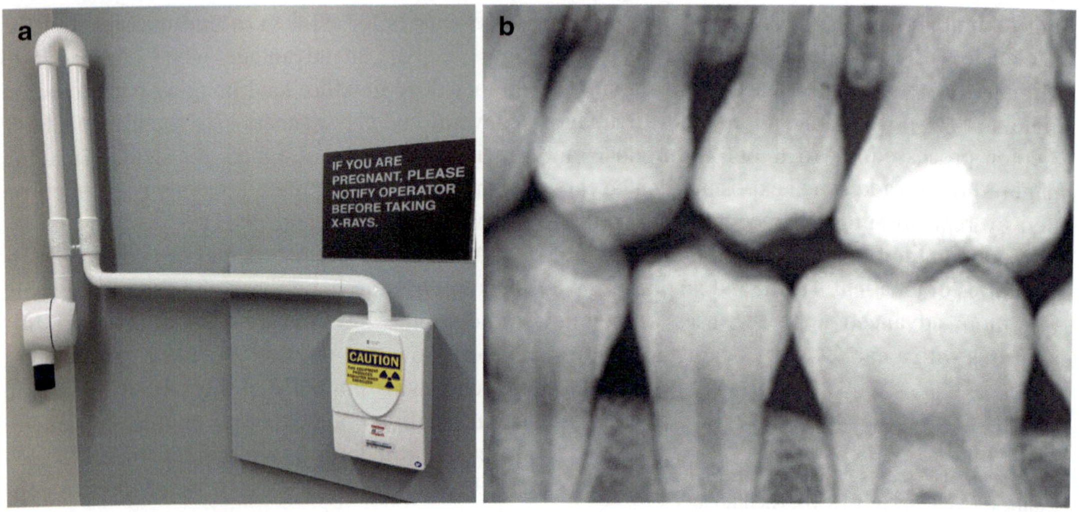

Fig. 4.1 A two-panel image: Panel (**a**) shows a dental X-ray machine mounted on a wall, with the x-ray tube at the end of an adjustable hinged arm that allows movement and positioning in several orientations. Panel (**b**) displays a dental X-ray image of teeth, showing the structure and alignment of several teeth

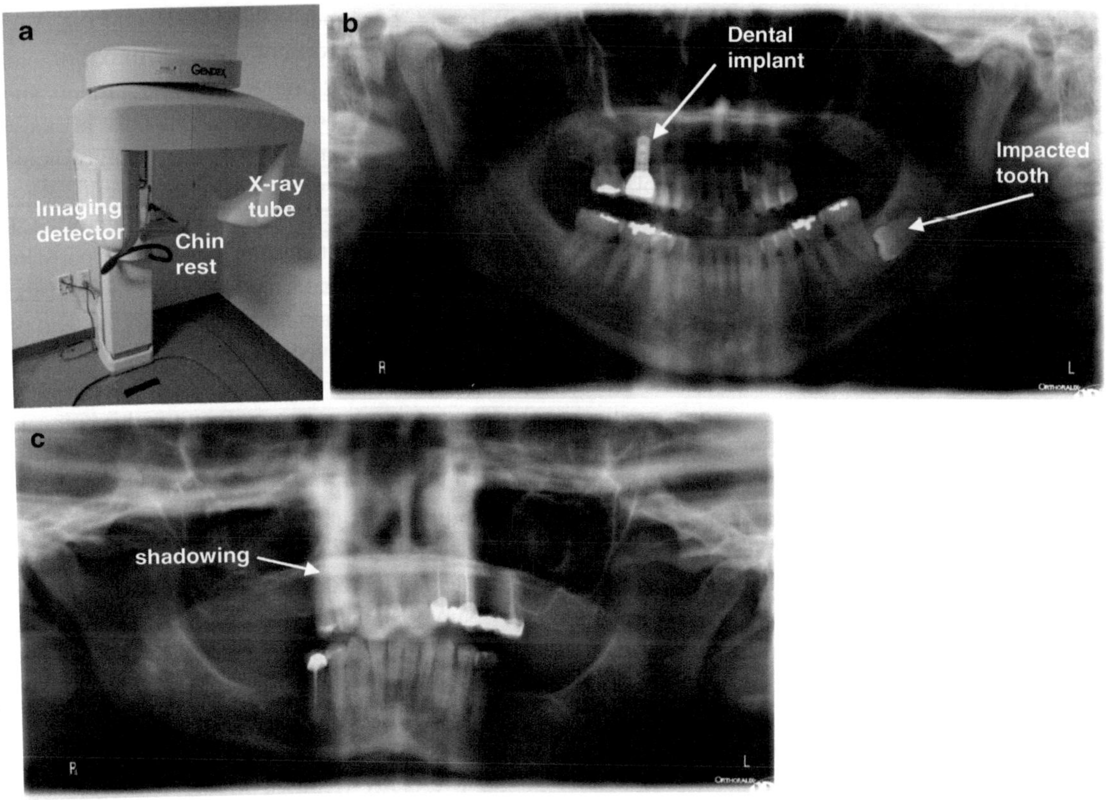

Fig. 4.2 (**a**) An example of dental panoramic machine with labeled parts; (**b**) a panoramic image of the jaw showing filings, dental implants, an impacted wisdom tooth, and missing teeth; (**c**) an image from another individual showing filings and missing teeth in both lower and upper jaws and an area of shadowing

Recent advances in digital detector technology have made digital x-ray detectors more widely available, replacing analog screen-film detectors. Digital devices include technologies based on photostimulable phosphors (PSPs) and charge-coupled devices (CCDs). Digital detectors enable near-instantaneous readout, reducing the time between image acquisition and display for dentist evaluation.

Intraoral dental radiographs are limited by a small field of view (FOV), making them unsuitable for evaluating maxillofacial trauma, and abnormal dental developments. Extraoral imaging, which uses a larger detector, can display a broader anatomical area, providing an advantage over intraoral imaging. For example, extraoral panoramic dental imaging can provide a wider FOV and an overall assessment of dental and jaw health.

Panoramic imaging devices consist of an x-ray tube and an x-ray detector mounted on a rotating head as shown in Fig. 4.2a. The patient stands with their head positioned between the x-ray tube and detector, resting their chin on a support. Once the patient is properly positioned, the x-ray tube produces a well-collimated x-ray beam that sweeps around the patient in a circular or elliptical path, depending on the imaging application selected. Typical panoramic x-ray techniques involve tube potentials (kVp) between 60 and 85 and currents (mA) ranging from 1 to 12 mA. Exposure durations may range from 5 to 20 s, depending on the manufacturer.

To improve the x-ray beam quality, manufacturers insert aluminum sheets into the output port of the x-ray device for filtration. A typical panoramic image of the jaw and teeth is shown in Fig. 4.2b, c, highlighting several anatomical features.

Panoramic images are ordered when dentists require comprehensive views of the teeth and their positions within the jawbone, such as after jaw or dental trauma. When planning dental surgery or implants a panoramic image may be ordered as part of the pretreatment protocol.

Although screen-film x-ray detectors can be used for panoramic imaging, advances in digital technology have led to widespread adoption of digital detectors, enabling immediate readout and reducing processing time. Panoramic dental machines may be installed in standard radiographic x-ray rooms, benefiting from existing radiation shielding.

Although panoramic dental imaging offers several advantages over intraoral dental imaging, the use of CT for dental imaging provides even greater benefits. These include image post-processing capabilities such as multi-planar reformatting (MPR) ability, maximum intensity projection (MIP), and three-dimensional (3D) rendering of the surface or volume. MPR allows for the reconstruction of multiple imaging views of the entire face, jaws, and teeth Fig. 4.3. 3D rendering enables the reconstruction of the various views to create a 3D representation of the anatomy under examination. This 3D visualization alone gives CT scanners a significant advantage over dental panoramic imaging. CT scanners are described in a separate chapter. Readers are encouraged to refer to that chapter for more comprehensive information.

When a CT scanner is used for dental imaging, a specialized CT protocol called a maxillofacial scan is employed for imaging trauma patients and planning for orthodontic surgery. This protocol can be tailored for either low-dose or high-image quality, depending on clinical requirements. With the availability of wider multi-detector CT (MDCT) scanners, it is now possible to perform wide-beam CT scans of the teeth and jaws. If the image receptor uses a flat panel detector instead of the conventional curved detectors typically found in CT scanners, it is referred to as a cone beam CT (CBCT) scanner. Some manufacturers have developed CBCT specifically designed for the use in dental offices, offering enhanced convenience and accessibility for dental imaging procedures.

CBCT machines are designed to allow the patient to be seated, standing, or in some rare cases, supine. There are several CBCT vendors on the market currently. The following list is taken from [7]:

1. NewTom 3G (QR, Verona, Italy)
2. CB Mercuray (Hitachi Medical of America, Twinsburg, OH)
3. Promax3D (Planmeca OY, Helsinki, Finland)
4. Prexion 3D (Terarecon, San Mateo, CA)
5. Galileos (Sirona, Charlotte, NC)
6. Classic i-CAT (Imaging Sciences International, Hatfield, PA)
7. Next Generation i-CAT (Imaging Sciences International)
8. Iluma (Imtec Imaging, Ardmore, OK)

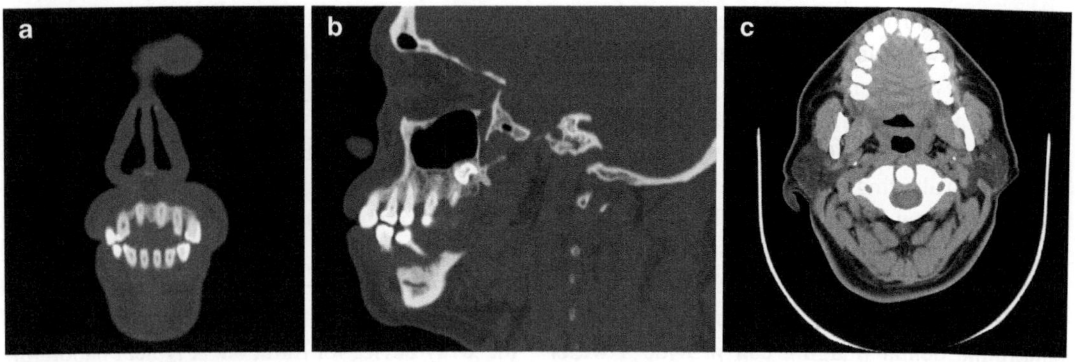

Fig. 4.3 CT scan images of a human skull in three views: (**a**) coronal view showing the nasal cavity and teeth alignment, (**b**) sagittal view displaying the side profile of the skull with teeth and nasal cavity, and (**c**) axial view illustrating the upper jaw and teeth arrangement. Each subfigure is labeled with letters **a**, **b**, and **c**

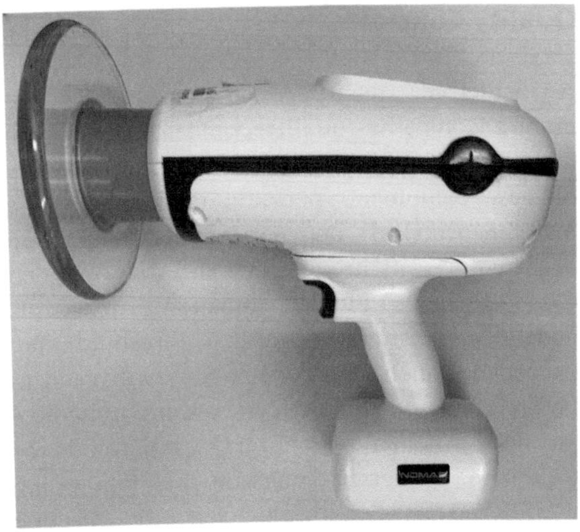

Fig. 4.4 A handheld medical imaging device showing a pistol grip handle with a trigger and a small display screen to show the selected KV and mA used for imaging

Another important area of dental imaging is the use of handheld portable devices (Fig. 4.4). Handheld dental devices are lightweight, rechargeable, ergonomically designed, allowing for use in a variety of clinical settings. Typically weighing less than 7 pounds, handheld devices often come with a charging cradle that plugs into a standard outlet. Their ergonomic design includes a removable battery enabling continuous operation with an extra battery on hand to prevent downtime. Due to their portability, handheld devices are ideal for imaging patients who are immobile or in remote locations where fixed units are not available, such as in nursing homes and home healthcare settings. They are also useful in specialized applications [15, 18] such as forensics, where crime victims can be imaged and analyzed immediately if a digital detector and readout display are available [16]. In a military campaign, handheld devices provide rapid imaging and diagnosis on the battlefield [19]. Veterinarians also may benefit from the use of a handheld device.

Cephalometric imaging is a diagnostic tool used for studying and measuring the human head, particularly in orthodontics and dentistry. It aids in assessing the size and positions of teeth, jaw, and cranial structures, making it essential for planning dental implants, braces, or maxillofacial surgeries [20–22]. Typically, a radiograph of the side of the face is captured and reviewed by the dentist for orthodontic planning. Unlike standard extraoral dental images, cephalometric imaging requires larger detectors capable of covering the entire head and facial regions. Digital or computed radiographic (CR) detectors may be used depending on their availability. Cephalometric imaging systems may be integrated with panoramic dental units or with CBCT units, offering versatile diagnostic capabilities. Various imaging projections are applied in cephalometric imaging, including lateral cephalometric, PA cephalometric, submentovertex, occipito-mental, and occipito-frontal views, among others. More details of these techniques as well as others can be found in the IAEA documents on Dental Radiology [4].

Quality Concerns

Image Quality/Diagnostic Accuracy

Image quality in dental imaging is influenced by the type of image receptor or detector used. Several x-ray detector technologies are currently available, including screen-film systems, photostimulable phosphor (PSP) plates, charge-coupled devices (CCDs), and complementary metal oxide semiconductor (CMOS) detectors. Detailed comparisons between these technologies as well as general dental imaging information can be found in references [23–25]. When screen film is used for imaging, faster film requires less x-ray exposure to achieve the required optical density. This reduces radiation exposure, making it a safer option. However, PSPs and CMOS receptors offer the added advantage of providing equal or better image quality with a fraction of the x-ray exposure. More information can be found in [26–28]. The types of detector technologies mentioned above are not exclusive to dental radiographic imaging and are also utilized in general radiographic imaging.

The diagnostic quality of images produced by panoramic dental imaging is different from that of other dental imaging modalities. Image quality can be compromised by soft tissues overlaying bone structures and the occurrence of ghosting artifacts. In addition, tomographic blur, inherent to the panoramic imaging technique, obscures anatomical features outside of the focal plane. Further challenges include variable magnification caused by the type of orbit, whether circular or elliptical, and overlapping of adjacent teeth, which can complicate accurate diagnosis.

Compared to dental panoramic images, CT maxillofacial scans provide more detailed information by avoiding the overlay of dental anatomy often seen in panoramic imaging. In addition, CT maxillofacials images can be reconstructed to display sagittal, coronal, and transverse views. The ability to produce thin millimeter slices and apply various reconstruction kernels allow for the visualization of fine anatomical details. Image quality in CBCT is also better due to sub-millimeter isotropic voxel resolution ranging from 0.4 mm to as low as 0.076 mm. Because of this, axial, sagittal, and coronal reformats achieve a level of spatial resolution that makes it easier to visualize tiny details when assessing implants [9].

Image quality of handheld dental images can be on par with those of fixed dental machines if digital image detectors are used for image acquisition. A study examining multiple handheld devices in combination with several digital imaging systems shows statistically good image quality for all systems [15]. A study comparing information yield from a fixed dental unit to a handheld unit found no significant difference in the number of details observed between the two types of devices [17]. In addition, handheld devices can produce images with little or no blurring from hand motion due to the use of motion stabilization. In fixed dental devices, use of a small anode focal spot size enables high-resolution images to be produced. Power is provided by a high-frequency high-kilovoltage DC generator that allows clear images to be produced at low patient dose. If film is to be used for image acquisition, then films with speeds of F or faster should be used to minimize acquisition time as this could lead to movement artifacts.

Quality Control

A dedicated quality assurance (QA) program encompasses quality control (QC), which includes acceptance testing and commissioning of new equipment, periodic testing, periodic maintenance (PM), and performance evaluation of the equipment throughout its lifespan. Beyond QC, there is also the determination of protocols and setting thresholds. When thresholds are exceeded, patient dose estimations will need to be done by a qualified expert, usually a medical physicist. Another aspect of a QA program is the training of workers and ensuring that policies are established and followed. Generally, routine quality control deals with the performance evaluation of the equipment after installation and is done on a regular timetable.

Quality control in dental imaging is no different from other radiographic systems. Specific tests for dental QC can be obtained in references [29, 30]. Daily dental QC includes both intraoral system constancy test and extraoral processor tests (for film system only). Film viewboxes (if applicable) require monthly checks. The quarterly QC program includes repeat image rate analysis, tube head-boom stability, film and chemical storage (if applicable), cleaning of cassettes and screens (if applicable). For digital image receptors, manufacturer's recommendations of QC testing should be followed. Manufacturers may have built in QC protocols designed to test digital detector performance on a daily, weekly, or monthly basis. In addition to detector tests, annual QC also includes lead apron checks (when appropriate), x-ray and light field alignment, and overall program review. Other routine tests involve daily system checks, x-ray tube performance checks, image quality checks, image display performance checks, and dosimetry. Additional tests include radiation safety surveys of equipment rooms. A radiation safety survey is recommended by the Conference of Radiation Control Program Directors (CRCPD) every 2 years. This is subject to state regulation. Some states require periodic QC of dental systems, which may be every 2 years or longer. Guidelines for carrying out acceptance testing and QC of dental imaging equipment are laid out in AAPM report No 175 [31].

Some tests done for dental radiographic devices can also be done for other dental devices. Specific dental modalities may require their own specialized QC tests and measurements. A qualified medical physicist should be consulted about QC of dental devices.

A specific test for dental panoramic imaging devices pertains to alignment of the x-ray beam with the slit at the image receptor. This can also be done for scanning-based cephalometric devices. For wide-beam cephalometric devices, the field size should be compared to nominal beam values and checked for alignment with the light field. The tests mentioned here do not represent an exhaustive list of all required tests. A qualified medical physicist should be consulted and retained to perform all required tests.

Regarding CBCT, guidelines have been published for QC procedures for cone beam imaging devices. A few of the publishing organizations are listed below:

- European Commission, Radiation Protection 172 (SEDENTEXCT guidelines) (EC, 2012)
- UK Health Protection Agency (HPA, 2010)
- German DIN 6868-161/DIN 6868-15
- Unified protocol for CBCT (not exclusive for dental) (EFOMP-ESTRO-IAEA, 2017)
- AAPM task group 261

Tests for CBCT include image quality tests and dosimetry tests. Image quality tests including image uniformity, geometric accuracy, Hounsfield number accuracy, spatial resolution, contrast, and noise are done on a periodic basis.

QC of CT machines used for dental imaging is done as part of a comprehensive QA program for CT scanners and will not be covered in this chapter. For quality control of CT imaging devices used for dental imaging, please see the chapter on computed tomography for a general QC of CT machines.

Handheld dental imaging devices should follow the same QA guidelines as radiographic dental machines. Other specifications for focus to skin distance (≥200 mm) and field size (≤40 × 50 mm) should be followed [32]. In addition to any standard tests required by the manufacturer, daily checks of battery levels and inspection of cracks in the equipment housing should be performed before daily use.

Safety Concerns: Strategies for Enhancing Patient Safety

Risks from Dental Radiographic Imaging

Dental bitewing and full-mouth radiographs result in low radiation doses that carry less risk than natural background radiation. Risk is calculated using effective dose. According to the NCRP 2006 report, natural background radiation from radionuclides and cosmic rays is 3100 microSieverts, while effective doses from bitewing studies are about 5 microSieverts. Full-mouth effective doses ranging from 34.9 to 170.7 microSieverts (μSv) have been reported [33]. Due to such low effective doses, the risks of cancer induction from dental radiographic imaging are consequently small.

Risks from Panoramic Imaging

As with other imaging modalities where x-rays are used, dental panoramic imaging poses certain risks that can be reduced either by using modern digital detectors or adjusting techniques. To characterize the magnitude of effective doses, some authors report effective dose differences between direct and indirect panoramic imaging systems [34]. Anthropomorphic male and female head phantoms were used for the study where doses were measured using thermoluminescent dosimeters (TLDs). Effective doses were derived using the International Commission on Radiological Protection (ICRP) 2007 recommendations [35]. Female phantom effective doses were found to be higher than male phantom effective doses. Effective doses are used to calculate cancer risks by utilizing the Biological Effects of Ionizing Radiation (BEIR) VII report guidelines. According to Ludlow [33], effective doses from panoramic studies ranges from 14.2–24.3 μSv. This is small compared to the 3100 μSv background radiation from naturally occurring radionuclides in our environment and from natural cosmic background radiation (NCRP 2006).

In a review of the literature concerning doses and risks in radiography, it was reported by several authors that incorporation of rare earth screen film combinations reduced doses compared to older technologies [36]. In addition, risks of high doses in panoramic imaging were associated with the use of older machines using circular scanning motion compared to elliptical motion. Furthermore, dose reduction can be achieved using field size reduction. This can lead to the reduction of absorbed dose by 85% and effective dose by 50% when the temporal-mandibular joints are excluded from the field.

It is generally not necessary to use leaded aprons or thyroid collars to protect patients during panoramic exams. Due to the placement of such thyroid collars where they can attenuate parts of the primary beam and obscure parts of the mandible, it is reasonable to suggest that no lead protection is needed during panoramic dental examinations.

Risks from Dental Maxillofacial Imaging

Risks of exposure from CT maxillofacials to patients are not different from the risks associated with a CT head scan. Because patients are typically imaged or scanned on regular CT scanners in the imaging department, doses displayed on the scanner console from CT maxillofacial image acquisitions are often in the same magnitude as doses displayed for a regular head scan, which is around 2 mSv. Nevertheless, patient risk is typically weighed against a medical benefit of acquiring the image. So in situations of emergency or trauma, the benefit of imaging a patient to determine their injuries outweighs the small risks of radiation induced injury or risks of cancer induction. Compared to the use of conventional CT in dental imaging to asses jaw health, CBCT has the potential to reduce radiation dose [37, 38]. In particular, low-dose CBCT can reduce absorbed dose to organs in the head and neck region that are affected by dental imaging of the jaws. In a study measuring the absorbed radiation dose to a Rando head phantom, it was found that the absorbed dose and effective dose were lower with the use of CBCT [10]. To reduce the risks of high doses, manufacturers of CT equipment provide imaging techniques that can be modified to meet the needs of imaging centers.

Strategies for Enhancing Patient Safety

The ALARA principle is the basis of radiation safety not only in dental imaging but also in all imaging involving ionizing radiation. It advocates for minimizing radiation exposure by using the lowest possible dose while still maintaining diagnostic quality images. Strategic examples include:

Using Digital Imaging Systems Digital radiographic systems allow image post-processing to improve quality even when the lowest exposures are used. They have wider dynamic ranges than traditional screen-film systems and can require significantly lower radiation dose to produce a diagnostic quality image.

Limiting Imaging to Region of Interest (ROI) Collimating to only the ROI limits exposure to adjacent tissues while still providing diagnostic quality images.

Ongoing Efforts to Improve Quality and Patient Safety

Currently, efforts to improve quality focus on using advanced imaging receptors such as digital detectors and dose reduction software (Dental CT). Digital detectors are more efficient and have wider dynamic ranges than screen-film systems. This allows lower x-ray exposure to be used with little or no penalty for image quality. Lower x-ray exposures lead to lower doses to patients for the imaging task at hand. Dental cone beam computed tomography (CBCT) scanners increasingly utilize pulse x-rays to reduce exposure [39]. By using pulsed x-rays, dental CBCT scanners have comparable exposures to panoramic dental scanners [40]. In addition, for CT maxillofacials done with modern CT scanners, there is the option to use dose reduction algorithms like dose modulation or automatic exposure compensation (AEC) that can reduce dose while maintaining image quality, or iterative reconstructions and AI/deep learning approaches that can be used to improve image quality at the same [41] or lower dose levels. Dose reduction algorithms in CT are discussed in a different chapter on CT imaging. Emerging technologies like photon counting detectors for CT can potentially improve image quality in dental CT while also reducing or keeping doses low [42–45]. While having advanced image receptors are helpful to improve quality and safety, following the proper regulations and guidelines ensures the equipment is properly maintained and functioning correctly when patients are scanned.

Regulations and Guidelines for Dental Imaging

Dental imaging, much like general radiographic x-ray imaging, is regulated under state radiation control programs based on the CRCPD publications. Regulations apply to both fixed units and handheld or portable units. These regulations cover, among other things, equipment performance evaluation (EPE) and radiation machine requirements. After installation, EPE for dental machines is required to be done every 4 years. The tests include timer accuracy, tube head stability, collimation, and entrance exposure limits for dental facilities.

Artificial Intelligence (AI)

The application of AI in dentistry typically involves its use to aid in diagnosis, decision-making, and predicting the prognosis for a treatment [41]. To identify the development of AI and evaluate its performance in these areas, a review of articles from various journals and electronic databases was conducted by using various keywords [46]. The authors report excellent performance of AI-based automated systems that mimic the precision and accuracy of trained specialists. In some studies, the authors found that AI outperformed specialists in terms of precision and accuracy. In specific areas of application, an AI system based on a convoluted neural network (CNN) was used to aid diagnosis of anatomical landmarks, pathologies, clinical effectiveness, and safety when used by dentists in a clinical setting [47]. Two groups of dentists participated in this study. On group was aided by AI and the other group was not. The authors found a statistically significant difference between groups, with an improvement in diagnostic capabilities for the aided group. Another area that has boosted the development of AI systems is in the use of 3D imaging techniques. A review focusing on current developments and performance of AI for 3D imaging in dentomaxillofacial radiology (DMFR) as well as intraoral and facial scanning has been conducted. This review aimed to provide a comprehensive understanding of current trends in AI developments in the field of 3D dental imaging [41]. Other comprehensive reviews are available [48–50].

Table 4.1 Resources for quality and patient safety in dental imaging

Dental imaging	
Dental radiography	**CRCPD Publication 01–04**: Quality control recommendations for diagnostic radiography, volume 1: Dental Facilities Acceptance Testing and Quality Control of Dental Imaging Equipment: The Report of AAPM Task Group 175 NCRP (2003). Report No. 145: Radiation Protection in Dentistry **IAEA** Report: Radiation Protection in Dental Radiology American Academy of Pediatric Dentistry, guideline on prescribing dental radiographs for infants, children, adolescents, and persons with special health care needs E.A.O. guidelines for the use of diagnostic imaging in implant dentistry 2011. A consensus workshop organized by the European Association for Osseointegration at the Medical University of Warsaw
CBCT	Guidelines to be published in NCRP Report No. 177
Handheld devices	Guidelines to be published in NCRP Report No. 177

NCRP Report No. 099: Quality Assurance for Diagnostic Imaging
ICRP Publication 73: Radiological Protection and Safety in Medicine

Resources for Quality and Patient Safety

Table 4.1 provides a summary of resources (e.g., QC recommendations, safety guidelines, etc.,) for quality and safety specifically for dental imaging. The goal of this table is to facilitate readers for quick access to those resources.

Chapter Summary

In summary, dental imaging techniques encompass fixed dental machines, handheld or portable machines, panoramic machines, CBCT, conventional CT, and cephalometric imaging. These methods provide low-dose assessments of dental health below the gum line while posing minimal radiation risk to patients. Panoramic imaging can be substituted with CT maxillofacial imaging for orthodontic planning due to its superior detail. CBCT devices serve as an alternative to conventional CT, offering lower doses, better image quality, and a smaller equipment footprint. Handheld dental devices are versatile, used in clinical settings, forensics, and remote locations, producing high-quality images comparable to fixed machines.

Quality and patient safety in dental imaging requires a balanced approach that minimizes radiation exposure while maintaining high diagnostic image quality. By following ALARA principles, applying appropriate justifications, using shielding when, optimizing imaging protocols, and leveraging technological advancements, dental professionals can protect patients from unnecessary radiation exposure while ensuring diagnostic accuracy. Commitment to quality and patient safety must remain a top priority, guided by current research and best practices as technologies evolve.

Glossary

AAPM American Association of Physicists in Medicine
ACR American College of Radiology
CCD Charge-Coupled Device
CRCPD Conference of Radiation Control Program Directors
CBCT Cone Beam Computed Tomography
CMOS Complementary Metal Oxide Semiconductor
FBP Filtered Backprojection
FDA Food and Drug Administration (USA)
FDK Feldkamp-Davis-Kress
ICRP International Commission on Radiological Protection
JCAHO Joint Commission on the Accreditation of Health Organizations
MIP Maximum Intensity Projection
MPR Multi-planar Reformat

NCRP National Council on Radiation Protection
PSP Photostimulable Phosphor
QA Quality Assurance
QC Quality Control
TLD Thermoluminescent Dosimeter
WHO World Health Organization

References

1. Vandenberghe B, Jacobs R, Bosmans H. Modern dental imaging: a review of the current technology and clinical applications in dental practice. Eur Radiol. 2010;20(11):2637–55.
2. Mol A. Imaging methods in periodontology. Periodontology. 2000;34(1):34–48.
3. Patel S, et al. New dimensions in endodontic imaging: part 1. Conventional and alternative radiographic systems. Int Endod J. 2009;42(6):447–62.
4. IAEA. RPOP dental radiology. 2017 [cited 2017].
5. Boeddinghaus R, Whyte A. Current concepts in maxillofacial imaging. Eur J Radiol. 2008;66(3):396–418.
6. De Vos W, Casselman J, Swennen G. Cone-beam computerized tomography (CBCT) imaging of the oral and maxillofacial region: a systematic review of the literature. Int J Oral Maxillofac Surg. 2009;38(6):609–25.
7. Ludlow JB, Ivanovic M. Comparative dosimetry of dental CBCT devices and 64-slice CT for oral and maxillofacial radiology. Oral Surg Oral Med Oral Pathol Oral Radiol Endod. 2008;106(1):106–14.
8. Mah JK, et al. Radiation absorbed in maxillofacial imaging with a new dental computed tomography device. Oral Surg Oral Med Oral Pathol Oral Radiol Endod. 2003;96(4):508–13.
9. Scarfe WC, Farman AG. What is cone-beam CT and how does it work? Dent Clin N Am. 2008;52(4):707–30.
10. Tsiklakis K, et al. Dose reduction in maxillofacial imaging using low dose cone beam CT. Eur J Radiol. 2005;56(3):413–7.
11. Patel S. New dimensions in endodontic imaging: part 2. Cone beam computed tomography. Int Endod J. 2009;42(6):463–75.
12. Goren A, et al. Radiation exposure with the NOMADTM portable X-ray system. Dentomaxillofac Radiol. 2008;37(2):109–12.
13. Mahdian M, et al. Using hand-held dental x-ray devices: using hand-held dental x-ray devices. J Am Dent Assoc. 2014;145(11):1130–2.
14. McGiff TJ, Danforth RA, Herschaft EE. Maintaining radiation exposures as low as reasonably achievable (ALARA) for dental personnel operating portable hand-held x-ray equipment. Health Phys. 2012;103(2):S179–85.
15. Pittayapat P, et al. Image quality assessment and medical physics evaluation of different portable dental X-ray units. Forensic Sci Int. 2010;201(1):112–7.
16. Pittayapat P, et al. Forensic oral imaging quality of hand-held dental X-ray devices: comparison of two image receptors and two devices. Forensic Sci Int. 2010;194(1):20–7.
17. Van Dis ML, et al. Information yield from a hand-held dental x-ray unit. Oral Surg Oral Med Oral Pathol. 1993;76(3):381–5.
18. Hermsen KP, Jaeger SS, Jaeger MA. Radiation safety for the NOMAD™ portable X-ray system in a temporary morgue setting. J Forensic Sci. 2008;53(4):917–21.
19. Coy J, Vandre RH, Davidson W. Use of the hand-held dental X-ray machine during joint operation, NATO exercise display determination-92. Mil Med. 1997;162(8):575–7.
20. Silva MAG, et al. Cone-beam computed tomography for routine orthodontic treatment planning: a radiation dose evaluation. Am J Orthod Dentofacial Orthop. 2008; 133(5): 640. e1–640. e5.
21. Farman AG, Scarfe WC. Development of imaging selection criteria and procedures should precede cephalometric assessment with cone-beam computed tomography. Am J Orthod Dentofacial Orthop. 2006;130(2):257–65.
22. Hilgers ML, et al. Accuracy of linear temporomandibular joint measurements with cone beam computed tomography and digital cephalometric radiography. Am J Orthod Dentofacial Orthop. 2005;128(6):803–11.
23. Parks ET. Digital radiographic imaging: is the dental practice ready? J Am Dent Assoc. 2008;139(4):477–81.
24. Parks ET, Williamson GF. Digital radiography: an overview. J Contemp Dent Pract. 2002;3(4):23–39.
25. Van Der Stelt PF. Filmless imaging: the uses of digital radiography in dental practice. J Am Dent Assoc. 2005;136(10):1379–87.
26. Grassl U, Schulze RKW. In vitro perception of low-contrast features in digital, film, and digitized dental radiographs: a receiver operating characteristic analysis. Oral Surg Oral Med Oral Pathol Oral Radiol Endod. 2007;103(5):694–701.
27. Svanaes D, Møystad A, Larheim T. Approximal caries depth assessment with storage phosphor versus film radiography. Caries Res. 2000;34(6):448–53.
28. White S, Yoon D. Comparative performance of digital and conventional images for detecting proximal surface caries. Dentomaxillofac Radiol. 1997;26(1):32–8.
29. CRCPD. CRCPD Publication 01–4: quality control recommendations for diagnostic radiography, volume 1: Dental Facilities, 2001, Conference of Radiation Control Program Directors.
30. NCRP. Report No. 099: quality assurance for diagnostic imaging, 1998.
31. AAPM. Acceptance testing and quality control of dental imaging equipment. 2016.
32. Faulkner K., et al. RP 162. Criteria for the acceptability of radiological equipment. 2012.
33. Ludlow JB, Davies-Ludlow LE, White SC. Patient risk related to common dental radiographic

examinations: the impact of 2007 International Commission on Radiological Protection recommendations regarding dose calculation. J Am Dent Assoc. 2008;139(9):1237–43.
34. Lee G-S, et al. Effective dose from direct and indirect digital panoramic units. Imaging Sci Dent. 2013;43(2):77–84.
35. ICRP. The 2007 recommendations of the international commission on radiological protection. ICRP publication 103. Ann ICRP. 2007;37(2–4)
36. Rushton VE, Horner K. The use of panoramic radiology in dental practice. J Dent. 1996;24(3):185–201.
37. Tam KC, Samarasekera S, Somer F. Exact cone beam CT with a spiral scan. Phys Med Biol. 1998;43:1015–24.
38. Siewerdsen JH, Jaffray DA. Cone-beam computed tomography with a flat-panel imager. Med Phys. 1999;26:2635–47.
39. Kiljunen T, et al. Dental cone beam CT: a review. Phys Med. 2015;31(8):844–60.
40. Gaêta-Araujo H, et al. Cone beam computed tomography in dentomaxillofacial radiology: a two-decade overview. Dentomaxillofac Radiol. 2020;49(8):20200145.
41. Hung K, et al. Current applications, opportunities, and limitations of AI for 3D imaging in dental research and practice. Int J Environ Res Public Health. 2020;17(12):4424.
42. Vanden Broeke L, et al. Feasibility of photon-counting spectral CT in dental applications—a comparative qualitative analysis. BDJ open. 2021;7(1):4.
43. Zanon C, et al. Potential benefits of photon-counting CT in DENTAL IMAGING: a NARRATIVE REView. J Clin Med. 2024;13(8):2436.
44. Sawall S, et al. Dental imaging in clinical photon-counting CT at a quarter of DVT dose. J Dent. 2024;142:104859.
45. Ruetters M, et al. Dental imaging using an ultra-high resolution photon-counting CT system. Sci Rep. 2022;12(1):7125.
46. Khanagar SB, et al. Developments, application, and performance of artificial intelligence in dentistry–a systematic review. J Dent Sci. 2021;16(1):508–22.
47. Ezhov M, et al. Clinically applicable artificial intelligence system for dental diagnosis with CBCT. Sci Rep. 2021;11(1):15006.
48. Carrillo-Perez F, et al. Applications of artificial intelligence in dentistry: a comprehensive review. J Esthet Restor Dent. 2022;34(1):259–80.
49. Ding H, et al. Artificial intelligence in dentistry – a review. Front Dent Med. 2023;4:1085251.
50. Schwendicke FA, Samek W, Krois J. Artificial intelligence in dentistry: chances and challenges. J Dent Res. 2020;99(7):769–74.

Bone Densitometry Imaging

5

Victor J. Weir

Key Points

1. DEXA.
2. X-ray radiation.
3. Quality concerns.
4. Safety concerns.
5. Quality assurance and quality control.
6. Regulations and guidelines.
7. Efforts to improve safety and quality.

Introduction

Osteoporosis and osteopenia commonly affect men and women aged 50 years or older, with approximately 55% of American men and women in this group experiencing reduced bone density [1]. These conditions increase the risk of fractures due to weakened bone strength. The World Health Organization (WHO) classifies osteoporosis and osteopenia based on T-scores, as shown in Table 5.1 by Maghraoui [2]. The T-score is a statistical measure used to compare an individual's bone mineral density (BMD) to the average BMD of a young healthy reference population of the same sex. It indicates how much a person's BMD deviates from the reference group's average, measured in standard deviations (SD) [3, 4].

Table 5.1 T-score for osteoporosis and osteopenia

Diagnosis	T-score
Normal	≥−1.0
Osteopenia	<−1.0, >−2.5
Osteoporosis	≤−2.5
Severe osteoporosis	≤−2.5, plus fragility fractures

More details as well as guidelines for the treatment and prevention of osteoporosis can be found in [1]. T-scores are derived from dual-energy x-ray absorptiometry (DEXA) measurements of bone mineral density (BMD) in the lumbar spine and femur. DEXA uses two x-ray energy levels to image a portion of the bone, subtracting soft tissue absorption to calculate BMD based on the differential absorption of x-ray energy by bone.

Over the years, DEXA has become a widely accepted and validated technique for assessing bone quality and body composition due to its availability and ease of use [2, 5–7]. Bone quality and strength are typically quantified by using BMD and bone mineral content (BMC), among other properties. Other techniques for measuring BMD include vertebral fracture assessment (VFA) using a densitometer [8] and quantitative computed tomography (qCT) [9–14]. Peripheral QCT (pQCT) and quantitative ultrasound (QUS) are also used for BMD assessment [15].

V. J. Weir (✉)
Department of Veterans Affairs, Central Virginia VA Healthcare Systems (CVHCS), Richmond VA Medical Center, Richmond, VA, USA
e-mail: victor.weir@va.gov

J. Zhang (ed.), *Quality and Patient Safety in Medical Imaging*,
https://doi.org/10.1007/978-3-031-89007-9_5

This chapter reviews the use of DEXA in measuring BMD and BMC for the diagnosis of osteoporosis and osteopenia. It also discusses advanced technologies such as quantitative computed tomography (qCT), emphasizing their role in assessing and managing bone loss. Key issues related to radiation dose and image quality are explored, with a focus on techniques to minimize dose and improve image quality in qCT. The chapter highlights emerging AI tools that support analysis and diagnosis in bone health management. It discusses the regulatory framework surrounding the use of DEXA and qCT.

Bone Densitometry Modalities

Dual-Energy X-Ray Absorptiometry (DEXA)

DEXA or dual x-ray absorptiometry (DXA) is an imaging modality used for assessing bone health through the measurement of BMD. BMD measurements help evaluate individuals for low bone density, a condition associated with increased fracture risk. BMD measurements can also be used for monitoring the effectiveness of treatment for osteoporosis. Because of its low costs and ease of use, DEXA is commonly used to assess bone density at central skeletal sites such as proximal femur and lumbar spine [16]. A guide to the use of DEXA has been published by [7]. Figure 5.1 shows a typical DEXA system.

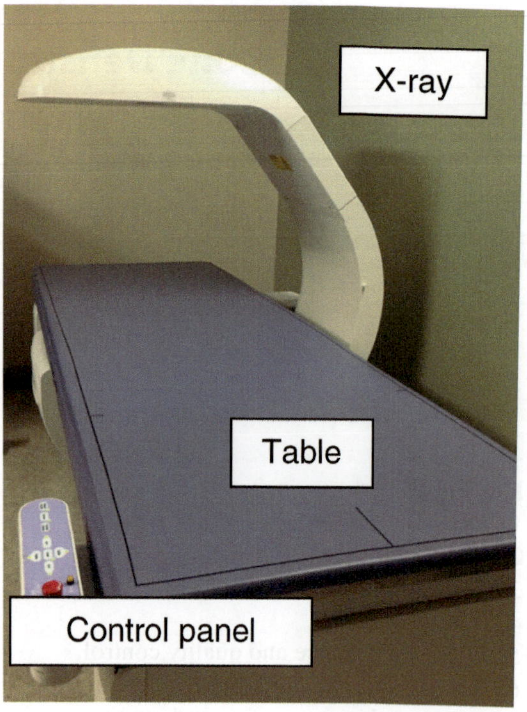

Fig. 5.1 A typical dual-energy x-ray absorptiometry (DEXA) imaging system showing the table and x-ray source

Clinical Indications of DEXA

The American College of Radiology (ACR) as well as other professional groups such as the International Society for Clinical Densitometry (ISCD), the National Osteoporosis Foundation (NOF), and the International Osteoporosis Foundation (IOF) [17], recommend healthy postmenopausal women aged 65 years and older be screened for osteoporosis [18] and that women at higher risk may be screened earlier. Men can be screened at 70 years of age and older if they have no risk factors. Men with risk factors can be screened earlier. Risk factors include dementia, old age, recent falls, alcohol abuse, low body weight, history of first degree fractures, estrogen deficiency at an early age (<45), and steroid use for more than 3 months [2].

DEXA could be contraindicated in patients for multiple reasons including the following [2]:

1. A recent study with gastrointestinal contrast.
2. Having a radionuclide study.
3. Severe degenerative changes or fracture deformity in the measured area.
4. Inability to attain the correct position and/or remain motionless for the measurement.
5. Extreme obesity or extremely low body mass index that may inversely affect the technique and the ability to obtain accurate and precise measurements.

Positioning for the Scan

Proper patient positioning is crucial for obtaining accurate and reliable DXA scan results. After completing the scan, an image is produced for the technologist to review. The main purpose of the image is to check that the patient is properly positioned before the patient leaves the testing center. If there are any concerns about positioning, the technologist should consult with the interpreting physician.

When a patient is properly positioned, the spine image appears straight, centered in the image field, and not rotated, with equal amounts of soft tissue on either side of the bone. The scan should extend high enough to include parts of the lowest vertebra with ribs (which is usually T12) and low enough to include the pelvic brim (interspace between L4 and L5 [2]. Figure 5.2 shows a representative

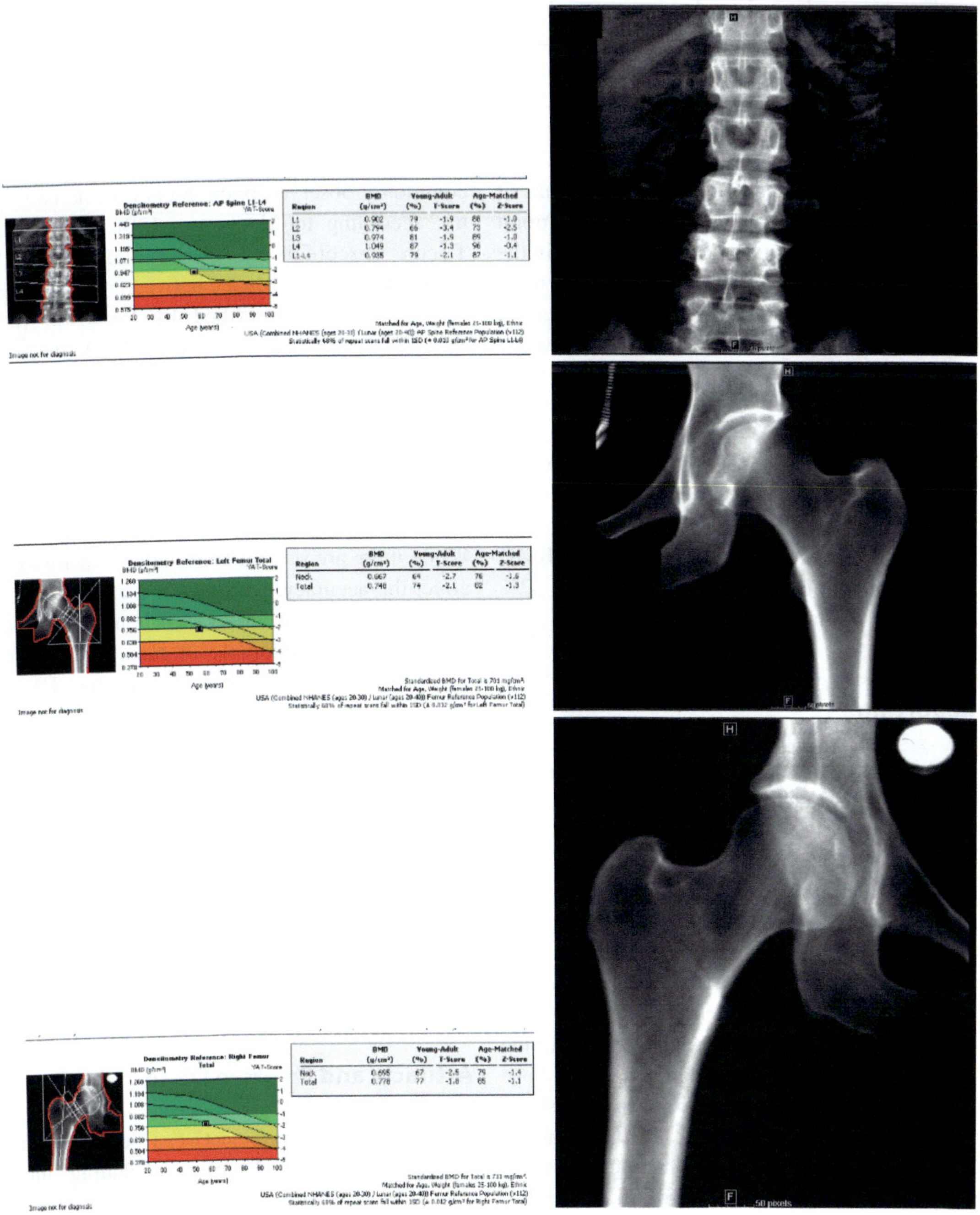

Fig. 5.2 Example of images and results from a DEXA bone density scan. The lumber spine and the pelvis regions are shown above together with the regions of interest (ROI) used for analysis

DEXA scan of the lumbar spine and pelvis, demonstrating proper patient positioning.

Measurement Site for BMD

Although BMD assessment is done for central lumbar spine and proximal femur, it can also be used for assessing bone density in the distal radius [10]. In particular, in adults, central DEXA measurement of the lumbar spine and proximal hip is recommended for osteoporosis diagnosis [5]. Only the central lumbar measurement is recommended for children 20 years of age or lower [19] due to variability in femoral maturity, leading to lack of reproducibility in the hip region [7]. The analysis of the bone is done by drawing regions of interest (ROIs) either manually or by an automatic software feature available on the DEXA machine. The ROIs used and the diagnostic criteria are well defined by organizations such as the WHO, International Atomic Energy Agency (IAEA) [5], and others. In obese patients, those with hyperparathyroidism, or those in whom the hip or the spine, or both, cannot be measured or interpreted, BMD may be measured in the forearm, using a 33% radius on the nondominant forearm [20].

Reporting

Analysis of BMD data leads to the calculation of a T-score for the adult patient based on database matches of race, age, and gender. The WHO has established definitions for the use of T-scores for the assessment of osteoporosis of the spine for DEXA, but not for qCT. However, manufacturers provide software, or third parties may provide T-score data for use with qCT. The use of T-scores is not helpful when BMD of children are compared to the BMD of the reference adult. T-scores underestimate the BMD of children because children have less bone mass than adults, leading to an overdiagnosis of osteopenia in children. After BMD measurements of children, it is important to compare the data to a reference BMD data base of the same race and age when calculating a z-score for the patient. While z-scores are used to diagnose low bone mass in young adults and children, T-scores are used to diagnose osteoporosis in adults [5]. Due to the lack of adequate data for BMD of all ethnic groups and men, the data pertains to white women.

Quality Concerns

There are several limitations of T-score measurements associated with DEXA scans. When T-scores are compared between lumbar spine and hip testing sites for individual patients, there is discordance between measurements. This is a commonly observed phenomenon in densitometry, according to Maghraoui [20]. It is called T-score discordance. Several causes for the occurrence of discordance between measurement sites have been described by Woodson [21]. When discordance is observed, DEXA measurements can be corroborated by measurements using other modalities like qCT.

Factors Affecting the Use of DEXA

While there are several confounding factors that affect the accuracy and precision of BMD measurements, an important factor is bone size, which varies with age, ethnicity or race, and gender. Moreover, experience has shown that DEXA tends to overestimate BMD in taller patients and underestimate BMD in shorter patients. This discrepancy arises from how DEXA calculates BMD, by using 2 dimensional bone area instead of 3 dimensional bone volume. As a result, BMD calculated by DEXA is often referred to as areal BMD (aBMD). This limitation is addressed by qCT, which uses bone volume for calculations, providing a more accurate assessment of bone density.

Artifacts and Errors in DEXA

DEXA BMD measurements can be affected by various artifacts and errors, including those caused by simulated weight loss or gain. A study examining simulated weight gain found that fat associated errors were more pronounced in

DEXA spine and hip BMD measurements compared to QCT trabecular spine BMD. This suggests that qCT may be more robust in assessing BMD in patients with changing body composition. The authors recommend exercising caution when interpreting BMD changes in individuals undergoing significant weight fluctuations [22].

A review of artifacts and incidental findings in DEXA imaging highlights the importance of recognizing abnormal findings even though DEXA is not primarily used for diagnostic imaging [23]. Various focal and diffuse osseous conditions can cause false increase or decrease in BMD readings. Furthermore, prior radionuclide administration has been associated with inaccurate BMD measurements, though the magnitude of the effect depends on the specific system and technical settings used during the scan [24]. Recognizing these potential sources of error is crucial for accurate interpretation of DEXA results.

Quantitative Computed Tomography (qCT)

qCT was first introduced in the 1970s as a quantitative tool for musculoskeletal imaging [25]. Subsequent developments established it as a tool for BMD measurement [9, 12, 26–28]. qCT uses standard CT technology combined with a calibration qCT phantom and analysis software to measure BMD. qCT can be performed using either conventional or asynchronous methods. For conventional qCT, a calibration phantom is placed beneath the patient during a CT scan (Fig. 5.3). The patient's ROIs in the bone are compared against corresponding ROIs in the calibration phantom for accurate BMD calculations. For asynchronous qCT, a calibration phantom is not required during the CT scan. Instead, calibration data is applied retrospectively using previously scanned phantom data, streamlining the process. ROIs are automatically placed for image data analysis. Because qCT is considered a screening examination, it can be done when a patient has other CT procedures. For example, CT colonography scans have been proposed as an opportunity to assess BMD simultaneously, adding clinical and economic value to colorectal cancer screening, as supported by research studies [14]. When analyzing data from qCT studies, commercially available software from Mindways™ (Mindways, Software Inc., Austin TX) is commonly used. Mindways™ also provides a phantom for use during qCT scans [13]. There are two major types of qCT phantom: the Cann-Geneat phantom and another phantom developed by Kalendar et al. [27].

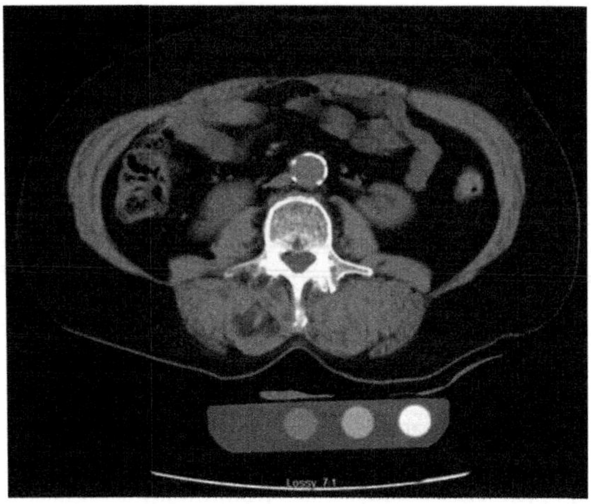

Fig. 5.3 A cross section of a patient abdomen acquired during a conventional qCT examination includes a calibration phantom under the patient during the scan

Comparing Results from qCT and DEXA

Although qCT and DEXA have pertinent differences in imaging methods and display of information, 2D for DEXA and 3D for qCT, it is expected that the basic information obtained from either modality should be consistent. Nevertheless, there is a significant detection rate difference between qCT and DEXA, with qCT having a higher detection rate than DEXA. Particularly, qCT may avoid the overestimation of BMD by DEXA associated with spinal degeneration, abdominal aortic calcifications, and other sclerotic lesions, and it may be more sensitive than DEXA in detecting osteoporosis in postmenopausal women [29]. Another study compared qCT and DEXA-derived areal bone mineral density and T-scores [30]. Other studies have found similar results when comparing DEXA and qCT. Studies of areal BMD using the CTXA Hip™ software (Mindways™ Software Inc. Austin TX) as well as DEXA have reported lower RMS errors for CT x-ray absorptiometry (CTXA). In particular, F-test revealed a significant difference between CTXA and DEXA at femoral neck (FN) and trochanter (TR) with $p < 0.05$. It was also found that qCT underestimated DEXA values at the TR, FN and intertrochanter (IT), and total hip (TH) regions. Nevertheless, appropriate adjustment of the qCT-derived aBMD values by using the National Health and Nutrition Examination Survey (NHANES) DEXA-derived reference data improved agreement and clinical utility [31]. Accuracy and precision of qCT compared to DEXA have been done for general-purpose qCT of the forearm using spiral whole-body CT scanners and DEXA. Overall accuracy and precision errors were consistent and generally less than 3% for BMD, bone mineral content (BMC), and volume [10].

DEXA and qCT Vendors

The two largest vendors of DEXA equipment are Hologic (Hologic, Inc., Bedford, MA, United States of America) and GE Lunar (GE Healthcare, Madison, WI, United States of America). GE manufactures popular models such as the Lunar Prodigy and Lunar DPX-L, both of which are widely used in clinical settings. These scanners are equipped with dedicated software and built-in QA tools for efficient patient scanning and system calibration.

In contrast, qCT can be performed using standard volumetric CT scanners commonly found in most medical facilities. For facilities conducting qCT, a quantitative tomography phantom is typically used to calibrate the scanner and ensure accurate BMD. If a phantom is not integrated into routine operations, external products such as Mindways™ (Mindways Software Inc., Austin, TX) can be used. This phantom can be scanned simultaneously with patients undergoing other CT procedures, allowing BMD analysis to be performed without a dedicated qCT scan.

Quality Assurance

Requirements for DEXA and qCT

It is critical that thorough QC under the guidelines of the ISCD [18] is performed if meaningful BDM data is to be obtained under qCT. Guidelines for performing QC are outlined in the article by Engelke et al. [15], which includes assessment of scanner stability, precision, and use of standardized protocols. Another precaution is to use the same standard protocol for the same individual patient for repeat visits.

Quality assurance for DEXA is also described in the International Atomic Energy Agency (IAEA) manual [5]. Scanner QC is done when patients are to be scanned or at least three times a week. Scanner QC is designed for several purposes, one of which is to detect changes in machine performance. The most common methods of QC are control tables, visual inspection of Shewhart chart, Shewhart rules, and cumulative sum chart (CUSUM). All these require scanning a phantom and establishing a baseline initially and regular scanning to establish longitudinal values [32]. Manufacturers of DEXA equipment typically provide a phantom as well as a programmed QC protocol that the technologist can run at regular intervals to assess the performance of the machine. After scanning the spine phantom according to specific guidelines, the results are analyzed automatically and added to a QC database stored on the machine.

qCT QA is typically performed using the Mindways™ (Mindways Software Inc. Austin TX) phantom. It includes several sections of materials where the Hounsfield Units (HU) in an ROI can be measured and compared to ROIs measured in a known standard. This can be done at intervals specified by the Midways manual. In those facilities where few qCT scans are done, the QA can be done at those times when a qCT scan for a patient is to be done.

Regulatory Issues in DEXA and qCT

Various regulations govern the use of DEXA and qCT in clinical practice. For DEXA, the regulations that apply to x-ray-based medical imaging also apply. These regulations mandate equipment performance evaluation (EPE) testing every 2 years, along with daily and weekly QC testing to ensure consistent performance and patient safety.

Some states enforce stricter regulations, requiring yearly EPE testing for DEXA systems. Additionally, the Joint Commission on the Accreditation of Health Organizations (TJC) mandates annual testing for certain types of x-ray equipment, including DEXA scanners, as part of its accreditation process. These regulatory requirements help maintain high imaging standards while ensuring that radiation exposure is kept within safe limits.

Safety Concerns

Patient Safety

Similar to other x-ray-based imaging modalities, DEXA uses ionizing radiation to generate images. This means the patient is exposed to low levels of ionizing radiation because of the procedure. Ionizing radiation gets absorbed in the body and is called absorbed dose. Absorbed dose is quantified as the energy in Joules (J) absorbed in a kilogram (Kg) of tissue and has the unit called Gray (Gy), with 1Gy = 1 J/Kg of tissue. It is used to calculate effective dose. Effective dose considers the type of radiation involved and the susceptibility of the organ that absorbed the radiation. It is measured in units of Sieverts (Sv). Effective dose in Sv is the dose in Gy multiplied by tissue weighting factors W_T and radiation weighting factors W_R. Effective dose is useful for assessing occupational and public exposures to radiation and to estimate cancer risks from the radiation. Patient doses in DEXA depend on the type of geometry employed, type of beam, whether fan beam, pencil beam or cone beam, as well as the acquisition mode used. Adult doses are on the order of 1–10 μSv for newer DEXA units although the choice of acquisition mode may lead to higher doses.

Doses from DXA are small when compared to natural background radiation. Natural background radiation averages about 2.4 mSv worldwide and 3.0 mSv for the USA. A DEXA dose is similar to what a patient will receive after being exposed to several days of natural background radiation [5].

When DEXA is justified, it is expected that the protocol be optimized to produce the necessary information using the lowest dose possible. Some of the factors influencing dose optimization include:

1. **Patient positioning:** Properly positioning the patient can reduce errors requiring the need for repeat scans. This is true for scans involving all ionizing radiation modalities.
2. **Technology:** Cutting-edge technological advancements like more sensitive image receptors and use of AI can help improve image quality while keeping radiation exposures low or even reducing exposures in some cases. Having modern DEXA machines that come with these enhancements can help minimize patient doses.
3. **Field of view (FOV):** By limiting the scanning FOV to the area of interest, the dose to other sensitive organs in the body can be avoided or reduced.

Due to the low doses used, beneficial diagnostic information obtained from DEXA scans outweighs the risk of radiation detriment. ICRP 45 [33] recommends that justifications be applied when scanning patients both for generic and individual cases. Particularly, issues related to certain patient groups require special attention:

1. **Scanning of children:** When scanning children, special care must be taken to ensure that the protocols used for scanning are optimized. A qualified expert should be consulted on how to optimize protocols available on each machine so it can be used for scanning children. Special consideration should also be given to alternative means of determining bone density, such as QUS. Patient or legal

guardians should be informed of the risks of ionizing radiation. This is important if younger patients are to be scanned and alternative nonionizing radiation methods will not provide the necessary diagnostic information.

2. **Scanning during pregnancy:** In clinical practice, there is very little reason to perform a bone density scan on a pregnant person. Postings should be available within the scanning area to prompt a woman to disclose her pregnancy. The "10-day rule", where a radiologic examination should only be performed within 10 days of the last menstrual period, should be used [32]. But if it is absolutely necessary to scan a pregnant patient, care should be taken to limit exposure to the fetus. The same principles of optimization and justification of the scan should be applied. In those instances where a pregnant patient is scanned, studies have shown that the dose to the fetus is very low even if the fetus is included in the primary beam [34]. Modern DEXA scanners are often programmed with patient-specific dose adjustments that take a patient's body mass index (BMI) into account. While covering the patient with protective lead shielding is not common during DEXA scans, if lead shielding is to be used, it may be placed over areas not being scanned to protect a fetus or sensitive organs. Care should be taken to ensure the use of lead protection does not compromise the scanning process in any way and does not interfere with the diagnostic information required.

Another issue of concern is scan or screening frequency. According to [32], *"Rarely are repeat studies justified more often than once a year at the spine and more often than every 2 years at the proximal femur."* Some modeling studies suggest using a screening interval based on age, baseline BMD, and a calculated project time to transition to osteoporosis. Two other studies found no benefit in predicting fractures from repeated bone measurement testing 4 to 8 years after the initial screening [35].

Artificial Intelligence (AI)

AI tools have the potential for enhancing various processes in radiology, not the least of which are improving diagnostic accuracy, increasing sensitivity, and aiding in decision-making. Recently, AI has become a useful tool for diagnosing orthopedic fractures from medical images [36], achieving comparable results to expert human readers and better results than non-expert humans [37]. Convolutional neural network (CNN) models can also be used for bone quality classification [38], while a machine learning approach can be used to predict bone mineral density of the lumbar spine [39]. In another application, researchers proposed using AI to pre-diagnose osteoarthritis that would allow patients to avoid the radiation of a DEXA scan [40]. Another application aims to use AI to find studies that predict the risk of hip fractures among patients in developing countries where patients may not have easy access to DEXA. In a review of various online Journal and research databases, several articles purporting to use AI in one form or another were identified. Because of the possibilities for error, the authors caution that any clinical use of AI should first involve identifying characteristics of the dataset and AI model used and performing appropriate validations [41].

Ongoing Efforts to Improve Quality and Safety

Efforts to improve quality and safety are related to QC of DEXA machines as described in various documents from both the IAEA and ISCD. Stable performance of DEXA machines is important for proper diagnosis of osteoporosis or osteopenia in patients. In qCT, efforts to improve quality and safety in CT also benefit qCT imaging which is performed on CT scanners. Currently, the American College of

Radiology (ACR) accredits CT scanners in hospitals and clinical centers in the USA. The accreditation process assesses the performance of CT scanners by requiring that CT scanners meet certain standards of dose and image quality for head and body scans for both adults and pediatric patients. Dose measurements for CT accreditation are collected by a qualified medical physicist.

Organizational Efforts

Organizations like the American Association of Physicists in Medicine (AAPM) and ISCD play a critical role in quality and safety for x-ray imaging. Regarding DEXA, the AAPM has appointed a task group (AAPM TG367) to address quality control (QC) testing for DEXA equipment. The report generated by this task group is in its final phase of completion and will be released soon. While the report focuses mainly on QC testing and the role of technologists and physicists, it includes a section on quality. In this section, it is recommended that a group consisting of at least one physician, physicist, and technologist collaboratively review the quality management program at least annually to ensure QC is performed at the recommended intervals and to identify and correct deficiencies (AAPM TG367 Draft report) [42].

Resources

Table 5.2 provides a summary of resources (e.g., QC recommendations, safety guidelines) for DEXA and qCT. Our goal is to facilitate quick access for readers to these resources.

Chapter Summary

In summary, DEXA is a low-dose imaging method used to assess BMD and BMC. It poses a very low risk of radiation injury to both patients and staff and is commonly used alongside other imaging modalities, such as qCT, to provide a more comprehensive evaluation of bone health. The radiation dose from a typical DEXA scan is comparable to the amount of radiation a person receives from several days of natural background exposure, making it a safe and effective tool for diagnosing and monitoring conditions like osteopenia and osteoporosis.

Table 5.2 Resources for quality and patient safety in bone densitometry imaging

ACR–SPR-SSR *Practice Guideline for the Performance of Dual-energy x-ray Absorptiometry (DXA)*
NHANES: *Dual Energy X-ray Absorptiometry (DXA) Procedures Manual*
IAEA Human Health Series No. 15 *Dual Energy X Ray Absorptiometry for Bone Mineral Density and Body Composition Assessment*
ISCD: International Society of Clinical Densitometry
US Preventive Services Task Force, **Screening for Osteoporosis: Recommendation Statement**
New USPSTF Recommendations for Osteoporosis Screening
The USPSTF recommends screening for osteoporosis with bone measurement testing to prevent osteoporotic fractures in women 65 years and older (JAMA. 2018;319(24):2521-2531. doi:10.1001/jama.2018.7498)
Guidelines Issued for Screening Men for Osteoporosis
The USPSTF concludes that the current evidence is insufficient to assess the balance of benefits and harms of screening for osteoporosis to prevent osteoporotic fractures in men (JAMA. 2018;319(24):2521-2531. doi:10.1001/jama.2018.7498).

ACR American College of Radiology, *NHANES* National Health and Nutrition Examination Survey, *SPR* Society for Pediatric Radiology, *SSR* Society for Skeletal Radiology, *IAEA* Dual Energy X Ray Absorptiometry for Bone Mineral Density and Body Composition Assessment, *IAEA* Human Health Series No. 15, *NCRP* National Council on Radiation Protection, *ICRP* International Commission on Radiological Protection qCT, in contrast, uses standard volumetric CT scanners to evaluate BMD by measuring bone volume rather than area, offering more accurate and three-dimensional assessments of bone structure. qCT can be integrated into routine CT scans, such as CT colonography, providing a dual diagnostic opportunity for patients. Although qCT involves higher radiation exposure compared to DEXA, advancements in image reconstruction and dose optimization techniques continue to improve its safety and clinical utility.

Following best practices, QA measures, and regulatory guidelines ensures the safe and effective use of these essential imaging technologies.

Glossary

AAPM American Association of Physicists in Medicine
ACR American College of Radiology
BMD Bone Mineral Density
BMC Bone Mineral Content
CRCPD Conference of Radiation Control Program Directors
DEXA Dual-energy X-ray Absorptiometry
FDA Food and Drug Administration (USA)
ICRP International Commission on Radiological Protection
IOF International Osteoporosis Foundation
ISCD International Society of Clinical Densitometry
JCAHO Joint Commission on the Accreditation of Health Organizations
NCRP National Council on Radiation Protection
NHANES National Health and Nutrition Examination Survey
NOF National Osteoporosis Foundation
pQCT Peripheral Quantitative Computed Tomography
QA Quality Assurance
QC Quality Control
qCT Quantitative Computed Tomography
QUS Quantitative Ultrasound
SPR Society for Pediatric Radiology
SSR Society for Skeletal Radiology
US Ultrasound
WHO World Health Organization

References

1. Cosman F, et al. Clinician's guide to prevention and treatment of osteoporosis. Osteoporos Int. 2014;25(10):2359–81.
2. El Maghraoui A. Interpreting a DXA scan in clinical practice. In: Dual energy X-Ray absorptiometry; 2011. p. 1.
3. Kling JM, Clarke BL, Sandhu NP. Osteoporosis prevention, screening, and treatment: a review. J Women's Health. 2014;23(7):563–72.
4. World Health Organization. Assessment of fracture risk and its application to screening for postmenopausal osteoporosis: report of a WHO study group [meeting held in Rome from 22 to 25 June 1992]. 1994.
5. AGENCY, I.A.E. Dual energy X ray absorptiometry for bone mineral density and body composition assessment, IAEA human health series. Vienna: International Atomic Energy Agency; 2011.
6. Baum T, et al. Automated 3D trabecular bone structure analysis of the proximal femur – prediction of biomechanical strength by CT and DXA. Osteoporos Int. 2010;21(9):1553–64.
7. Lorente-Ramos R, et al. Dual-energy X-ray absorptiometry in the diagnosis of osteoporosis: a practical guide. Am J Roentgenol. 2011;196(4):897–904.
8. McCloskey EV, et al. Vertebral fracture assessment (VFA) with a densitometer predicts future fractures in elderly women unselected for osteoporosis. J Bone Miner Res. 2008;23(10):1561–8.
9. Cann CE, Genant HK, Kolb FO, Ettinger B. Quantitative computed tomography for the prediction of vertebral body fracture risk. Bone 1985. 6(1e7).
10. Engelke K. Quantitative computed tomography (QCT) of the forearm using general purpose spiral whole-body CT scanners : accuracy, precision and comparison with dual-energy X-ray absorptiometry (DXA). 2009.
11. Engelke K, et al. Quantitative computed tomography (QCT) of the forearm using general purpose spiral whole-body CT scanners: accuracy, precision and comparison with dual-energy X-ray absorptiometry (DXA). Bone. 2009;45(1):110–8.
12. Genant HK, et al. Quantitative computed tomography of vertebral spongiosa: a sensitive method for detecting early bone loss after oophorectomy. Ann Intern Med. 1982;97(5):699–705.
13. Link TM, Lang TF. Axial QCT: clinical applications and new developments. J Clin Densitom. 2014;17(4):438–48.
14. Ziemlewicz TJ, Binkley N, Pickhardt PJ. Opportunistic osteoporosis screening: addition of quantitative CT bone mineral density evaluation to CT colonography. J Am Coll Radiol. 2015;12:1036–41.
15. Engelke K, et al. Clinical use of quantitative computed tomography and peripheral quantitative computed tomography in the management of osteoporosis

in adults: the 2007 ISCD Official Positions. J Clin Densitom. 2008;11(1):123–62.
16. Hui SK, et al. Assessing the clinical utility of quantitative computed tomography with a routinely used diagnostic computed tomography scanner in a cancer center. J Clin Densitom. 2011;14(1):41–6.
17. Baddoura R, et al. An audit of bone densitometry practice with reference to ISCD, IOF and NOF guidelines. Osteoporos Int. 2006;17(7):1111–5.
18. Leib ES, et al. Official positions of the International Society for Clinical Densitometry. J Clin Densitom. 2004;7(1):1–5.
19. Baim S, et al. Official positions of the International Society for Clinical Densitometry and executive summary of the 2007 ISCD Pediatric position development conference. J Clin Densitom. 2008; 11(1):6–21.
20. Maghraoui AE. Interpreting a DXA scan in clinical practice, Dual energy X-ray absorptiometry, PAE. Maghraoui, 2012, InTech, https://doi.org/10.5772/30574. https://www.intechopen.com/books/dual-energy-x-ray-absorptiometry/interpreting-a-dxa-scan-in-clinical-practice.
21. Woodson G. Dual X-ray absorptiometry T-score concordance and discordance between hip and spine measurement sites. J Clin Densitom. 2000;3(4): 319–24.
22. Yu EW, et al. Simulated increases in body fat and errors in bone mineral density measurements by DXA and QCT. J Bone Miner Res. 2012;27(1):119–24.
23. Martineau P, Bazarjani S, Zuckier LS. Artifacts and incidental findings encountered on dual-energy X-ray absorptiometry: atlas and analysis. In: Seminars in nuclear medicine. Elsevier; 2015.
24. Mueller B, O'Connor MK. Effects of radioisotopes on the accuracy of dual-energy X-ray absorptiometry for bone densitometry. J Clin Densitom. 2002;5(3):283–7.
25. Genant HK, Boyd D. Quantitative bone mineral analysis using dual energy computed tomography. Investig Radiol. 1977;12:545–51.
26. Cann CE, Genant H. Precise measurement of vertebral mineral content using computed tomography. J Comput Assist Tomogr. 1980;4(4):493–500.
27. Kalender WA, Koltz E, Suess C. Vertebral bone mineral analysis: an integrated approach. Radiology. 1987;164:419–23.
28. Kalender WA, Suess C. A new calibration phantom for quantitative computed tomography. Med Phys. 1987;9:816–9.
29. Li N, et al. Comparison of QCT and DXA: osteoporosis detection rates in postmenopausal women. Int J Endocrinol. 2013;2013:5.
30. Khoo BCC, et al. Comparison of QCT-derived and DXA-derived areal bone mineral density and T scores. Osteoporos Int. 2009;20(9):1539–45.
31. Wang M-C, Dixon LB. Socioeconomic influences on bone health in postmenopausal women: findings from NHANES III, 1988–1994. Osteoporos Int. 2006;17(1):91–8.
32. Bonnick SL. Bone densitometry in clinical practice. Springer; 1998.
33. ICRP. Developing a Unified Index of Harm, in ICRP Publication 451985, Ann ICRP.
34. Lloyd T, et al. Radiation dose from DXA scanning to reproductive tissues of females. J Clin Densitom. 1998;1(4):379–83.
35. Viswanathan M, et al. Screening to prevent osteoporotic fractures: updated evidence report and systematic review for the US Preventive Services Task Force. JAMA. 2018;319(24):2532–51.
36. Nissinen T, et al. Detecting pathological features and predicting fracture risk from dual-energy X-ray absorptiometry images using deep learning. Bone Rep. 2021;14:101070.
37. Zhang X, et al. Diagnostic accuracy and potential covariates of artificial intelligence for diagnosing orthopedic fractures: a systematic literature review and meta-analysis. Eur Radiol. 2022;32(10):7196–216.
38. Gonzalez M, et al. Bone quality classification of dual energy X-ray absorptiometry images using convolutional neural network models. Int J Adv Comput Sci Appl. 2024;15(6)
39. Kirilov N, Kirilova E, Krastev E. Using machine learning to predict bone mineral density from dual-energy X-ray absorptiometry images of the lumbar spine. In: CEUR workshop proceedings, 2933. 2021.
40. Aksoy FG, Akdoğan V, Korkmaz M. Pre-diagnosis of Osteoartritis before DEXA with the help of artificial neural networks. Artif Intell Theory Appl. 2021;1(1):76–82.
41. Cha Y, et al. Effect of artificial intelligence or machine learning on prediction of hip fracture risk: systematic review. J Bone Metabo. 2023;30(3):245.
42. Frimeth J, et al. AAPM TG367 draft report on quality control in DEXA. 2024.

Further Reading

Binkovitz LA, Henwood MJ. Pediatric DXA: technique and interpretation. Pediatr Radiol. 2007;37(1):21–31. https://doi.org/10.1007/s00247-006-0153-y.

Donlon CM, Chou SH, Yu CY, LeBoff MS. Accounting for surgical confounding factors affecting dual-energy X-ray absorptiometry in a large clinical trial. J Clin Densitom. 2022;25(2):127–32, ISSN 1094-6950. https://doi.org/10.1016/j.jocd.2021.06.002, https://www.sciencedirect.com/science/article/pii/S1094695021000433.

Sheu A, Diamond T. Bone mineral density: testing for osteoporosis. Aust Prescr. 2016;39(2):35–9. https://doi.org/10.18773/austprescr.2016.020.

Ultrasound

6

Gary Ge, Brent Pressman, Adrian Dawkins,
and Jie Zhang

Introduction

Ultrasound imaging employs sound waves to generate images of internal body structure. It is portable, relatively inexpensive, and accurately displays anatomic images in real time. In addition, it is noninvasive and does not utilize ionizing radiation. Over the millions of diagnostic examinations performed since the introduction of ultrasound in the early 1950s, there have been no proven harmful effects [1]. As such, when the diagnostic results would be comparable, using ultrasound over x-ray-producing modalities represents a primary consideration for patient safety.

The range of clinical applications for ultrasound is continually expanding alongside an increasing number of patients undergoing examinations. New techniques with higher acoustic output levels have been introduced. If used without care, diagnostic ultrasound could produce detrimental effects. As ultrasound technology has become more sophisticated, it is essential to ensure the highest level of patient safety and diagnostic quality.

G. Ge (✉) · B. Pressman · A. Dawkins · J. Zhang
Department of Radiology, University of Kentucky, Lexington, KY, USA
e-mail: gyge222@uky.edu; bpr229@uky.edu; ada226@uky.edu; jnzh222@uky.edu

This chapter aims to address essential quality and safety concerns related to diagnostic ultrasound systems. Quality and safety associated with sonographer's skill and experience are beyond the scope of the chapter, as are therapeutic applications. The objectives of this chapter include:

- Present fundamental principles of ultrasound and associated intrinsic safety issues (e.g., potential bioeffects, hazards related to specific equipment, and relative risks associated with clinical applications).
- Describe quality control of the equipment to ensure quality and enhance patient safety.
- Discuss current efforts to improve image quality and patient safety.

Fundamental Principles

Ultrasound refers to sound waves with frequencies exceeding the upper threshold of human hearing (approximately 20 kHz in healthy young adults). Medical diagnostic ultrasound, or sonography, is an imaging modality that utilizes ultrasound waves to generate images of structures within the body for the diagnosis and treatment of various diseases and conditions. During an ultrasound procedure, a transducer, or ultrasound

J. Zhang (ed.), *Quality and Patient Safety in Medical Imaging*,
https://doi.org/10.1007/978-3-031-89007-9_6

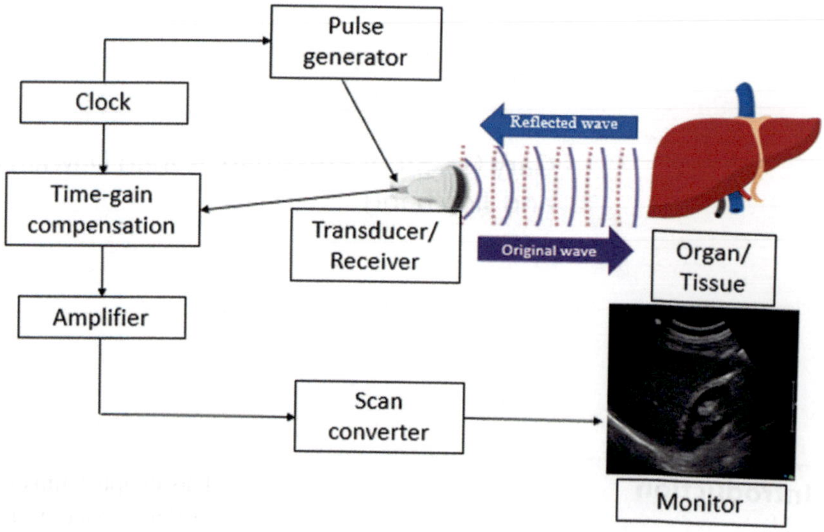

Fig. 6.1 A diagram showing how an ultrasound image is formed

probe, emits longitudinal ultrasound waves through an active element composed of piezoelectric materials. These waves are transmitted into the body, and the active element then "listens" for echoes reflected off interfaces between different tissue types due to their different acoustic properties. These echoes are then processed and displayed as images on a video monitor, revealing details about the inner structure of the body. Figure 6.1 shows a diagram of how an ultrasound unit forms an image. The frequency, density, focus, and aperture of the ultrasound beam can vary. Higher frequencies produce high-resolution images but with lower penetration depth, while lower frequencies penetrate more deeply but with inferior resolution.

Applications

Most ultrasound examinations are conducted using a transducer positioned externally with a water-based gel, known as a coupling agent, applied between the skin and the transducer to improve wave transmission. Figure 6.2 illustrates a typical ultrasound system along with a representative body image. Generally, low-frequency curvilinear probes are most suitable for imaging deep structures, while high-frequency linear probes are better for superficial anatomy. Beyond these, a variety of transducer probes are available, allowing operators to switch between different configurations to better visualize different anatomic regions. Examples include transvaginal ultrasound, endoscopy, and intravascular ultrasound, each presenting both overlapping and distinct safety considerations. Obstetric ultrasound is another prevalent diagnostic examination that combines both transabdominal and transvaginal techniques to evaluate the fetal-maternal interface, carrying its own specific hazards.

Ultrasound has also assumed significant roles in interventional procedures, where "ultrasound guidance" has become the standard of care. In such examinations, ultrasound serves as an important auxiliary function, assisting the interventionalist in visualizing the primary activity occurring beneath the skin, such as ensuring accurate needle placement during thyroid aspiration biopsies. Unlike typical diagnostic examinations, where dedicated sonographers perform the scanning, the interventionalist operates the probe in these procedures.

Another category of interventional sonography is "therapeutic ultrasound," in which acoustic power is increased by several orders to produce direct biological effects, such as fracturing large kidney stones into passable fragments in shockwave lithotripsy. These comprise a

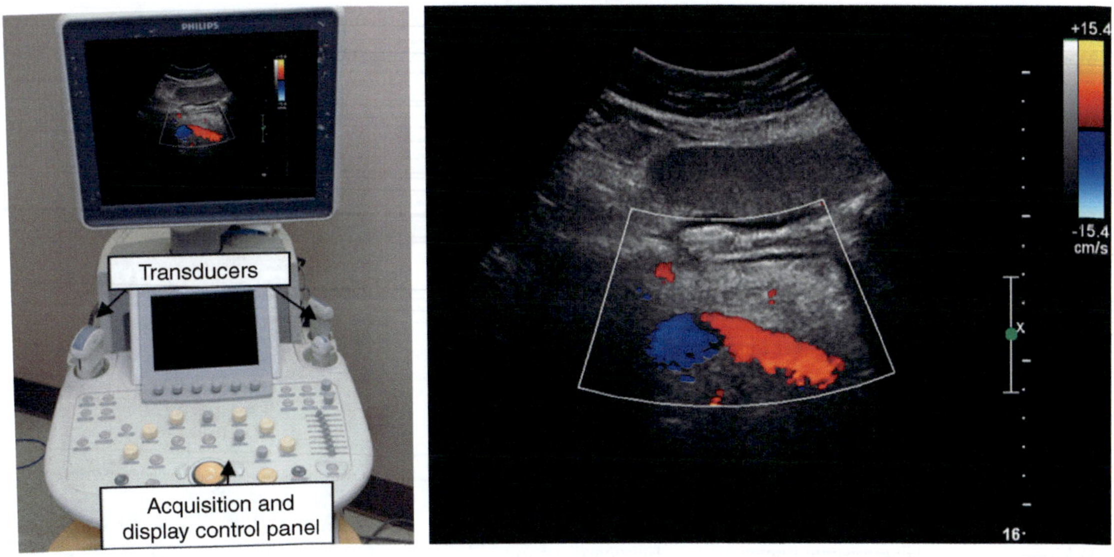

Fig. 6.2 An ultrasound imaging system (left) and grayscale ultrasound abdominal image with Doppler vascular ultrasound of the hepatic vasculature (right)

minority of total examinations and intentionally exceed the safety thresholds established for diagnostic ultrasound, underscoring the potential impact of high-power sound waves.

Imaging Modes

Ultrasound imaging can present information to the operator using several different display modes. All modes are based on the principle that anatomy and pathology can be differentially characterized by echoed sound waves. A-mode is a one-dimensional, non-imaging mode that displays amplitudes resembling an electrocardiogram tracing rather than a traditional ultrasound image. This imaging mode is not typically used in general clinical settings, though it can provide diagnostic value in specific scenarios, such as in ophthalmic ultrasound. The most widely used mode in diagnostic radiology is B-mode (**B**rightness-**Mode**), which typically displays 2D anatomical images or cine sequences. In this mode, grayscale levels are related to the amplitude of reflected sound waves. B-mode can also be converted into 3D and 4D surface renderings, commonly used for fetal visualization in obstetric examinations.

Another commonly used mode is Doppler ultrasound, which evaluates the changes in frequency of returning sound waves to quantify fluid velocity, usually that of blood. Doppler is used in conjunction with B-mode. For example, duplex ultrasound overlays a color-coded representation of fluid velocity and direction onto the standard 2D grayscale ultrasound. By convention, red indicates motion toward the probe, while blue signifies motion away from it. In this mode, incident sound waves can be transmitted in either a pulsed (pulse wave, PW) or continuous (continuous wave, CW) pattern. PW Doppler and modes derived from them are among the most acoustically powerful techniques in diagnostic ultrasound, highlighting significant safety considerations.

Additional modes include harmonic imaging, which is a nonlinear mode that receives echoes of a frequency that is an integer multiple (typically 2N) of the incident or "fundamental" frequency. This mode uses intrinsic differences in harmonic frequencies between tissues to form images rather than differences in spectral reflection used in B-mode. Despite these distinctions, harmonic imaging produces 2D grayscale images that closely resemble those generated by B-mode. Harmonic imaging has advantages over B-mode,

Table 6.1 Summary of commonly used ultrasound modes with a characteristic monitor display

Mode	Characteristics	Clinical application	Display
B Mode (Brightness)	Standard 2D grayscale planar imaging Linear Based on amplitude of echo	Part of most clinical examinations	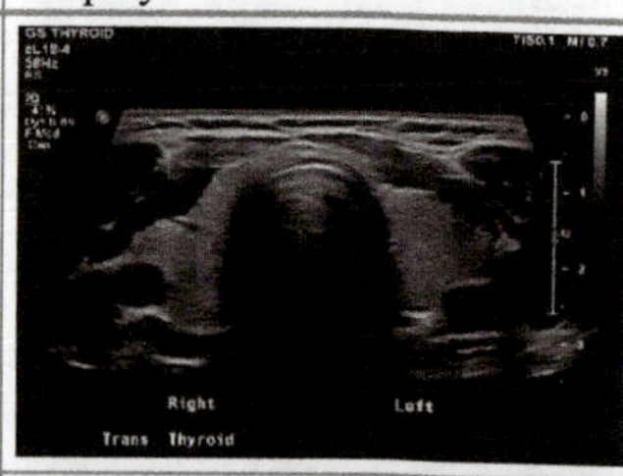
Harmonic Imaging	Alternative to 2D grayscale planar imaging Non-linear Based on induced harmonic frequencies of tissues	Lymph nodes Thyroid	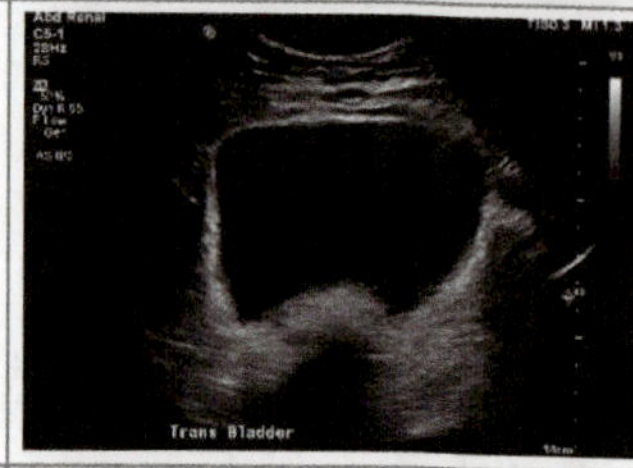
M Mode (Motion)	1D grayscale linear anatomic imaging Displays translocation of anatomy along a single line	Echocardiogram Fetal heart tones (manual calculation)	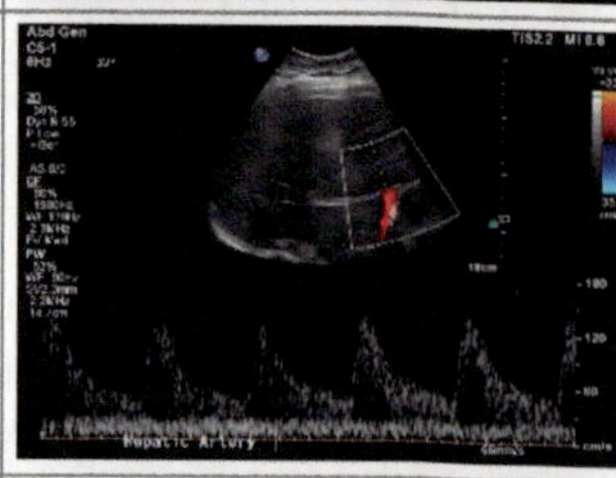
Doppler Mode	Typically color overlaid on 2D grayscale Based on changes in frequency with red toward transducer and blue away by default	Vascular examinations Adjunct to renal ultrasound	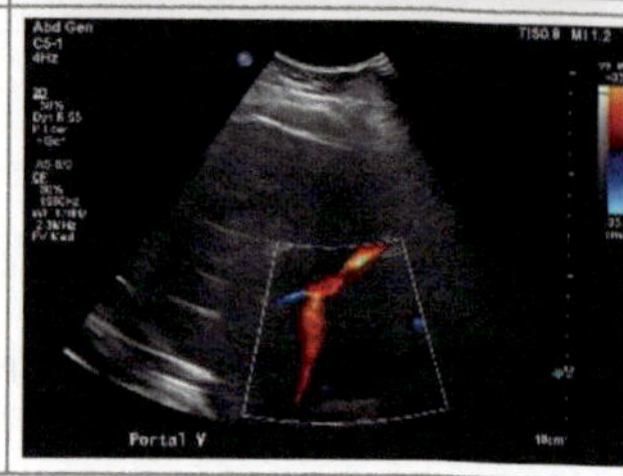

which include improved contrast-to-noise ratio and mitigation of certain artifacts, making it applicable in specific clinical scenarios [2]. A summary of ultrasound modes can be found in Table 6.1.

Safety Concerns

Concerns regarding ultrasound safety primarily focus on biological damage that may directly harm or kill an organism, as well as teratogenic effects that could adversely affect offspring [3–16]. To date, human studies have not identified potential risks associated with ultrasound exposure [14–16]. Accordingly, large-scale industry-wide efforts, such as the Image Gently campaign, advocate for the preferential use of ultrasound over other imaging modalities when diagnostic utility is equivalent [17]. Ultrasound is generally considered the safest imaging modality, as it avoids the ionizing radiation associated with CT, fluoroscopy, and nuclear medicine, as well as the risks of electromagnetic interactions with metallic foreign bodies or medical devices during MRI.

Ultrasound's safety record prompted the FDA to relax regulatory limits on acoustic power in 1992 to improve diagnostic quality. The change increased the spatial peak temporal average (SPTA) acoustic output limit for diagnostic ultrasound to 720 mW/cm^2. In exchange for these allowable higher outputs, the FDA mandated the inclusion of two on-screen safety indices: the Mechanical Index (MI) and the Thermal Index (TI). However, there are no requirements for monitoring acoustic outputs during product sales or subsequent use [18]. While image quality has improved significantly, it is crucial to remain vigilant about safety considerations.

Thermal Concerns

Ultrasound waves can be reflected, refracted, scattered, or absorbed. Reflected waves contribute to the formation of the ultrasound image, while absorbed waves are converted to heat. Increased tissue temperature can accelerate chemical reaction rates, disrupt cellular cycles, and has been experimentally proven to be teratogenic. Ethical constraints prevent the use of human models in prospective studies to determine toxic and lethal thermal dosing thresholds for ultrasound. Therefore, teratogenicity has been assessed and extrapolated from animal models [19–21]. Reports indicate that temperatures in animals, such as guinea pig fetuses and mice, can rise by up to 5 °C during ultrasound exposure [14, 15, 22]. Biological effects have been observed to correlate predictably with time and temperature, forming the basis of the thermal dose concept [20]. Like dosing in pharmacology, thermal dose estimates the risk of adverse bioeffects.

While animal studies have shown potential thermal risks associated with ultrasound, these results are not indicative of the possible risks in human clinical settings. For example, many of the animal studies investigate full-body heating, whereas clinical examinations typically involve focal heating, which can be dissipated effectively through perfusion [21]. Nevertheless, these studies provide conservative estimates of potential thermal bioeffects in ultrasound and have been used to inform guidelines and regulations.

Thermal Index

The only feedback mechanism available to sonographers for estimating tissue heating is TI, which should be displayed and monitored during examinations. TI is the ratio of acoustic power being produced to the power required to raise tissue temperature in the beam area by 1 °C. Worst-case conditions are typically assumed, such as a stationary probe, which is not representative of typical clinical scenarios, leading to conservative estimates [23].

Guidance on acceptable TI values for prenatal and postnatal patients has been provided by various international organizations, including the American Institute of Ultrasound in Medicine (AIUM), the British Medical Ultrasound Society (BMUS), and Health Canada. While there are differences between organizational guidelines, they all provide a reasonable margin for error before thermal bioeffects would be observed [24].

It is also important to note the three TI settings available to display: Thermal Index in Soft Tissue (TIS), Thermal Index for Bone (TIB), and Thermal Index for Craniul Bone (TIC). For postnatal examinations, TIC should be selected when imaging the cranium. If non-cranial bone is prominent in the scan field, TIB is appropriate, while TIS should be selected for predominantly soft tissue fields. For prenatal examinations, TIS is recommended until 10 weeks after the last menstruation, after which TIB should be used [25]. Improper selection could result in misleading values and the potential for excessive heating.

Minimizing Thermal Risk

The factors influencing tissue heating during ultrasound examinations can be categorized into equipment-dependent and tissue-dependent factors.

Equipment-Dependent Factors

- *Dwell Time*: The duration the probe remains in contact with a specific area is user dependent and contributes linearly to thermal dose [26]. Awareness of scan duration and operator experience can help mitigate thermal exposure.
- *Power*: The main contributing factor in both thermal and mechanical bioeffects. Different ultrasound modes produce varying acoustic outputs, summarized in Table 6.2, in the fol-

Table 6.2 Trends in mean power before and after the FDA relaxed regulations for equipment manufacturers. Note that B- and M-mode have increased in mean power to near equivalence with continuous wave (CW) Doppler while pulse wave (PW) Doppler and color Doppler (derived from PW) have decreased over this [27]

	Mean power (mW)	
Mode	1992–1997	2005–2010
B- and M-mode	26	59
CW Doppler	51	67
PW Doppler	134	90
Color Doppler	156	115

lowing descending order of power: Color Doppler (derived from PW Doppler) > PW Doppler > CW Doppler > B-mode/M-mode. Following changes to the FDA regulations, most modes have experienced significant increases in power, particularly B-mode, which is now comparable to CW Doppler. In contrast, the mean power of PW Doppler has decreased [27].

- *Frequency*: Lower frequencies allow for greater depth of field, increasing the probability of heat generation due to acoustic absorption. Scanning deeper than necessary results in higher thermal doses and decreased axial resolution.
- *Field Width*: A wider field increases the scan area and heat generation, which increases thermal dose.
- *Transducer Heat*: During an examination, the transducer generates heat that can be conducted to the patient, contributing to overall heating that is not accounted for in the TI. This may require special attention in specific scenarios, such as transvaginal ultrasound, where a larger surface area promotes conduction and limits heat dissipation [28].

Tissue-Dependent Factors

- *Tissue Composition*: The absorption of ultrasound and subsequent heat generation in tissue related to their composition. The absorption coefficient increases with protein content, with collagen exhibiting high specific absorption [9]. Accordingly, tissues such as skin, tendon, and spinal cord have relatively high absorption values (approximately 1 dB/cm/MHz), potentially leading to undesirable thermal effects. Tissues like the brain, liver, and kidney have moderate protein density and absorption coefficients (0.2–0.6 dB/cm/MHz). Fluids have minimal absorption (~0.003 dB/cm/MHz) [14]. Fetal tissues, especially bone and brain, are particularly vulnerable during ultrasound exposure, as collagen and bone possess the highest acoustic absorption coefficients.
- *Tissue Perfusion*: Movement of fluids through tissue transfers heat through conduction, which can remove heat from the imaging volume [29].

Mechanical Concerns

In addition to thermal bioeffects, ultrasound applications also involve nonthermal mechanical interactions, including cavitation and streaming [9]. Cavitation is a phenomenon that occurs when alternating pressure waves interact with microbubbles. At low peak pressures, they oscillate stably (non-inertial cavitation), but above a certain threshold, they can implode violently, causing extreme local temperature increases and intense microjets, potentially leading to cell injury and the generation of reactive free radicals [30, 31].

Cavitation occurs in the presence of gas-fluid interfaces, which occur naturally in the respiratory and digestive tracts and artificially during contrast-enhanced ultrasound (CEUS), where microbubbles are injected to assess perfusion. Hence, CEUS represents the highest risk for mechanical damage in diagnostic ultrasound, a topic explored further in this chapter.

In non-contrast settings, bioeffects related to cavitation have been observed in animal models. Reports indicate that cavitation-associated effects, such as pulmonary capillary hemorrhage, can occur under clinically relevant scanning conditions [32, 33]. Similar effects have been noted during low-power therapeutic lithotripsy during in vivo studies, although no such incidents have been reported during clinical examinations [23].

Mechanical Index

Like the TI, the MI is the only metric available to the sonographer for monitoring the risk of mechanical bioeffects. The MI quantifies the potential for ultrasound-induced inertial cavitation in fluid, such as blood, under worst-case conditions [23]. The FDA has set the upper limit for MI at 1.9 [34]. A more conservative limit of 1.0 is recommended for obstetric examinations and 0.4 for contrast-enhanced studies [35, 36].

Strategies for Minimizing Mechanical Risk

The factors influencing in vivo cavitation are still not well understood. Known conditions conducive to cavitation include the presence of viable nucleation sites and high peak rarefactive pressures, which are determined by high power and low frequency. Although the lung and gastrointestinal tract are theoretical sites for cavitation, they are not expected to present a significant risk during typical examinations [37].

Special Clinical Scenarios

Point-of-Care-Ultrasound (POCUS)

Point-of-care ultrasound has become increasingly popular in clinical settings because ultrasound is relatively inexpensive, easy to use, and safe. The flexibility of ultrasound also enables its use in a variety of hospital departments to perform a wide array of tasks [38–40]. However, the rapid adoption of POCUS lacks the level of oversight that would otherwise ensure consistent training of operators and use of the technology. Currently, there are minimal guidelines for the application, training, or credentialing of POCUS users. Some healthcare systems have developed their own policies, but these can vary widely across facilities and specialties. These inconsistencies can result in varying levels of user proficiency and raises the risk of inappropriate ultrasound use.

In order to address this growing issue, implementation of high-level administrative guidelines to standardize the training, credentialing, and imaging techniques used by POCUS operators. There has been increasing attention paid to these efforts at the institutional and organizational levels, though regulatory support has not yet emerged [41–45]. A coordinated approach is vital for maximizing the benefits of POCUS while ensuring patient safety and effective utilization.

Transvaginal Ultrasound

Transvaginal ultrasound (TVUS) is a widely used clinical examination with a robust safety profile, though there are several unique considerations. The main advantage of TVUS over transabdominal ultrasound is the increased resolution due to reduced distance between the probe and pelvic anatomy, particularly in obese patients. The primary special safety concern associated with TVUS is the prevention of disease transmission between patients, necessitating rigorous probe disinfection and barrier application. Transvaginal probes, which contact potentially non-intact mucous membranes, are classified as "semi-critical" medical devices, situated between "non-critical" (e.g., devices for external skin contact) and "critical" (e.g., devices for endovascular procedures) devices. This designation mandates high-level disinfection, which ensures the destruction or removal of all microbes except bacterial spores. Low-level sterilization likely increases the risk of probe-related disease transmission, although no proven cases of TVUS-associated transmission have been reported in the United States [46]. Protective measures include the use of disposable gloves by the sonographer and probe covers for the transducer, both of which must be replaced between patients [46, 47].

Obstetric Ultrasound

In industrialized countries, nearly all pregnancies undergo at least one ultrasound examination, raising significant concerns regarding safe scanning practices and potential effects of ultrasound on development. Epidemiologic studies assessing low birth weight, delayed speech, dyslexia, non-right-handedness, visual acuity, and visual biometry (objective anatomic measurements) have revealed no demonstrable adverse effects.

The The American College of Radiology (ACR), AIUM, and the American College of Obstetricians and Gynecologists (ACOG) have collaborated to develop unified guidelines for obstetric ultrasound examinations. The first trimester examination is recommended to confirm a viable intrauterine pregnancy, while the second/third trimester scan, known as the "anatomy scan," is recommended to assess specific metrics related to maternal and fetal health. Additional limited examinations may be warranted for monitoring known conditions or risks but are not considered routine. Typically, a transabdominal examination is performed, with transvaginal ultrasound reserved for cases where visualization is suboptimal via the transabdominal approach [48].

During prenatal examinations, the TI and MI should be monitored and minimized. Scans should be conducted by proficient sonographers to reduce dwell time [26]. The TIS should be displayed up to 10 weeks of gestation, after which the TIB should be used to reflect fetal bone development [25]. Doppler ultrasound should not be routinely used in the first trimester, save for the maternal vessels, and the AIUM only recommends assessing fetal heart rate using M-mode [49]. 3D and 4D ultrasound techniques are derived from B-mode imaging and therefore do not introduce additional risks. However, "souvenir scanning" and other nonmedical uses are discouraged, as they contradict the principle of ALARA.

Transcranial Ultrasound

Transcranial ultrasound is the first-line diagnostic tool for identifying intracranial complications associated with premature birth, which accounted for 12% of all US births in 2010 [50]. Safety concerns primarily focus on the high absorption coefficient of cranial bone along with the sensitivity of developing brain tissue to temperature changes. The absorption of ultrasound energy by bone is over 30 times that of soft tissue. As such, the TIB should always be used for these examinations.

Transcranial scans are performed through the fontanelle, resulting in two significant implications. First, the ultrasound beam is essentially stationary rather than sweeping as in conventional examinations, leading to continuous thermal exposure. Second, the small anatomic window requires a narrow insonation beam, causing normal tissue to behave as if it were non-perfused and limiting the benefits of convective cooling [51–53]. These scanning conditions require transcranial scans to be monitored carefully to avoid potential bioeffects. A relative increase of 4 °C sustained for 5 min is often advocated as the upper limit of safety, which has been shown in transcranial animal studies [52, 54, 55]. Despite the theoretical risks, no bioeffects have been documented in clinical practice.

Risk mitigation strategies focus on minimizing dwell times, frequency, and power settings (e.g., Doppler mode). Ensuring appropriate indications for the examination is also prudent, though typically straightforward. In premature neonates, the risk-to-benefit ratio remains highly favorable, given the long safety record and the critical importance of identifying intracranial hemorrhage and hydrocephalus.

Pediatric Ultrasound

Given the very low risk to patients associated with ultrasound, organizations such as Image Gently have recommended for the use of ultrasound whenever possible. Because image formation occurs concurrently with the examination protocol, patients are not required to remain still during the procedure. This is in contrast to modalities such as MRI, which may require that pediatric patients receive sedation to prevent motion during the scanning process. Another benefit to pediatric patients and family members is ultrasound procedures can be performed safely in the immediate presence of other people, easing the anxiety of a clinical procedure.

While ultrasound is highly recommended for pediatric patients, there are still guidelines that should be followed to ensure patient safety. According to AIUM guidelines, prenatal ultra-

Table 6.3 Reasonable maximum limits for scan time as a function of TI with summarization of prenatal (left) and postnatal times (right) values [24, 25]

Prenatal		Postnatal	
TI range	Max scanning time (min)	TI range	Max scanning time (min)
> 3.0	NOT	> 6.0	NOT
2.5 < TI ≤ 3.0	< 1	5.0 < TI ≤ 6.0	< 0.25 (15 s)
2.0 < TI ≤ 2.5	< 4	4.0 < TI ≤5.0	< 1
1.5 < TI ≤ 2.0	< 15	3.0 < TI ≤4.0	< 4
1.0 < TI ≤ 1.5	< 30	2.5 < TI ≤3.0	< 15
0.7 < TI ≤1.0	< 60	2.0 < TI ≤2.5	< 60
TI ≤ 0.7	NO	1.5 < TI ≤2.0	< 120
		TI ≤ 1.5	NO
These guidelines apply to obstetric (including gynecologic examinations when pregnancy is possible), neonatal transcranial, and neonatal spinal ultrasound examinations. For obstetric examinations, monitoring the TIS is recommended up to 10 weeks from the last menstrual period (LMP), after which the TIB should be used		These guidelines apply to adult transcranial, general abdominal, peripheral vascular, and neonatal (excluding head and spine) ultrasound examinations, as well as other scanning procedures excluding the eye	

sound can be reasonably assumed to be indefinitely safe with a TI < 0.7 and should not exceed 3.0 for any amount of time. For postnatal examinations, a TI < 1.5 is considered indefinitely safe and should not exceed 6.0 for any amount of time. TI values falling between these thresholds are deemed safe for finite periods, as outlined in Table 6.3.

The use of contrast-enhanced ultrasound, which will be covered in more detail later in this chapter, carries additional risk that should be considered for pediatric patients. Currently, there have been no findings that have indicated severe adverse effects stemming from the use of ultrasound contrast [56–58].

Ophthalmic Ultrasound

Ophthalmic ultrasound assesses the anatomy and vasculature of the eye. B-mode ultrasound is used for visualizing the posterior chamber, while Doppler ultrasound is employed to evaluate vascular structures. However, ophthalmic ultrasound diverges significantly from conventional ultrasound practices, with notable implications for safety.

First, standard probes in diagnostic radiology typically operate at a maximum frequency of 15 MHz, whereas ultrasound biomicroscopy (UBM) probes, used for high-resolution visualization of the anterior chamber, typically operate in the 50–70 MHz range. Second, while A-mode ultrasound is largely obsolete in conventional diagnostics, it serves specific purposes in ophthalmology, such as characterizing anatomy prior to cataract surgery. Third, the coupling gel used in standard ultrasound contains irritants for the eye, so ophthalmic tear gel is employed instead [59]. Regulatory standards for ophthalmic ultrasound are considerably more stringent than those for regular sonography, with FDA limits established at a spatial-peak temporal average intensity (ISPTA) of 50 mW/cm^2 (vs 720 mW/cm^2), a TI of less than 1.0 (vs 6.0), and a MI of less than 0.23 (vs 1.9) [20]. However, the proximity of the eye allows for highly detailed, safe examinations at high frequency and low power settings.

Ultrasound Elastography and Attenuation Imaging

Imaging-based elastography is a relatively new technology that assesses mechanical properties of tissue, particularly tissue "stiffness," by delivering a strong ultrasound pulse and measuring the resulting strain on the tissue [60]. This enables the evaluation of reduced elasticity associated with conditions like cirrhosis, potentially eliminating the need for invasive biopsies [61, 62].

Elastography techniques generally assess tissue stiffness indirectly by measuring the speed of shear waves as they propagate through tissue. This can be determined because shear-wave speed correlates with tissue stiffness (i.e., shear waves travel faster in stiffer tissues and slower in softer tissues). Typically, elastography reports one of several parameters, such as shear-wave speed, complex shear modulus, and Young's modulus, and may also provide parametric maps, known as "elastograms."

Similar in concept to elastography, attenuation imaging is also a relatively new technique that quantifies tissue composition and mechanical properties. Designed primarily to detect and quantify liver steatosis, the technique creates a map of the attenuation coefficients within the target tissue volume [63, 64]. This method can prevent biopsies, which had previously been the gold standard for diagnosis and staging of liver steatosis.

Artificial Intelligence in Ultrasound

Beyond conventional imaging techniques, recent developments in machine learning and AI have begun to make an impact in clinical ultrasound. The availability of clinical images within hospital databases has enabled AI model training and has resulted in a variety of useful clinical advancements [65]. For ultrasound imaging, AI tools contribute to improvements in image quality and patient safety with techniques to enhance image resolution, improve beamforming, and navigate users toward standard scan planes during imaging [66–68]. Clinically, AI-based image analysis tools can be used to improve and speed diagnosis, which can reduce patient exposure to ultrasound. For instance, there have been applications to assist in lesion detection and provide cancer risk assessment in breast imaging, determine abnormal fetal anatomy in obstetric imaging, and assess cardiac performance based on heart wall motion [69–73].

Artifacts in Ultrasound

Ultrasound artifacts are discrepancies in imaging that can affect the interpretation of ultrasound studies. Understanding these how artifacts are formed and how they can be mitigated is important for accurate diagnosis and effective patient management. Importantly, ultrasound artifacts do not always degrade image quality, as some artifacts are useful indicators of specific conditions [74–79]. Figure 6.3 contains some examples of ultrasound artifacts.

Below is a summary of common ultrasound artifacts that can arise during conventional 2D imaging:

- Acoustic enhancement: Increased signal beyond fluid-filled structures due to lower attenuation of ultrasound in fluid.
- Acoustic shadowing: Loss of signal behind highly reflective structures caused by wave reflection or absorption.
- Comet tail artifact: Series of closely spaced echoes following a strong echogenic focus, such as small calcifications.
- Mirror image artifact: Misrepresentation of structures due to ultrasound waves reflecting off highly reflective surfaces.
- Refraction artifact: Incorrect localization of structures caused by bending of ultrasound pulses due to non-perpendicular angles of incidence.
- Reverberation artifact: Depth misinterpretation from repeated reflections between strong parallel reflectors.
- Ring down artifact: Closely spaced structures that propagate downward, produced from resonating gas bubbles.
- Side lobe artifacts: Misleading echoes from secondary beams reflecting off structures outside the primary beam, complicating image interpretation.
- Speckle artifact: Granular image appearance due to ultrasound waves scattering off small structures.
- Speed displacement artifact: Depth miscalculations when ultrasound waves travel through tissues with varying propagation speeds.

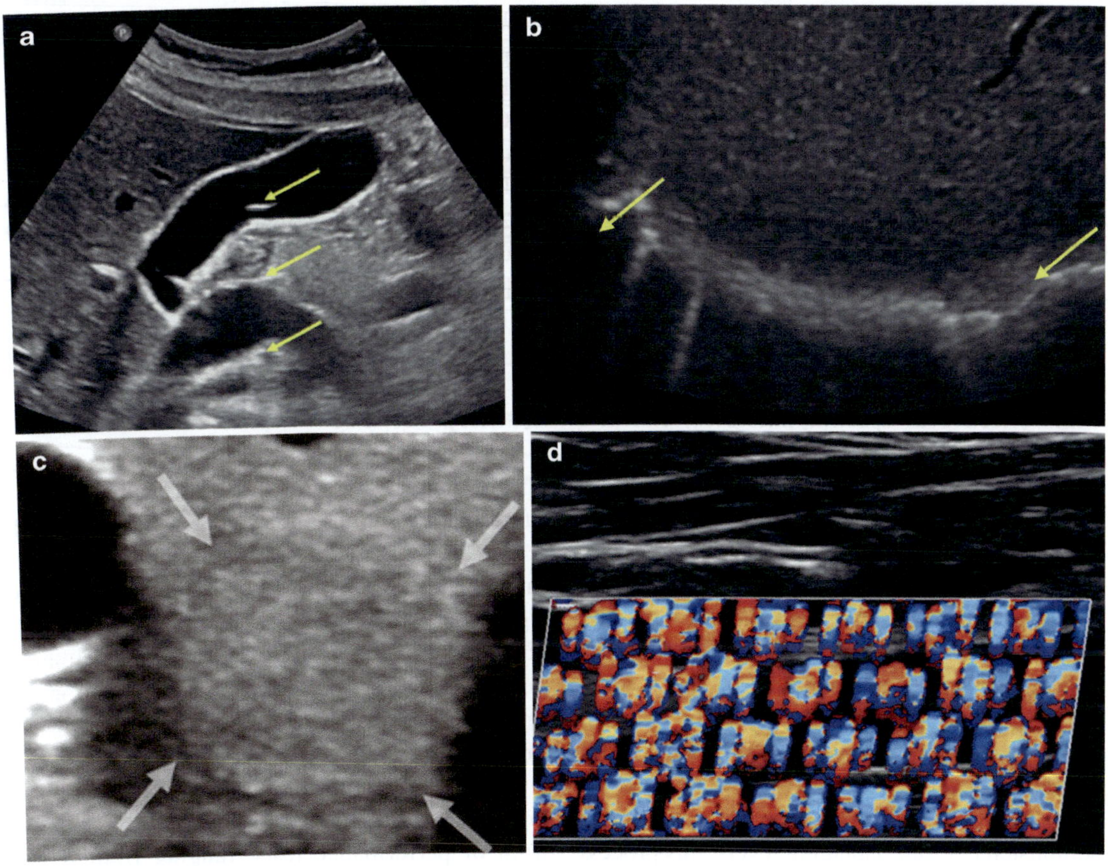

Fig. 6.3 Examples of ultrasound artifacts. (**a**) Reverberation artifact caused by repeated echoes generated between reflective surfaces. (**b**) Shadowing on the left of image and speed displacement on right of image. (**c**) Reverberation artifact causing thyroid pseudo-nodule. (**d**) Electronic artifact in Doppler image caused by external device interference

There are artifacts that are specific to Doppler ultrasound, typically caused by misidentifying sources of motion within the imaging volume:

- Aliasing: Misrepresentation of blood flow due to inadequate sampling when velocities exceed the Nyquist limit.
- Blooming artifact: Extension of color Doppler signals due to low spatial resolution and high gain, obscuring diagnostic details.
- Color Bruit artifact: Turbulent blood flow creates mixed color signals.
- Color flash artifact: Spurious color signals from tissue motion that may mimic true blood flow.
- Twinkling artifact: Alternating colors behind reflective objects, such as stones or air.

Contrast in Diagnostic Ultrasound

Ultrasound contrast agents, similar to those used in CT and MRI, enhance the visualization of blood relative to surrounding tissue. This is achieved by injecting a spectrally reflective medium that effectively reflects sound waves back to the transducer, resulting in brighter images of structures of interest against the darker background anatomy. Current CEUS agents consist of stabilized microbubbles slightly smaller than red blood cells, allowing them to traverse pulmonary capillaries following venous injection, enabling arterial phase imaging. Additionally, unlike standard Doppler techniques, CEUS can provide insights into end tissue perfusion. These contrast agents can be used across various ultrasound modes, including B-mode, harmonics, and Doppler. Clinical applications include echocardiography and characterization of liver lesions and hypervascular tumors in other organs [80]. CEUS offers real-time imaging advantages over CT and MRI, particularly in patients with contraindications to these modalities, such as contrast allergies or renal insufficiency.

While these agents are generally safe when administered correctly, adverse bioeffects can arise under specific conditions. Microbubbles, while effective as spectral interfaces, can also serve as sites for cavitation as discussed previously. Direct evidence of cavitation in myocardium has been reported via broadband noise emission during contrast-enhanced echocardiography [81]. Additional cavitation-related phenomena have also been documented. Shear stresses (those perpendicular to the ultrasound wave) can damage adjacent cell membranes under high-pressure and low-frequency conditions. For example, capillary rupture and petechial hemorrhage have been reported at MIs exceeding the threshold for inertial cavitation. Notably, when administered at sub-damaging levels, this process can enhance cell permeability, leading to research into its potential for improved drug delivery. Premature ventricular contractions (PVCs) have been observed during contrast-enhanced echocardiography; however, these are typically transient and do not result in significant sequelae [23, 30, 31]. Although anaphylactoid-like reactions are a known risk, they are exceedingly rare and even less frequently life-threatening [82].

To minimize cavitation and related complications, guidelines from the AIUM and the European Federation of Societies for Ultrasound in Medicine and Biology (EFSUMB) recommend the following when using contrast ultrasound agents:

- Minimize MI.
- Limit scan time.
- Minimize contrast dose.
- Use higher-frequency transducers when possible.
- Be prepared to treat anaphylactoid reactions.
- Caution for microvascular damage during ocular, cranial, and neonatal examinations.
- Do not perform shockwave lithotripsy within 24 hours of ultrasound contrast administration. Follow agent-specific package inserts [36, 82, 83].

Quality Control

Ultrasound is used across various healthcare settings and disciplines and is generally considered a safe imaging modality. However, inadequate maintenance of ultrasound equipment can lead to significant clinical risks, including compromised patient or operator safety and degraded image quality, which may result in misinterpretation of images. Thus, proper maintenance through routine quality assurance (QA) is essential.

The quality control (QC) process for diagnostic ultrasound equipment encompasses a spectrum of performance tests, ranging from basic assessments to advanced measurements [84–96]. Basic tests include evaluating the geometric accuracy of the instrument, maximum sensitivity of the scanner, and fidelity of hard copy records. Higher-level tests involve measurements of spatial resolution, image uniformity, and characterization of grayscale transfer properties.

Typically, basic tests are conducted by clinical personnel. A multipurpose ultrasound phantom, such as the CIRS Model 040GSE (CIRS, Virginia, USA), can be used for basic ultrasound QC (Fig. 6.4). Geometric accuracy encompasses depth calibration, digital caliper readout accuracy in both horizontal and vertical dimensions, scan registration accuracy, image distortion assessment, and externally referenced position registration accuracy. Sensitivity (visualization depth) refers to the weakest echo signal that an ultrasound instrument can detect and display sat-

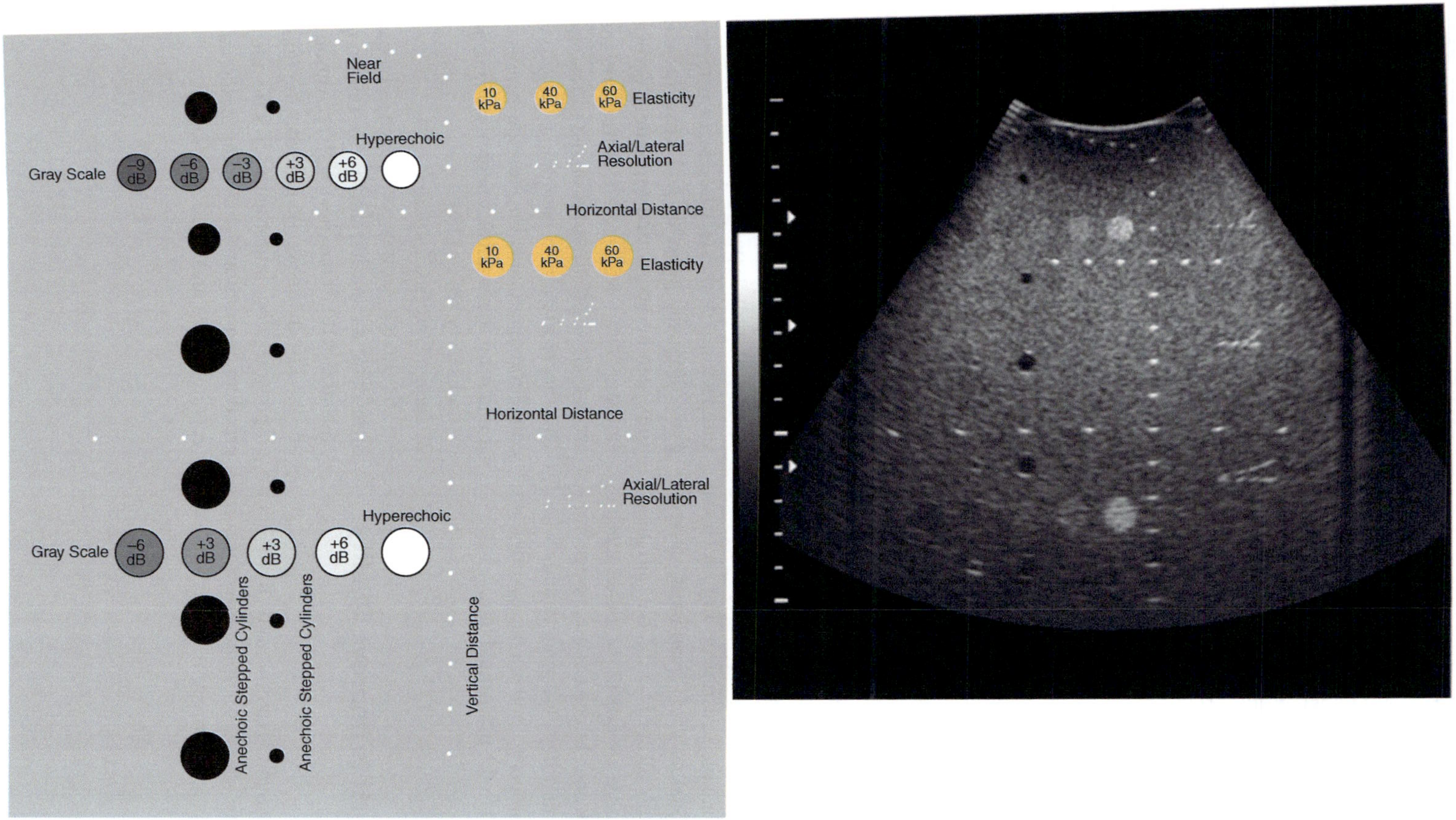

Fig. 6.4 Diagram of a multipurpose multi-tissue ultrasound phantom (left) and an associated phantom image (right). The phantom is used to test dead zone, horizontal and vertical distance accuracy, depth of penetration, image uniformity, system resolution (axial and lateral), anechoic mass resolution, grayscale contrast resolution, and elasticity targets

isfactorily. Image uniformity testing assesses the accuracy of sensitivity controls, ensuring consistent brightness across varying depths.

Additional performance evaluations of ultrasound scanners include assessments of spatial resolution, which refers to elevational, lateral, and axial resolution, as well as quantitative assessments of grayscale display properties.

The ACR ultrasound accreditation program mandates the evaluation of at least the following items:

1. System sensitivity and/or penetration capability.
2. Image uniformity.
3. Assurance of electrical and mechanical safety and cleanliness.
4. Photography and other hard copy recording.

Ultrasound QC should be performed semiannually. Hard copy output quality tests are recommended at least monthly, as specified by the hard copy equipment manufacturer. There is no designated phantom for these tests; users may select any commercially available test object. For electrical and mechanical safety and cleanliness, assessments should ensure all cords and cables are intact, transducers are free of cracks or delamination, transducers are cleaned after each use, image monitors are clean, air filters are maintained, wheel locks function properly, and all accessories are securely attached to the ultrasound unit.

Ongoing Efforts to Improve Quality and Safety

Diagnostic ultrasound examinations have been perceived as "safe" based on epidemiological literature and the lack of apparent deleterious outcomes. However, with the FDA-sanctioned increase in acoustic output to enhance diagnostic capabilities, there is a rising potential for harmful bioeffects resulting from misuse. Therefore, precautions must be implemented to ensure the appropriateness of ultrasound examinations and devices.

Federal/Organizational Efforts

Numerous regulations and guidelines exist concerning the safety and quality of diagnostic ultrasound, alongside ongoing initiatives such as the ACR accreditation program and the Image Gently campaign.

1. *ACR Accreditation*

   The ACR has established specific requirements for physician and technologist qualifications, although the involvement of a physicist is preferred but not mandatory. QC may be conducted by a medical physicist or service engineer. Different types of ultrasound, including antepartum, trimester-specific obstetrics, and gynecological, general, and vascular examinations, can be accredited separately or in combination. The ACR also offers a separate accreditation program for breast ultrasound [87]. This accreditation represents a peer-reviewed, educationally focused evaluation process aimed at ensuring the highest standards of image quality and safety [87, 88].
2. *Image Gently Campaign*

   The Image Gently campaign advocates for ultrasound as an alternative to x-ray imaging to minimize radiation exposure [97]. Although data on its effectiveness is limited, the campaign emphasizes the importance of safe ultrasound practices, particularly regarding potential bioeffects in fetuses and small children.

Clinical Efforts

Ultrasound is considered an established and safe modality, and as such it has received less focus in clinical practice compared to x-ray imaging, where significant efforts have been made to reduce radiation exposure. Proponents of ultrasound often argue that its 60-year history shows no biological effects at diagnostic levels. However, advancements in ultrasound technology necessitate a reevaluation of safety protocols. Modern ultrasound scanners are sophisticated devices that generate more echo information and processing options than previous iterations. Increased pressure output from diagnostic ultrasound scanners raises concerns about potential damage, such as inertial cavitation [98].

To enhance quality and safety, clinical efforts should involve physics support for quality assurance. This role includes verifying the proper operation of scanners and providing technical consultation to ensure appropriate usage, both of which are crucial for patient safety. Recent initiatives also focus on the safe use of higher exposure levels than currently permitted by the FDA to achieve improved resolution and deeper penetration [99]. As new technologies continue to emerge rapidly, further clinical efforts are anticipated to ensure the safe application of ultrasound.

Industry Efforts

In terms of safety, manufacturers adhere strictly to FDA limits on acoustic outputs as indicated by the TI and MI. Specific requirements are outlined in relevant references [18, 100, 101]. For quality improvements, a notable recent advancement involves replacing lead zirconate titanate (PZT) ceramics with lead-based piezoelectric single crystals in ultrasound transducers. This transition enhances transducer bandwidth and sensitivity, leading to significant performance benefits, particularly in penetration and imaging resolution [102].

Resources for Quality and Safety

Table 6.4 summarizes key resources, including quality control (QC) recommendations and safety guidelines for ultrasound imaging. This table aims to provide readers with quick access to essential resources.

It is important to note that most organizations do not operate as enforcement agencies. Regulatory bodies responsible for enforcing the implementation of these recommendations and guidelines include the FDA, Nuclear Regulatory Commission (NRC), Environmental Protection Agency (EPA), Occupational Safety and Health Administration (OSHA), and agreement States.

Table 6.4 Resources for quality and safety of diagnostic imaging modalities

AAPM Report No. 8: Pulse Echo Ultrasound Imaging Systems: Performance Tests and Criteria
AAPM Report No. 65: Real Time B-mode Ultrasound Quality Control Test Procedures
AAPM Report No. 128: Quality Assurance Tests for Prostate Brachytherapy Ultrasound Systems
ACR–AAPM: Technical Standard for Diagnostic Medical Physics Performance Monitoring of Real Time Ultrasound Equipment
ACR: Breast Ultrasound Accreditation Program
ACR: Ultrasound Accreditation Program
NEMA UD 2-2004 (R2009): Acoustic Output Measurement Standard for Diagnostic Ultrasound Equipment, Revision 3
AIUM: Methods for Measuring Performance of Pulse-Echo Ultrasound Imaging Equipment, 1990
AIUM: Quality Assurance Manual for Gray-Scale Ultrasound Scanners. 1995
AIUM: Methods for Measuring Performance of Pulse-Echo Ultrasound Imaging Equipment, Part II: Digital Methods, Stage 1. 1995
AIUM: Mechanical Bioeffects from Diagnostic Ultrasound: AIUM Consensus Statements
AIUM: Acoustic Output Labeling Standard for Diagnostic Ultrasound Equipment: A Standard for How Manufacturers Should Specify Acoustic Output Data, Revision 1
AIUM: Ultrasound Biosafety Considerations for the Practicing Sonographer and Sonologist
AIUM: Medical Ultrasound Safety, Third Edition
AIUM: Performance Criteria and Measurements for Doppler Ultrasound Devices: Technical Discussion—2nd Edition
AIUM: Routine Quality Assurance for Diagnostic Ultrasound Equipment
IEC: Ultrasonics-Field Characterization-Test Objects for Determining Temperature Elevation In Diagnostic Ultrasound Fields
IEC: Particular Requirements for the Basic Safety of and Essential Performance of Ultrasonic Medical Diagnostic and Monitoring Equipment (i.e., Output Display Standards)
FDA (2019): Marketing Clearance of Diagnostic Ultrasound Systems and Transducers
NCRP Report No. 099: Quality Assurance for Diagnostic Imaging
NCRP (2002). Report No. 140: Exposure Criteria for Medical Diagnostic Ultrasound.

AAPM: American Association of Physicists in Medicine
ACOG American College of Obstetricians and Gynecologists
ACR: American College of Radiology
AIUM: American Institute of Ultrasound in Medicine
BMUS: British Medical Ultrasound Society
CRCPD: Conference of Radiation Control Program Directors
FDA: US Food and Drug Administration
IAEA: International Atomic Energy Agency
ICRP: International Commission on Radiological Protection
IEC: International Electrotechnical Commission
WFUMB: World Federation for Ultrasound in Medicine and Biology

Chapter Summary

This chapter presents both fundamental principles and associated intrinsic safety issues of diagnostic ultrasound. While it is beyond this chapter's scope to comprehensively cover all details within ultrasound, it is hoped that the major topics are addressed, and references within should provide more detailed explanations. We expect that this chapter provides essential information on quality and safety of ultrasound. Other quality and safety issues (e.g., informatics, communication issues) beyond imaging modality equipment itself are discussed in other chapters in this book.

References

1. (AIUM), A.I.o.U.i.M. Prudent use and clinical safety. AIUM Official Statements 4/1/2012 [cited 2018 6/9/2018]; Available from: http://www.aium.org/officialStatements/34
2. Desser TS, Jeffrey RB. Tissue harmonic imaging techniques: physical principles and clinical applications. Semin Ultrasound CT MR. 2001;22(1):1–10.
3. Hellman LM, et al. Safety of diagnostic ultrasound in obstetrics. Lancet. 1970;1(7657):1133–4.
4. Hershkovitz R, Sheiner E, Mazor M. Ultrasound in obstetrics: a review of safety. Eur J Obstet Gynecol Reprod Biol. 2002;101(1):15–8.
5. Jakobsen JA, et al. Safety of ultrasound contrast agents. Eur Radiol. 2005;15(5):941–5.

6. Merritt CR. Ultrasound safety: what are the issues? Radiology. 1989;173(2):304–6.
7. Merritt CR, Kremkau FW, Hobbins JC. Diagnostic ultrasound: bioeffects and safety. Ultrasound Obstet Gynecol. 1992;2(5):366–74.
8. Natori M. Ultrasound safety: overview and what we do need in daily clinics for a safe use of diagnostic ultrasound. Int Congr Ser. 2004;1274(0):125–8.
9. NCRP, Report No. 140: exposure criteria for medical diagnostic ultrasound. 2002.
10. Shankar H. Ultrasound guidance: concerns and safety issues may have some answers. Anesthesiology. 2010;112(6):1537–8.
11. Tucker LB, Gentry WR, Thomas EA. Ultrasound safety. Phys Occup Ther Pediatr. 2009;12(2–3):77–96.
12. Nyborg WL. Biological effects of ultrasound: development of safety guidelines. Part II: general review. Ultrasound Med Biol. 2001;27(3):301–33.
13. Ziskin MC, Barnett SB. Ultrasound and the developing central nervous system. Ultrasound Med Biol. 2001;27(7):875–6.
14. Barnett SB, et al. The sensitivity of biological tissue to ultrasound. Ultrasound Med Biol. 1997;23(6):805–12.
15. Barnett SB, et al. International recommendations and guidelines for the safe use of diagnostic ultrasound in medicine. Ultrasound Med Biol. 2000;26(3):355–66.
16. AIUM. Medical ultrasound safety. 2nd ed. American Institute of Ultrasound in Medicine; 2009.
17. Image Gently and Ultrasound. [cited 2018 6/9/2018]; Available from: https://www.imagegently.org/Procedures/Ultrasound
18. FDA. Information for manufacturers seeking marketing clearance of diagnostic ultrasound systems and transducers, T.U.S.F.a.D. Administration, Editor. 1997.
19. Edwards MJ. Hyperthermia as a teratogen: a review of experimental studies and their clinical significance. Teratog Carcinog Mutagen. 1986;6(6):563–82.
20. Miller MW, et al. Hyperthermic teratogenicity, thermal dose and diagnostic ultrasound during pregnancy: implications of new standards on tissue heating. Int J Hyperth. 2002;18(5):361–84.
21. O'Brien WD Jr. Ultrasound-biophysics mechanisms. Prog Biophys Mol Biol. 2007;93(1–3):212–55.
22. Bosward KL, et al. Heating of Guinea-pig fetal brain during exposure to pulsed ultrasound. Ultrasound Med Biol. 1993;19(5):415–24.
23. Abbott JG. Rationale and derivation of MI and TI--a review. Ultrasound Med Biol. 1999;25(3):431–41.
24. Harris GR, et al. Comparison of thermal safety practice guidelines for diagnostic ultrasound exposures. Ultrasound Med Biol. 2016;42(2):345–57.
25. (AIUM), A.I.o.U.i.M. Recommended maximum scanning times for displayed thermal index (TI) values. AIUM Official Statements 10/30/2016 [cited 2018 6/12/2018]; Available from: http://www.aium.org/officialStatements/65
26. Bly S, et al. RETIRED: obstetric ultrasound biological effects and safety. J Obstet Gynaecol Can. 2005;27(6):572–80.
27. Cibull SL, Harris GR, Nell DM. Trends in diagnostic ultrasound acoustic output from data reported to the US Food and Drug Administration for device indications that include fetal applications. J Ultrasound Med. 2013;32(11):1921–32.
28. Calvert J, et al. Surface heating by transvaginal transducers. Ultrasound Obstet Gynecol. 2007;29(4):427–32.
29. Kolios MC, Sherar MD, Hunt JW. Large blood vessel cooling in heated tissues: a numerical study. Phys Med Biol. 1995;40(4):477–94.
30. Dalecki D. Mechanical bioeffects of ultrasound. Annu Rev Biomed Eng. 2004;6:229–48.
31. Miller DL, et al. Bioeffects considerations for diagnostic ultrasound contrast agents. J Ultrasound Med. 2008;27(4):611–32; quiz 633–6.
32. Child SZ, et al. Lung damage from exposure to pulsed ultrasound. Ultrasound Med Biol. 1990;16(8):817–25.
33. Tarantal AF, Canfield DR. Ultrasound-induced lung hemorrhage in the monkey. Ultrasound Med Biol. 1994;20(1):65–72.
34. Guidance for Industry and FDA Staff – Information for manufacturers seeking marketing clearance of diagnostic ultrasound systems and transducers – sections 4 through 6 and appendix A through H. 2018 02/07/2018 [cited 2018 6/13/2018]; Available from: https://www.fda.gov/RegulatoryInformation/Guidances/ucm089001.htm
35. NCRP. Exposure criteria for medical diagnostic ultrasound: 1. Criteria based on thermal mechanisms., N.C.o.R.P.a.M. (NCRP), Editor. 1992: Bethesda (MO)
36. (AIUM), A.I.o.U.i.M. Statement on Mammalian biological effects in tissues with gas body contrast agents. AIUM Official Statements 3/25/2015 [cited 2018 6/11/2018]; Available from: Statement on Mammalian biological effects in tissues with gas body contrast agents.
37. Duck FA. Hazards, risks and safety of diagnostic ultrasound. Med Eng Phys. 2008;30(10):1338–48.
38. Calderon Martinez E, et al. Point-of-care ultrasound for the diagnosis of frequent cardiovascular diseases: a review. Cureus. 2023;15(12):e51032.
39. Lin J, et al. Point-of-care ultrasound in airway evaluation and management: a comprehensive review. Diagnostics (Basel). 2023;13(9)

40. Nakashima Y, et al. Point-of-care ultrasound in musculoskeletal field. J Med Ultrason (2001). 2022;49(4):663–73.
41. Gaudreau-Simard M, et al. Start spreading the news: a deliberate approach to POCUS program development and implementation. Ultrasound J. 2023;15(1):13.
42. Hsieh A, et al. Handheld point-of-care ultrasound: safety considerations for creating guidelines. J Intensive Care Med. 2022;37(9):1146–51.
43. Miller DL, et al. Diagnostic ultrasound safety review for point-of-care ultrasound practitioners. J Ultrasound Med. 2020;39(6):1069–84.
44. Schlaepfer CH, et al. Current utilization and perceptions of formal education of point-of-care ultrasound in urology. Urology. 2024;184:8–14.
45. Shokoohi H, et al. Point-of-care ultrasound stewardship. J Am Coll Emerg Physicians Open. 2020;1(6):1326–31.
46. Leroy S. Infectious risk of endovaginal and transrectal ultrasonography: systematic review and meta-analysis. J Hosp Infect. 2013;83(2):99–106.
47. (AIUM), A.I.o.U.i.M. Guidelines for cleaning and preparing external- and internal-use ultrasound probes between patients, safe handling, and use of ultrasound coupling gel. AIUM Official Statements 3/25/2018 [cited 2018 6/17/2018]; Available from: http://www.aium.org/officialStatements/57
48. ACR-AIUM-acog practice guidelines for the performance of antepartum obstetrical ultrasound, Revised 2007 (Res. 25). 2007, ACR Standards: Reston.
49. (AIUM), A.I.o.U.i.M. Statement on measurement of fetal heart rate. AIUM Official Statements 10/30/2016 [cited 2018 6/10/2018]; Available from: http://www.aium.org/officialStatements/43
50. Blencowe H, et al. National, regional, and worldwide estimates of preterm birth rates in the year 2010 with time trends since 1990 for selected countries: a systematic analysis and implications. Lancet. 2012;379(9832):2162–72.
51. Duggan PM, et al. The influence of variations in blood flow on pulsed doppler ultrasonic heating of the cerebral cortex of the neonatal pig. Ultrasound Med Biol. 2000;26(4):647–54.
52. Barnett SB. Intracranial temperature elevation from diagnostic ultrasound. Ultrasound Med Biol. 2001;27(7):883–8.
53. Lalzad A, Wong F, Schneider M. Neonatal cranial ultrasound: are current safety guidelines appropriate? Ultrasound Med Biol. 2017;43(3):553–60.
54. WFUMB Symposium on Safety of Ultrasound in Medicine. Conclusions and recommendations on thermal and non-thermal mechanisms for biological effects of ultrasound. Kloster-Banz, Germany. 14–19 April, 1996. World Federation for Ultrasound in Medicine and Biology. Ultrasound Med Biol. 1998;24(Suppl 1):i–xvi, S1–58.
55. Horder MM, et al. In vivo heating of the Guinea-pig fetal brain by pulsed ultrasound and estimates of thermal index. Ultrasound Med Biol. 1998;24(9):1467–74.
56. Darge K, et al. Pediatric contrast-enhanced ultrasound: shedding light on the pursuit of approval in the United States. Pediatr Radiol. 2021;51(12):2128–38.
57. Ntoulia A, et al. Contrast-enhanced ultrasound: a comprehensive review of safety in children. Pediatr Radiol. 2021;51(12):2161–80.
58. Schreiber-Dietrich DG, et al. Contrast enhanced ultrasound in pediatric patients: a real challenge. Z Gastroenterol. 2014;52(10):1178–84.
59. Kendall CJ, et al. Diagnostic ophthalmic ultrasound for radiologists. Neuroimaging Clin N Am. 2015;25(3):327–65.
60. Tang A, et al. Ultrasound elastography and MR elastography for assessing liver fibrosis: part 1, principles and techniques. Am J Roentgenol. 2015;205(1):22–32.
61. De Robertis R, et al. Noninvasive diagnosis of cirrhosis: a review of different imaging modalities. World J Gastroenterol. 2014;20(23):7231–41.
62. Geng XX, et al. Transient elastography in clinical detection of liver cirrhosis: a systematic review and meta-analysis. Saudi J Gastroenterol. 2016;22(4):294–303.
63. Lin SC, et al. Noninvasive diagnosis of non-alcoholic fatty liver disease and quantification of liver fat using a new quantitative ultrasound technique. Clin Gastroenterol Hepatol. 2015;13(7):1337–1345.e6.
64. Jesper D, et al. Ultrasound-based attenuation imaging for the non-invasive quantification of liver fat – a pilot study on feasibility and inter-observer variability. IEEE J Transl Eng Health Med. 2020;8:1800409.
65. Zhang J, Dawkins A. Artificial intelligence in ultrasound imaging: where are we now? Ultrasound Q. 2024;40(2):93–7.
66. Athreya S, et al. Enhancing ultrasound image quality across disease domains: application of cycle-consistent generative adversarial network and perceptual loss. JMIR Biomed Eng. 2024;9:e58911.
67. Li K, et al. Autonomous navigation of an ultrasound probe towards standard scan planes with deep reinforcement learning. In: 2021 IEEE International Conference on Robotics and Automation (ICRA); 2021.
68. Tenajas R, et al. Recent advances in artificial intelligence-assisted ultrasound scanning. Appl Sci. 2023;13(6):3693.
69. Austin S, Haase D, Hamera J. Advances in trauma ultrasound. Emerg Med Clin North Am. 2023;41(1):131–42.
70. Huang Q, Zhang F, Li X. Machine learning in ultrasound computer-aided diagnostic systems: a survey. Biomed Res Int. 2018;2018:5137904.
71. Shen Y-T, et al. Artificial intelligence in ultrasound. Eur J Radiol. 2021;139:109717.
72. Wu M, et al. Advanced ultrasound and photoacoustic imaging in cardiology. Sensors. 2021;21(23):7947.

73. Zhang J, et al. Advances in the application of artificial intelligence in fetal echocardiography. J Am Soc Echocardiogr. 2024;37(5):550–61.
74. Baad M, et al. Clinical significance of US artifacts. Radiographics. 2017;37(5):1408–23.
75. Feldman MK, Katyal S, Blackwood MS. US artifacts. Radiographics. 2009;29(4):1179–89.
76. Le HT, et al. Imaging artifacts in echocardiography. Anesth Analg. 2016;122(3):633–46.
77. Prabhu SJ, et al. Ultrasound artifacts: classification, applied physics with illustrations, and imaging appearances. Ultrasound Q. 2014;30(2):145–57.
78. Quien MM, Saric M. Ultrasound imaging artifacts: how to recognize them and how to avoid them. Echocardiography. 2018;35(9):1388–401.
79. Ricci V, Soylu AR, Özçakar L. Artifacts and artistic facts: a visual simulation for ultrasound training. Am J Phys Med Rehabil. 2019;98(6):521–5.
80. Perera RH, et al. Ultrasound imaging beyond the vasculature with new generation contrast agents. Wiley Interdiscip Rev Nanomed Nanobiotechnol. 2015;7(4):593–608.
81. Porter TR, et al. Myocardial cavitational activity during continuous infusion and bolus intravenous injections of perfluorocarbon-containing microbubbles. J Am Soc Echocardiogr. 2001;14(6):618–25.
82. Piscaglia F, et al. The EFSUMB guidelines and recommendations on the clinical practice of contrast enhanced ultrasound (CEUS): update 2011 on non-hepatic applications. Ultraschall Med. 2012;33(1):33–59.
83. Barnett SB, Duck F, Ziskin M. Recommendations on the safe use of ultrasound contrast agents. Ultrasound Med Biol. 2007;33(2):173–4.
84. AAPM. Pulse echo ultrasound imaging systems: performance tests and criteria. American Association of Physicists in Medicine; 1980.
85. AAPM. AAPM Report No. 65: real time B-mode ultrasound quality control test procedures. American Association of Physicists in Medicine; 1998.
86. NCRP. Report No. 099: quality assurance for diagnostic imaging. 1998.
87. ACR. Breast ultrasound accreditation program requirements. American College of Radiology.
88. ACR. Ultrasound accreditation program requirements. American College of Radiology.
89. Dudley NJ, et al. A review of two alternative ultrasound quality assurance programmes. Eur J Ultrasound. 2001;12(3):233–45.
90. Hedrick WR, Hykes DL. Quality control for real-time ultrasound equipment. J Diagn Med Sonogr. 2016;13(2):68–75.
91. Madsen EL, et al. Performance testing of transrectal US scanners. Radiology. 1994;190(1):77–80.
92. AIUM. Methods for measuring performance of pulse-echo ultrasound imaging equipment. American Institute of Ultrasound in Medicine; 1990.
93. AIUM. Quality assurance manual for gray-scale ultrasound scanners. American Institute of Ultrasound in Medicine; 1995.
94. AIUM. Methods for measuring performance of pulse-echo ultrasound imaging equipment, Part II: digital methods, stage 1. American Institute of Ultrasound in Medicine; 1995.
95. AIUM. Performance criteria and measurements for doppler ultrasound devices: technical discussion. 2nd ed. American Institute of Ultrasound in Medicine; 2002.
96. AIUM. Routine quality assurance for diagnostic ultrasound equipment. American Institute of Ultrasound in Medicine; 2008.
97. The Alliance for Radiation Safety in Pediatric Imaging. ImageGently Web site: http://www.pedrad.org/associations/5364/ig/. [cited 2012 April 3rd].
98. Holland CK, et al. Direct evidence of cavitation in vivo from diagnostic ultrasound. Ultrasound Med Biol. 1996;22(7):917–25.
99. Karagoz I, Kartal MK. Improving image quality of diagnostic ultrasound by using the safe use time model with the dynamic safety factor and the effect of the exposure time on the image quality. Ultrasonics. 2012;52(1):93–102.
100. AIUM. Acoustic output labeling standard for diagnostic ultrasound equipment: a standard for how manufacturers should specify acoustic output data, revision 1. American Institute of Ultrasound in Medicine; 2008.
101. NEMA. NEMA UD 2-2004: acoustic output measurement standard for diagnostic ultrasound equipment, revision 3. National Electrical Manufacturers Association; 2009.
102. Jie C, Panda R. Review: commercialization of piezoelectric single crystals for medical imaging applications. In: Ultrasonics symposium, 2005. IEEE; 2005.

Magnetic Resonance Imaging

7

William F. Sensakovic

Abbreviations

ABMRS	American Board of Magnetic Resonance Safety
ADC	Apparent Diffusion Coefficient
ACR	American College of Radiology
DWI	Diffusion-Weighted Imaging
EPI	Echo Planar Imaging
ETL	Echo Train Length
FEG	Frequency Encode Gradient
FDA	US Food and Drug Administration
Gd	Gadolinium
GRE	Gradient (Recalled) Echo
ICNIRP	The International Commission on Non-Ionizing Radiation Protection
IEC	International Electrotechnical Commission
IMRSER	The Institute for Magnetic Resonance Safety, Education, and Research
MRI	Magnetic Resonance Imaging
NEX	Number of Excitations (Acquisitions)
PDW	Proton Density Weighted
PEG	Phase Encode Gradient
PNS	Peripheral Nerve Stimulation
rBW	Receiver Bandwidth
RF	Radiofrequency
SAR	Specific Absorption Rate
SE	Spin Echo
SNR	Signal-to-Noise Ratio
SSG	Slice-Select Gradient
T1W	T1 Weighted
T2W	T2 Weighted
T2*W	T2* Weighted

W. F. Sensakovic (✉)
Department of Radiology, Mayo Clinic,
Phoenix, AZ, USA

Telerad Physics Teaching, LLC, Phoenix, AZ, USA

Introduction

Magnetic resonance imaging (MRI) is one of the most useful and most complicated modalities in modern radiology. MRI does not share basic scientific principles (and associated intuitions) with other modalities such as radiography, computed tomography, mammography, and fluoroscopy. Complex trajectories of the dancing proton spins, confusing pulse sequence diagrams, and equations that veer into quantum mechanics can quickly scare those with a more casual interest and obscure clinically useful information in a thicket of lengthy equations.

The objectives of this chapter are as follows:

- Present fundamental principles of MRI.
- Discuss how scanner hardware and acquisition parameters impact image quality.
- Discuss pertinent safety issues related to magnetic resonance (MR) imaging.

J. Zhang (ed.), *Quality and Patient Safety in Medical Imaging*,
https://doi.org/10.1007/978-3-031-89007-9_7

Basics of Magnetic Resonance Imaging

All magnets have two poles: North and South. Connecting the North and South poles are magnetic field lines. The protons in our body each have a property called spin that allows them to generate a magnetic field. In atoms with even numbers of protons, the proton magnetic fields oppose each other and cancel out, but a net field remains in atoms with odd numbers of protons. Since atoms typically are oriented randomly, the fields from all the protons of such atoms in a sample (piece of human tissue) still cancel each other out. However, if a person is placed in a strong external static magnetic field (like an MRI scanner), then the atoms (and thus their proton magnetic fields) will slightly align with the external field (about four protons per million) and create, for the purposes of this discussion, a net magnetic field. This net magnetic field is typically denoted by M and called the net magnetic moment. The more the protons are aligned, the larger the magnetic moment will be. The human body is made primarily of water and fat which both contain hydrogen. Hydrogen has one proton and thus a magnetic field. Thus, in MR imaging of the human body, it is typically hydrogen atoms bound to various molecules that are imaged. The stronger the external field, the stronger the net magnetic moment will become because more protons will align with the external field. Magnetic field is measured in either Tesla or Gauss (1 T = 10,000 G). While the Earth's field is only 0.5 G, MR scanners typically use 1.5 T or 3 T fields. The external static magnetic field is typically depicted as pointing in the "Z" direction (oriented in the craniocaudal direction relative the patient lying headfirst in the gantry) and is denoted by B_0 (Fig. 7.1). The external field is generated by a coil of superconducting wire that acts as a giant electromagnet. Since superconducting wire is used, the entire coil must be immersed in liquid helium and cannot be switched on and off (B_0 is always on) [1].

The net magnetic moment created by the aligned protons must be manipulated so that it can be measured and transformed into an image. A basic principle of physics is that a changing magnetic field will create an electric field and vice versa. Thus, to measure the net magnetic moment, an antenna (coil) is set up in or attached to the MRI scanner. Next, the proton field must be forced to "change" so that it induces an electric field (and thus an electric current) in the antenna. The individual protons in the external field are not stationary but rotate (precess) at a specific frequency called the Larmor frequency (the stronger the external field, the higher the Larmor frequency). Unfortunately, the net magnetic moment does not naturally rotate but stays fixed in the direction of the external field. The net proton magnetic moment is typically denoted by M_z in this orientation (Fig. 7.1). If the protons are hit with a magnetic field also oscillating at the Larmor frequency, then the oscillating field can push them and, in the process, push the net magnetic moment so that it is pointing perpendicular to the external field and rotating about it (at the Larmor frequency). The net magnetic moment is typically denoted by M_{xy} in this transverse orientation (Fig. 7.1). The oscillating field that pushes the protons is radiofrequency and denoted by Radiofrequency (RF) or B_1. The resonance in magnetic resonance imaging refers to the fact that the B_1 field must oscillate at the proton's rotational frequency (Larmor frequency) in order to push them into the xy-plane and cause the net magnetization to change (rotate) so it can be detected by the antenna. Conceptually think of pushing someone on a swing. They must be pushed at a specific interval (resonant frequency) in order to make them go higher, the same is true for pushing the protons using the RF field.

The rotating net magnetization (Mxy) can be detected and measured by the antenna, but the antenna does not have the ability to create an image from this alone because it picks up a single signal from the entire body (at the Larmor frequency). To make an image, the MRI machine must be able to localize the strength of the signal from each little piece of the body. This is accomplished by slightly changing (increasing or decreasing) the magnetic field in a known way along various directions (x, y, and z). This change in external field strength with position is called a

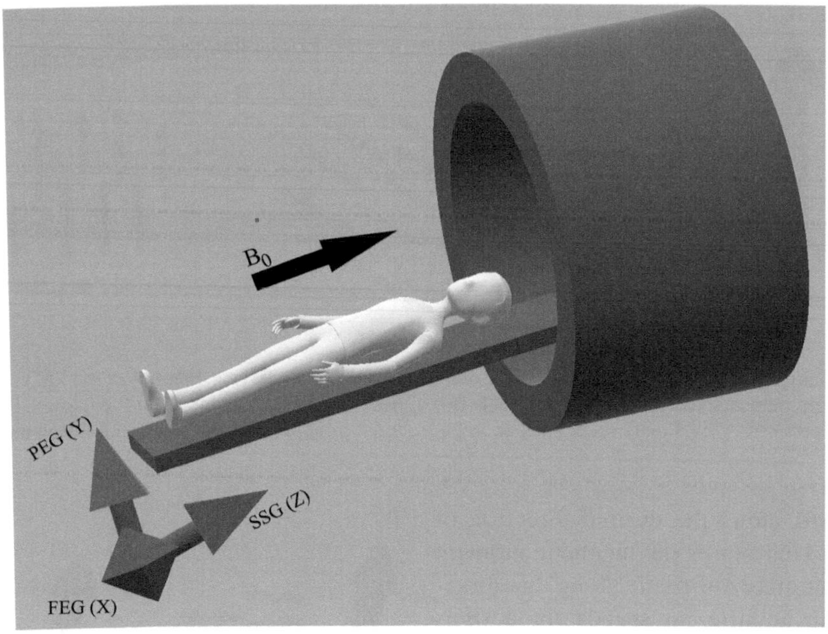

Fig. 7.1 Canonical directions for magnetic fields and gradients. The main magnetic field (B0), slice-select gradient (SSG), and Z direction are perpendicular to the magnet bore. The frequency encode direction (FEG) and X direction are parallel to the bore face and table top. The phase encode direction (PEG) and Y direction are parallel to the bore face and perpendicular to the table top. The net magnetization begins aligned with B0 (Mz) and is tipped into the xy-plane (Mxy) where it rotates about Z. This setup will create transvers slices through the patient anatomy

gradient and typically has a strength of a few mT/m (i.e., it is 1000× weaker than B_0). The Larmor frequency changes with external field strength, thus the gradient means that each piece of the body sends out a signal with a slightly different frequency along the direction of the gradient. When such signals are detected by an antenna, the Fourier transform can be applied to determine how strong the signal is from each frequency and thus determine how strong the signal is from each part of the body along the direction of the gradient (since each piece of the body emits at its own specific frequency). This is called frequency encoding and the gradient used is called the frequency encoding gradient (FEG). While this method localized the signal along one direction, other slightly different tricks are necessary to localize the signal in all three directions before applying the Fourier transform to make the final image set (Fig. 7.1).

When images are acquired in 2D mode (slice by slice), three types of gradients are required for localization: slice-selection (SSG), phase encoding (PEG), and frequency encoding (FEG) [1] (Fig. 7.1). The principle of the FEG was discussed in the previous paragraph. The SSG creates a "slice" of the patient in the following way. A gradient is first applied along a direction perpendicular to the desired slice direction (so field strength would change in the craniocaudal direction to acquire transverse slices). An RF pulse is then applied to the patient. Only those protons with Larmor frequencies near the RF pulse frequency will be rotated into the xy-plane and thus only signals from those protons will be detected by the antenna. The gradient essentially keeps the signal from being detected if the protons do not rotate (precess) near the RF frequency. Changing the RF frequency changes the position of the slice. The RF pulse has a finite bandwidth (range of frequencies), and increasing this bandwidth will increase the thickness of the slice.

The PEG is needed to localize the signal in the third dimension (the SSG and FEG are localizing it in the other two dimensions). The PEG is created by temporarily turning a gradi-

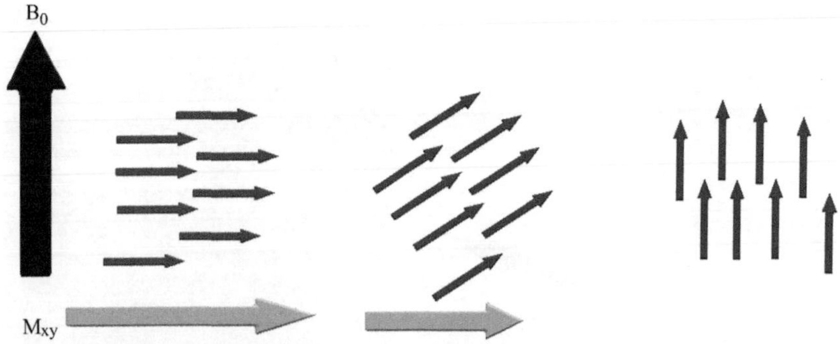

Fig. 7.2 Spin-lattice relaxation. The proton spins from a piece of tissue are perpendicular to the external field (B0) after a 90° RF pulse. As they slowly relax back to alignment, the transverse magnetization (Mxy) decreases (as does the signal strength from the tissue). The time characteristic of spin-lattice relaxation for each tissue is called T1

ent on and off along the desired direction of localization. This causes the magnetic moment from different pieces of tissue along that direction to rotate at different speeds for a short amount of time. When the PEG is turned off, the magnetic moments again rotate at the same frequency, but they are all pointing in slightly different directions (different phases). This difference in phase can be detected and used to distinguish signal at different positions. To properly localize the signal using the PEG, it is necessary to have as many phase encoding steps as there are rows in the image. Thus, the PEG is applied, data is collected, and then the process is repeated with a new PEG (slightly different strength). It is repeated as many times as there are rows in the image.

The protons do not simply stay put once rotated by B1 into the xy-plane, nor do they stay in phase with each other (within the little pieces we measure) to keep the signal large. Instead, the net magnetic moment slowly rotates back to align with B_0. This rotation is termed spin-lattice relaxation (Fig. 7.2). The amount of time it takes to realign to the main field is characteristic of each material (tissue), and T1 represents how long it takes for the net magnetic moment in that tissue to realign 63% with the external field. The more aligned the net magnetic moment is with the external field (i.e., the larger M_z and thus smaller M_{xy}), the weaker the signal.

Protons in M_{xy} do not all stay in phase (pointing in the same direction). Instead, the protons

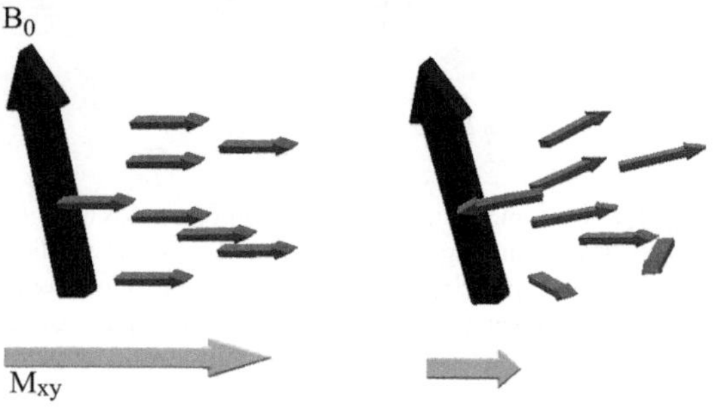

Fig. 7.3 Spin-spin relaxation. The proton spins from a volume of tissue are perpendicular to the external field (B0) and in phase after a 90° RF pulse. As they dephase, the transverse magnetization (Mxy) decreases (resulting in a loss of signal strength from the tissue). The time characteristic of spin-spin relaxation for each tissue is called T2. If the relaxation is also caused by magnetic field inhomogeneities, then the characteristic time is called T2*

push each other and cause dephasing (pointing in different directions). This is called spin-spin relaxation (Fig. 7.3). The amount of time it takes to lose 63% of Mxy from dephasing is called the T2 time. This time is also characteristic of each specific tissue. The more dephasing that occurs before the signal is measured, the weaker the signal will be when collected. T2 dephasing always decreases Mxy (and thus the signal) about an order of magnitude faster than T1 relaxation.

In summary, hydrogen in the body has protons (spins) that act like little magnets. The MR scanner causes the magnets to slightly align with B_0 to create M_z. The MR scanner applies the SSG and an RF pulse to localize signal from desired slice and rotate M_z to become M_{xy}. The MR scanner applies PEGs to localize signal from one of the dimensions of the slice and an FEG to localize signal from the other dimension of the slice. The MR scanner "reads out" the signal during the FEG application with an antenna (coil). The strength of the signal from each small piece of the patient is proportional to Mxy generated in that piece of the patient. Mxy (and thus the signal strength collected from that tissue) depends on how many protons there are in the piece of tissue, how much T2 dephasing occurs, and how much T1 relaxation occurs. If multiple slices are needed, then the process is repeated, with a slightly different RF frequency to localize a new slice. An image of each slice is created by applying a 2D Fourier transform to the collected signal. Typically, strong signals are mapped as bright pixels in the image and weak signals are mapped as dark pixels in the image.

The high contrast between different tissues is the single most important property of MRI. MRI is not the highest resolution modality, and it has a relatively large amount of noise. It has many artifacts and generally takes a long time to acquire images. However, using different pulse sequences allows different tissues to have very different signal strengths. The ability to manipulate the protons to differentiate and highlight certain types of tissue (e.g., pathology) is what makes MRI so useful clinically.

Spin Echo (SE) Imaging

In the above summary of basic MRI imaging, an important detail was left unspoken. Mz is rotated to become Mxy by applying a RF pulse that rotates the protons 90°. Once rotated into the xy-plane, the signal instantaneously begins to decrease due to T1 and T2 relaxation. It is not possible to apply the necessary gradients and collect the signal fast enough to record the signal before it decays away. Instead, the signal is allowed to decay away due to T2 dephasing, and then another RF pulse is applied to rotate all the spins 180° (essentially flips them upside-down). This is important because the dephasing that was occurring now moves in the opposite direction rephrasing Mxy (making the signal stronger) before again dephasing in the opposite direction. The signal from this rephrase-dephase is called an echo, and since it was created by flipping the protons (spins) by 180°, it is called a spin echo [2].

If almost all Mxy is allowed to return to Mz before rotating it back to Mxy, and if the signal is acquired quickly, not much T2 dephasing has occurred, then the signal from each tissue type will only depend on the number of spins aligned to the external field. This is called proton-density or spin-density weighting (PDW). Tissues with many hydrogen protons that can be rotated will be bright, while tissues with few hydrogen protons that can be rotated will be dark (Fig. 7.4).

On the MR machine, the amount of time to wait for Mxy to return to Mz before applying another 90° RF pulse is called the repetition time (TR). Similarly, the amount of time to wait for spins to dephase before acquiring the signal is called the echo time (TE). A long TR time means that enough time will pass that all Mxy will rotate back to Mz regardless of the type of tissue. In some sense, any change in the signal due to T1 differences between tissues is eliminated by long TR settings. A short TR setting would mean some tissues fully recover to Mz, while others will not. As a result, when rotated again into Mxy, the tissues that did not fully recover to Mz previously will have a lower signal when rotated into Mxy. Thus, a short TR will encode T1 differences into the signal strength. If the signal is acquired immediately before much dephasing occurs (short TE), then the image is T1 weighted (T1W). Tissues with short T1 values will be bright (strong signal), while tissues with long T1 values will be dark (weak signal) on T1W images (Fig. 7.4).

On the MR scanner, the amount of time to wait for Mxy to dephase before collecting the signal is called the echo time (TE). A short echo time means that little dephasing will occur for most tissue types, and thus T2 dephasing will have no impact on signal strength regardless of

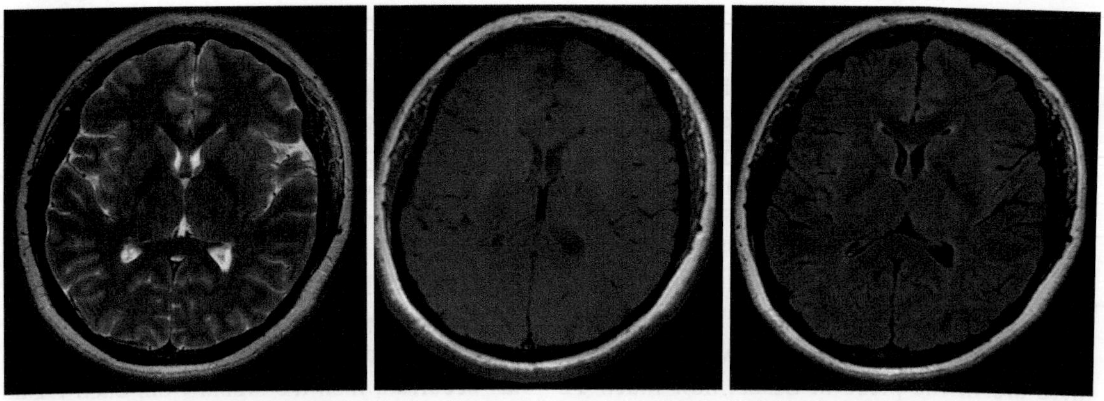

Fig. 7.4 Contrast weighting. Left: T2-weighted image of the brain. Note that long T2 tissues such as cerebrospinal fluid are bright. Middle: proton density weighted image. Note the low contrast due to similar proton density in the various tissues. Right: T1-weighted image. Note that long T1 tissues such as the cerebrospinal fluid are dark

the tissue. A long TE means that some time has been allowed for spins to dephase. Tissues with a short T2 will dephase faster than those with a long T2. As a result, the T2 time will be encoded into the brightness of the signal and create a T2-weighted image (T2W). Tissues with a short T2 dephase more and thus have smaller Mxy, a smaller signal, and darker pixels in the T2W image. Tissues with a long T2 dephase less and thus have larger Mxy, a larger signal, and brighter pixels on T2W images (Fig. 7.4).

In SE imaging, the signal is typically acquired long before TR finishes and, as a result, there is a lot waiting for Mxy to sufficiently relax to Mz (at the end of TR), which extends the acquisition time. True SE imaging is rarely used in current clinical practice due to its long acquisition times. Instead, a variant called fast or turbo spin echo imaging is used clinically. In fast SE imaging, the signal is acquired for a PEG and then, instead of waiting for TR, a new PEG is applied, a 180° RF pulse is applied, and another signal is acquired. In this way, time is not wasted simply waiting for TR to finish for each applied PEG. In SE imaging, the dead time between successive excitations is instead used to acquire additional phase-encoding lines, improving scan efficiency. The number of PEGs to fit into each TR is called the echo train length (ETL). Since multiple signals are now acquired per TR, it means that multiple TEs are used. The effective TE, typically in the center to the echo train, determines the image contrast weighting [3] (Table 7.1).

Table 7.1 Spin echo and fast spin echo contrast weighting parameters. T1 values are appropriate for 1.5 T

	TR (ms)	TE (ms)
T1W	Short (<500)	Short (<30)
T2W	Long (~2000)	Long (~90)
PDW	Long (~2000)	Short (<30)

Abbreviations: *T1W* T1 weighted, *T2W* T2 weighted, *PDW* proton density weighted

Basic Gradient Recalled Echo (GRE)

The dephasing that reduces Mxy (and thus signal) can come from spin-spin interactions that are characteristic of the tissue; however, they also come from imperfections in B0 (inhomogeneities). If B0 is not the same everywhere in the patient, then some protons will precess faster than other protons due to the B0 inhomogeneities. This increases dephasing and decreases signal strength. The time for this dephasing (that includes effects from B0 inhomogeneities) is denoted by T2* and is partially characteristic of the tissue and partially characteristic of the homogeneity of the local magnetic field. T2* dephasing reduces signal in an order of magnitude faster than T2 dephasing alone.

In SE imaging, the RF pulse that flips protons 180° also makes protons go through the inhomogeneities once in one direction and again in the opposite direction (after the flip). The net effect of the inhomogeneity is essentially canceled in this way, and thus SE imaging elimi-

Table 7.2 Gradient echo contrast weighting parameters. T1 values are appropriate for 1.5 T

	TR (ms)	TE (ms)	Flip angle (°C)
T1W	Short (<50)	Short (<5)	Large (~70)
T2W	Long (~200)	Long (~25)	Small (<15)
PDW	Long (~200)	Short (<5)	Small (<15)

Abbreviations: *T1W* T1 weighted, *T2W* T2 weighted, *PDW* proton density weighted

nates T2* dephasing (leaving only T2). In gradient recalled imaging (GRE), there is no 180° RF pulse like in SE and fast SE imaging. GRE imaging is about speed, and for many of the sequences, the focus is acquiring data as fast as possible (high temporal resolution). In GRE, a gradient is applied to speed the natural spin dephasing, and then the gradient is reversed to make an echo. In this case, the protons do not traverse the same inhomogeneities twice in opposite directions, and thus the T2* effect is not canceled. Since T2* dephases much more quickly than T2, it is T2* weighting (T2*W) that is created with a long TE in GRE sequences. A short TE will still eliminate T2* (and T2) encodings in the signal in a manner similar to a short TE in SE imaging.

In SE imaging, an RF pulse rotates protons 90°, and thus all Mz become Mxy. GRE imaging rotates the protons less than 90°. This has three consequences. First, the signal from GRE is weaker than SE because only a portion of Mz becomes Mxy and generates a signal. Second, the smaller flip angle (rotation angle) in GRE means that there will always be some Mz ready to flip into Mxy and that it takes less time for an appreciable amount of Mxy to recover to Mz. This means it is not necessary to wait as long for Mz recovery, so TR can be shortened (which reduces imaging time). Third, the flip angle becomes another parameter controlling contrast weighting (like TR and TE). When the flip angle is very small, all tissues recover Mz quickly, and there is little difference in signal due to different T1 times, thus small flip angles minimize T1 weighting. Conversely, larger flip angles allow for larger signal variations due to different T1 times characteristic of different tissues; thus, a larger flip angle is necessary to encode different T1 times into the contrast and produce T1-weighted images [1].

This section has only scratched the surface of the large variety of GRE techniques that can be applied. It mainly focused on spoiled gradient GRE sequences. There are several other techniques, called steady state, that utilize the residual transverse magnetization from the smaller flip angles to create new types of echoes (i.e., stimulated echoes and refocused previous echoes) to create new types of contrast. Though a thorough explanation of these is beyond this section, one of the most important of these is the balanced steady-state free procession technique. This has gained wide usage in clinical practice (especially in MR angiography) and is characterized by a contrast weighting of T2/T1. This produces bright blood that stands out against most other tissues except fat and other fluids (e.g., cerebrospinal fluid; Table 7.2).

Flow

Depending on the specific acquisition parameters used, flowing blood can be either dark (low signal) or bright (high signal). SE images acquired in 2D deliver black blood contrast. This occurs because the 90° and 180° RF pulses only hit blood protons in the designated slice. Since the blood is flowing, the same bit of blood is never hit by both RF pulses, and thus no echo (signal) is created by the blood. GRE images acquired in 2D deliver bright blood contrast. This occurs because the echo is created from gradients, not the RF pulse. Because the gradients creating the echo are applied throughout the patient (not just the single slice), an echo is formed by the blood (bright signal).

Flow that moves along a gradient "sees" a changing magnetic field. This means that the protons dephase because each proton sees a changing magnetic field (inhomogeneity). The more different field strengths the protons see, the more dephasing there is. In other words, the faster the protons move (the more inhomogeneity they see), the weaker the signal from the flow (due to increased dephasing). This loss of signal can be partially compensated for by using flow compensation (gradient moment nulling) [3].

In GRE imaging, there is typically residual Mxy because TR is very short (there is no time for Mxy to fully relax to Mz). As a result, the protons become partially saturated (i.e., have a low signal) because not as much signal is available the next time the RF pulse is applied. Fresh blood flowing into the slice is not partially saturated and thus will give an abnormally bright signal compared to surrounding stationary tissue in the slice that is partially saturated. This is called flow-related enhancement. This enhancement is the basis of time-of-flight angiography methods. In these methods, a GRE sequence is applied to suppress signal from stationary tissues in a slice. Fresh blood coming in will not be suppressed, and thus when the signal is acquired, it will look very bright next to the suppressed stationary tissues. These sequences are typically T1W, and it is important to be aware that bright T1W tissues may still retain enough signal to be visible in time-of-flight angiograms [3]. Another clinical caveat involves the measurement of stenosis from time-of-flight angiograms. Since turbulent flow, such as is found around a stenosis, increases dephasing, the blood around a stenosis can display little or no signal. Since a stenosis also displays little or no signal, it is important to realize that the signal void visualized on the image is not necessarily the true size of the stenosis, but a combination of dephased blood and the true stenosis. Thus, measurement of stenosis size on time-of-flight angiography can overestimate the true size [4, 5].

Diffusion

Water molecules typically move with a random direction and velocity as they bounce off of each other and surrounding atoms. Since each molecule moves in a random direction at a given speed, the net effect is that water will spread out. To visualize this, think of a drop of dye placed in a cup of clear water. Each molecule of dye moves in a random direction, and since no direction is preferred, the drop expands (diffuses) in all directions (isotropic) until it uniformly mixes in the cup. If there is some sort of physical barrier, then the diffusion will be anisotropic and move more in the direction of least resistance (parallel to the barrier). The goal of diffusion MR sequences is to identify abnormal diffusion caused by disease processes or damage.

The basic principle of diffusion imaging utilizes a bipolar gradient [3]. Essentially, a gradient is applied to the tissues of interest and dephase the signal from the tissues. A second gradient is then applied that is the opposite of the first gradient. This second gradient reverses the dephasing in stationary tissue. However, any molecules that moved along the gradient (diffusing water) and dephased due to the changing magnetic field will not have their dephasing exactly reversed by the second gradient (because they are in a different position). Diffusing water will have a darker signal the faster it moves along the gradient direction, and the stationary tissue will not be affected. Thus, a dark signal in a diffusion-weighted (DW) image indicates faster diffusion in the direction of the bipolar gradient. The gradient strength, time between poles of the gradient, and the length of time each gradient is applied are controlled by the b-value parameter. This parameter can be conceptualized as the amount of time it takes for free water to diffuse 1mm^2. High b-values are more sensitive to diffusion but have a worse signal-to-noise ratio. Since the image only shows diffusion in the direction of the gradient, three bipolar gradients must be applied, one at a time, to get a full 3D rendering of the diffusion. A DW image is typically T2W, and thus artifacts and the natural T2-weghitings of tissues can make determination of fast and slow flows difficult [6] (Fig. 7.5).

DW imaging does not give a quantitative measurement of diffusion. The apparent diffusion coefficient (ADC) image was partially created to combat this problem. The ADC image is created by taking two (or more) DW images obtained at

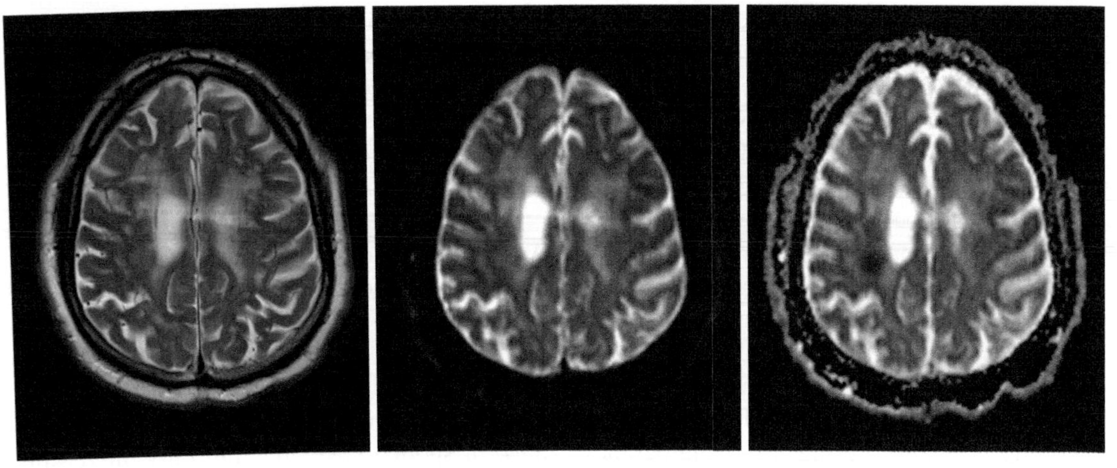

Fig. 7.5 Diffusion. Left: T2-weighted image of the brain. There is a slight hyperintensity in the right corona radiata. Note the relatively high resolution and signal-to-noise ratio of the image. Middle: diffusion-weighted image. There is still a slight hyperintensity in the right corona radiata that could be shine-through or could indicate restricted diffusion. Note the low resolution due to smaller matrix size and other factors. Right: apparent diffusion coefficient image. There is now a hypointensity in the right corona radiata confirming restricted diffusion

different b-values (typically 0 and 1000) and fitting them to an empirical model of diffusion. By fitting the model, the apparent diffusion coefficient can be determined. It is "apparent" because secondary factors such as perfusion, partial volume, and artifacts as well as the assumption of Gaussian diffusion model all mean it is only an approximation of the true diffusion coefficient. ADC images display bright pixels in tissues with high diffusion and dark pixels for tissues with low (restricted) diffusion [6–8] (Fig. 7.5).

Diffusion is measured along the direction of the gradients chosen by the user. If bipolar gradients along all three dimensions are applied, then diffusion along each dimension can be recorded. Advanced image processing and model fitting can be used to fit glyphs to the diffusion pattern in each pixel giving an indication of strength, direction, and other properties. If the direction of strong flow is connected between glyphs, then tracts of diffusion can be visualized. This is referred to as tractography and is typically used to visualize the structure of the brain since water molecules will typically diffuse more quickly along axons than across them. It is important to note that it is not actually the axon tracts that are visualized, but the diffusion of water, which typically diffuses parallel to the axon tracts [6–8].

Contrast-Enhanced Imaging

Although the major advantage of MRI is the wide range of tissue contrasts available depending on the pulse sequence used, there are still times when it is not possible (or very difficult) to acquire the necessary clinical information without the aid of external agents. The main contrast agent used in MR imaging is gadolinium (Gd). Unlike contrast in x-ray modalities, it is not the contrast agent that is visualized. Indeed, if this were the case, then a toxic amount of Gd would be necessary for visualization. Instead, Gd impacts the local protons by temporarily binding with them and relaxing them. Each Gd atom relaxes millions of water protons. As a result, protons in the area of Gd have a decreased T1 time. Thus, Gd-infused areas appear bright on T1W images (Fig. 7.9). The Gd also increases dephasing and thus reduces T2 times, but the effect is much smaller than the T1 shortening at typical concentrations and B0 used in clinical imaging [9].

The multitude of Gd-based contrast agent types are due to the molecules that are bound to the Gd. Depending on the structure of these molecules, the efficacy of the Gd can be enhanced (by more quickly exchanging and relaxing protons in the local area). Similarly, the molecular structure can be designed to interact in the body in a specific manner. Gadoxetate disodium begins in the vascular and extravascular space, but is designed to be taken up by hepatocytes through the organic anion transporting polypeptide [10]. The result is an order of magnitude increase in hepatic uptake as compared to other Gd contrast agents. Gadofosveset trisodium is a blood pool agent specifically designed to bind with serum albumin. This binding means that contrast agent will stay intravascular longer and thus will demonstrate increased concentration (and enhancement) during MR angiography studies [11].

Spatial Resolution

The spatial resolution of an image relates to the ability to distinguish small objects or object placed closely together. When spatial resolution is not sufficient, then the object will appear blurred and that blurring may be so severe as to render the object invisible or in the case of two closely placed indistinguishable objects [1]. In MRI, several acquisition parameters directly and indirectly impact spatial resolution. Pixel size and slice thickness determine the volume of anatomy occupying a single element in our image. Large pixels and slice thicknesses provide lower resolution because each pixel contains more anatomy (Fig. 7.5). Pixel size, measured in mm/pixel, can be reduced (resolution improved) by either increasing the matrix size (more pixels per unit area) or by reducing the field of view (same number of pixels, but they cover a smaller amount of anatomy). Similarly, increasing slice thickness decreases the spatial resolution since each slice encompasses a larger amount of anatomy. Using fewer large pixels or slices decreases noise and decreases acquisition time as well. In 3D imaging, the entire volume is acquired instead of each slice individually. Acquiring in 3D mode often results in more uniform and smaller slice thicknesses and thus improves out-of-plane resolution. SNR is often typically improved as well. The major trade-off is longer acquisition time, though specialized pulse sequences attempt to reduce this disadvantage.

Contrast

As discussed earlier, the ability to assign desired contrast to different tissues is the strength of MRI. Contrast depends on the specific pulse sequence used. In SE and some GRE imaging, TR controls the amount of T1 weighting found in the image (shorter TR giving more T1 weighting). In spoiled GRE imaging only, increasing the flip angle will increase the T1 weighting in the image. TE controls the amount of T2 weighting in SE imaging and T2* weighting in some GRE imaging. Longer TE gives increased T2 (or T2*) weighting to the image. If TR and TE are set to minimize both T1 and T2 weightings, then the contrast will be primarily determined by the proton spin density of each tissue. Tradeoffs to long TR include impact on some artifacts and increased acquisition time. A long TE will reduce signal strength and thus SNR. Tissues with low proton density will have a low signal (low SNR).

Several modifiers exist to manipulate the contrast of specific parts of the image. Gadolinium contrast media decreases T1 and thus increases the T1 weighting of local tissue. Tradeoffs include induction of artifacts and safety issues. Subtraction and saturation methods can be used to suppress all signals except one and are typically used in angiography. In one method, spins in a specific area are nulled. This might be all tissues except the flowing blood to make time-of-flight imaging of blood stand out. It could also be a local band of saturation applied to arteries flowing up into the brain to null the arterial blood signal so a venogram can be created (or vice versa for an angiogram). An image before contrast media injections can also be subtracted from an image after contrast media injection. In this case, only tissues that uptake the contrast media will demonstrate a signal in the subtracted image. The trade-off is possible motion artifacts and increased noise due to the image subtraction.

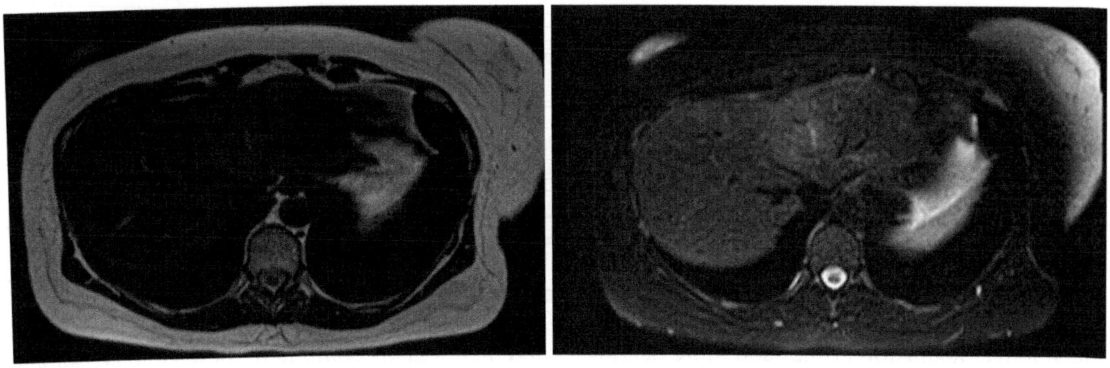

Fig. 7.6 Chemical fat saturation. Left: T2-weighted abdominal image. Right: fat saturated T2-weighted abdominal image. Breast fat at the periphery of the image is not saturated. This is due to a change in the local fat Larmor frequency from B0 inhomogeneities away from the center of the bore as well as bilateral breast implants that cannot be visualized on this section

Specific tissues can be nulled (zero signal) using several methods including inversion recovery, chemical saturation, and Dixon's method. Inversion recovery methods use the T1 time of the tissue to null it. First, a 180° pulse is applied to the patient. When the tissue to be nulled relaxes to the xy-plane, a typical SE image is acquired. The 90° RF pulse that begins the SE sequences causes the Mxy of the tissue to flip back along the negative z-axis and thus give no signal. Since other tissues have other T1 times, they still emit a signal (thus only the tissue of interest is nulled). When the tissue of interest is fat, then the sequence is referred to as short tau inversion recovery (STIR), and when the tissue of interest is cerebrospinal fluid, the sequence is called fluid attenuation inversion recovery (FLAIR). Inversion sequences are robust to inhomogeneities that impact other nulling methods but increase tissue heating and increase scan time. Chemical saturation relies on the idea that protons rotate at slightly different frequencies depending on their local environment (e.g., fat protons have a different Larmor frequency than muscle protons). This difference is exploited by the MR scanner, which creates an RF pulse tuned only to the specified tissue. The RF pulse saturates the tissue of interest, so it does not give off a signal. Saturation methods are generally fast, but increase tissue heating and fail if there is any inhomogeneity in the magnetic field that alters the Larmor frequency of the tissue to be nulled [12] (Fig. 7.6). The Dixon method relies on the Larmor frequency of protons in different local environments as well. Specifically, it attempts to acquire images where Mxy of fat protons is in phase with the Mxy of water protons (in-phase) and when Mxy of fat protons are at an opposing phase with Mxy of water protons (out-of-phase). Some image processing then allows for the creation of fat-only (nulling water) and water-only (nulling fat) images [13]. Methods of fat suppression are often necessary when imaging flow and diffusion as they can cause false signals that distort the image or mimic disease. Further, suppression is typically used to ensure lesions are not missed due to the bright background signal of surrounding fat.

Signal, Noise, and Signal-to-Noise Ratio

Detectability is typically proportional to the signal-to-noise ratio (SNR). A higher SNR means it is more likely to detect a signal. SNR is increased by increasing the tissue signal, decreasing the image noise, or both. A long TR allows more time for spins to recover, and thus typically more net magnetization is available to create a strong signal when Mz is flipped into Mxy. The tradeoff is that long TR impacts both contrast weighting and acquisition times as well as some artifacts. Similarly, a large flip angle means more of Mz is converted to Mxy to create a strong signal. The tradeoff is that a large flip angle increases tissue heating and affects contrast weighting. Both a large pixel size or slice thickness both allow more protons into each pixel. Thus, there is higher signal and higher SNR. The tradeoff is decreased resolution due to the size of the pixels. SE imaging uses a larger flip angle and longer TR which gives it a higher SNR than GRE imaging in general. The tradeoff is that SE imaging has much longer acquisition times and more heating. When parallel imaging is applied to decrease acquisition time (see below), there is generally a decrease in SNR that is proportional to the square root of the speed increase factor (reducing acquisition time by four reduces SNR by half). Image subtraction is used to suppress background tissue to improve contrast (typically in breast imaging and angiography), but the subtraction method increases image noise and thus lowers SNR [3].

The operator can set the number of acquisitions (excitations or NEX), which essentially tells the MR machine how many images of the same slice to create and then average together. Because signal adds linearly, but noise adds in quadrature the result of setting NEX to 4 is that the signal quadruples, the noise doubles, and the SNR doubles. The tradeoff is that tissue heating also increases as does acquisition time (4×) [1]. Another parameter the operator controls is receiver bandwidth which is the range of frequencies the machine acquires when measuring a signal. A higher receiver bandwidth (rBW) generally means the machine collects more frequencies when recording the signal, but the signal strength is not impacted. However, there is noise in all the new frequencies that the machine is listening to and thus it increases. Specifically, cutting rBW to one fourth doubles the SNR. The tradeoff is that the minimum TE available increases impacting contrast, and chemical shift artifact becomes more severe [14].

The receive coil type and the number of coil channels greatly impact the SNR. In general, signal strength quickly increases as distance from patient to coil decreases, hence surface and anatomy specific coils provide better signal than the coils embedded in the MR scanner (body coil), which is far from the patient. A coil can only "see" anatomy inside its diameter; thus, it must be large enough to encompass the anatomy. However, the larger the coil, the more is the noise, and it can also "see," and thus smaller diameters will reduce image noise. A tradeoff in using small coils is that they can only "see" to a depth about 50–75% of their diameter, thus very small coils are only used on superficial anatomy [15]. Since multiple coils can be made into arrays and their signals combined, there is an advantage for both signal and noise when using arrays of small coils, and the decreased penetration depth no longer is an issue as the array of coils essentially acts as a single large coil [16]. Such arrays also facilitate the use of parallel imaging. The number of elements that can be activated in an array depends on the number of channels available. A channel is all the electronics needed to take the output of a coil and turn it into an image. In general, having more channels available facilitates the use of more advanced coil arrays that improve SNR, but at a significant increase in monetary cost [17].

Acquisition Time

MRI acquisition time is generally much longer than x-ray modalities. Studies routinely last 30 minutes or more depending on the imaging sequences. When acquisition time is long, the possibility of motion artifact and patient discomfort increase (in addition to lowering overall patient throughput in the clinic). Several acquisition parameters can be altered to reduce scanning time. Each pixel in the PEG direction requires the spins to be flipped into Mxy and then relax to Mz before again being flipped. If the number of pixels in the PEG direction is halved, then the amount of time to acquire the scan is also halved with the tradeoff of reduced resolution. Thus, to minimize acquisition time, it is important that the field of view be set as small as possible to minimize the number of pixels in the PEG direction. Unlike computed tomography, MRI images can be rectangular. The advantage of this is that when imaging structures that are larger in one dimen-

Table 7.3 Quality metrics relevant to MR scanning

	Explanation	Typical tradeoffs
Contrast	Difference in gray level between tissues of interest	Acquisition time, SNR
Spatial resolution	Ability to visualize small details	SNR, acquisition time
SNR	The ability to detect a signal (object of interest)	Acquisition time, resolution
Acquisition time	Time required to image the patient	SNR, spatial resolution, contrast, artifacts

Abbreviations: *SNR* signal-to-noise ratio

sion than another (e.g., arm), the phase encode direction can be a set along the smaller dimension so that fewer pixels are needed in the PEG direction to make the image. Partial Fourier techniques exploit some data symmetries to acquire fewer PEG steps and thus decrease acquisition time with the tradeoff of lower SNR. Conversely, averaging multiple acquisitions to improve SNR will proportionally increase acquisition time. Thus, a NEX of 4 doubles the SNR and quadruples scan time [3].

When acquiring the signal during each PEG step, most of the time is spent waiting for Mxy to relax to Mz. TR determines how long we wait until beginning on the next PEG step. Halving the TR will halve the total acquisition time with the tradeoff that it alters the image contrast and reduces the SNR. Instead of reducing TR, the time waiting can be put to use. Using the multi-slice technique, the scanner will move onto one or more other slices and begin acquisition while waiting for TR in the current slice. In this manner, multiple slices are simultaneously acquired, and thus total scan time is reduced. In Fast Spin Echo (FSE) imaging, increasing the echo train length will proportionally decrease the acquisition time. The tradeoff is that long echo train lengths add T2 weighting to the image, increase blur, and reduce SNR [1, 3]. MR scans may be acquired in 2D or 3D. Acquiring images in 3D substantially increases acquisition time. This is because in 3D acquisition, the SSG is replaced by a second PEG. Further, 3D is often applied to acquire isotropic voxels and thus typically will use more pixels in the z direction. As a result, the acquisition time is typically longer, but resolution and SNR are both improved.

New coil technology and pulse sequences have substantially reduced scan times. Parallel imaging uses signals from multiple coils in an array to decrease scan time. In general, if the acceleration factor is 4, the scan time will be quartered with the tradeoff that SNR is halved [18]. GRE sequences use small flip angles and lack a 180° pulse. In addition, they use gradients to speed up dephasing and then rephrasing of spins. These factors generally make GRE sequences much faster than even fast SE with the tradeoff that SNR is often worse, artifacts are worse, and contrast weightings are different than those seen in SE imaging. Typically, the fastest acquisitions are single shot versions of echo planar imaging (EPI) [3, 19]. Though there are many different sequences that have been developed, EPI typically involves starting with a traditional 90° and then 18° SE sequence; however, once this is performed, a series of gradients step through all the PEG steps and create all gradient echoes necessary to make the image. The TR is effectively infinite because there is never a second 90° pulse (the entire image is acquired in a single shot). EPI is excellent for cardiac imaging and is employed in diffusion and functional imaging where the many images that need to be acquired that would otherwise make scan time with other sequences too long to be of use. The tradeoff for using EPI sequences is low SNR and severe artifacts including ghosting and geometric distortion (Table 7.3).

Artifacts

Image artifacts are essentially unwanted signals that are visualized in the image. These may mimic or mask disease states and generally degrade image quality. Knowledge of typical artifacts and their causes is crucial to avoid misdiagnosis.

Patient Driven

The FEG is used to localize a signal to a particular part of the body. As a result, anything that alters the expected proton Larmor frequency will confuse the machine and cause it to misplace the signal spatially. Chemical shift (first kind) occurs because protons in fat rotate at a different frequency than water. As a result, the fat signal can be shifted several pixels along the FEG direction. This can be mitigated by applying fat suppression, increasing rBW, and decreasing the matrix size [20].

Susceptibility artifact appears as a sudden and unnatural signal decrease or void. This occurs because spins are dephased so rapidly that no Mxy is left when the signal is supposed to be read out. Causes of the dephasing are typically implants. Susceptibility artifact will also occur at complex interfaces such as between the toes where air, bone, and tissue of complex shape are all positioned closely to each other. Fast SE (and SE) sequences display much less severe susceptibility than GRE or EPI sequences (Fig. 7.7). Utilizing a short TE, high rBW, and thin slices also help. Susceptibility artifacts are also less severe on low-B0 MRI scanners [20, 21].

The MR scanner assumes that the patient is stationary during the entire scan. If the patient moves, then "ghosts" of the moving patient will extend across the image in the FEG direction. Motion is typically mitigated by speeding up image acquisition. Signal suppression bands can be applied to null signal from the moving body part (e.g., chest wall during breathing) if it does not obscure tissue of interest. For cardiac and respiratory motion, gating may also be employed [22]. The artifact can also be redirected away from tissue of interest by switching the PEG and FEG directions [1, 20]. Finally, special acquisition sequences called propeller or blade sequences acquire signals using a complex scanning pattern that can be processed to partially correct for a moving patient [23–25].

Cross-excitation artifact occurs when two scans of the same piece of anatomy at different angles happen in quick succession. If the time between the two scans is small, then Mz will not have fully recovered from the first scan and a band of signal void will occur in the second image. This often occurs in the lumbar spine because the scan is oriented to be perpendicular to the spine, but the spine bends, so the same tissue posterior to the spine may be imaged twice in quick succession and at different angles. Once identified as a problem, the protocol can be altered to allow for sufficient recovery from the first scan before the second is acquired [26].

The magnetic field from a proton has a specific pattern called a dipole pattern. If protons are near a stranded tissue with a strong orientation (tendon or nerves), then the water molecules may weakly bond to the tissue. If the stranded tissue is oriented at a specific angle (~ 55°) to B0, then the bound water molecules will be oriented, so each water molecule feels the minimum possible magnetic field from the neighboring water molecules. As a result, spin-spin interactions decrease and T2 times artificially increase. This results in an artificially bright signal that may mimic disease. This can be mitigated by reorienting the patient so they are at a different angle with B0 or by using long TE so the increased T2 does not have an appreciable effect [27].

Machine Driven

Truncation (Gibbs Ringing) occurs when the body has high-intensity sharp image edges (transitions from dark to bright or vice versa in adjacent pixels) that the image cannot reproduce. It is a consequence insufficient sampling (Fig. 7.7). The result is a repetition of the edge with rapidly decreasing intensity. This is especially important in the spine where it may mimic lesions. Truncation artifact can be mitigated by increasing the matrix size and image processing [20, 21].

K-space errors (also called herringbone, corduroy, and spike) cause a regular pattern of light and dark signal overlaid on the image. This error is typically the consequence of an electrical error placing a single high amplitude signal (spike) in the raw k-space data. The Fourier transform turns this spike into the pattern described above. Although this may occur if there are loose con-

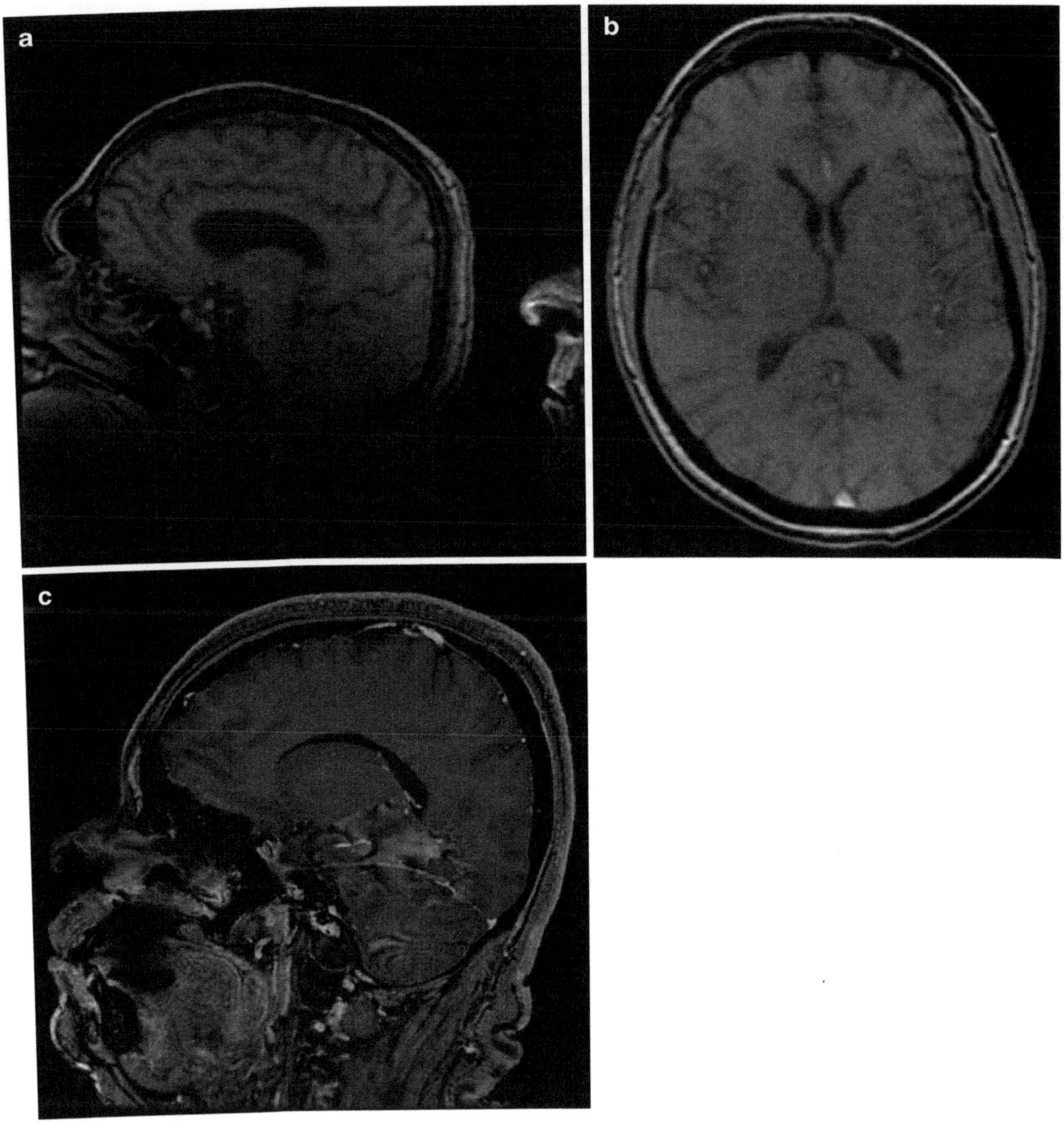

Fig. 7.7 Artifacts. (**a**) Wrap-around artifact. Note that this means the phase encode direction is along the anteroposterior (left-right in the image). (**b**) Moire artifact. Note the curved zebra-like appearance in the cerebellum as well as other areas of the image. (**c**) Truncation. Note the repeated edge of the brain whose intensity gradually diminishes with distance from the edge

nection (e.g., the receiver coil), typically the only way to fix the problem is to identify and replace the source of the spikes, which is often a broken piece of electronics [20, 21].

Zipper artifact occurs because an external signal with a frequency near the Larmor frequency of the body is detected. This external RF signal is mistakenly assumed to be from the body and is incorporated into the image. It typically appears as one or more bright dotted/noisy lines. If the contaminating source is external to the room, then the artifact can be fixed by checking the electromagnetic shielding that surrounds the MR scan room. In this case, the door is often the cause (either shielding degradation or accidentally not closed during scanning). If the source is

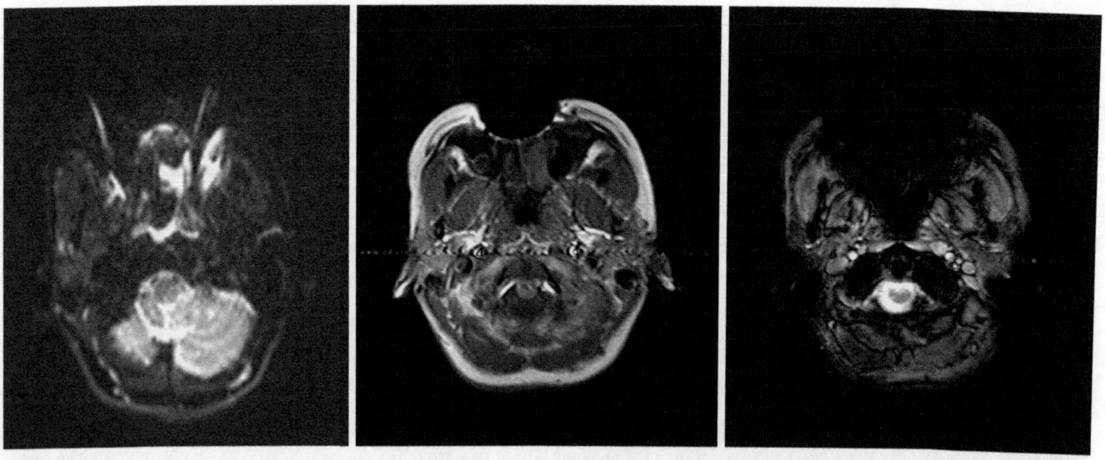

Fig. 7.8 Susceptibility artifact due to permanent metal retainer. Left: echo planar image demonstrates severe susceptibility and geometric distortion due to the metal artifact. Middle: the artifact is minimized using spin echo sequences. Note there is also pulsation artifact running horizontal through the middle of the image. Right: gradient echo sequences demonstrate a large artifact due to the lack of 180° refocusing RF pulse

inside the room, then it must be identified and removed. Flickering fluorescent lights and damaged electrical equipment are common culprits [20, 21].

Geometric distortion typically occurs when gradients applied are not linear due to some machine error or degradation. This results in anatomy in the image being shrunk, expanded, or otherwise distorted due to improper localization. Strong local distortions to the magnetic field, such as from an implant, can also cause local distortion. If gradients are the issue, then the machine will need to be serviced. It should be noted that EPI sequences are particularly susceptible to geometric distortion due to the rapid changing of gradients that is required to make the image quickly [20, 21].

If the field of view is smaller than the patient's anatomy, then wraparound artifact may occur (Fig. 7.7). This is visualized as part of the anatomy that should have been outside the image wrapping around and appearing on the opposite side of the image. Suppressing the signal of the exterior tissue, increasing the field of view, or activating the "no-phase wrap" feature will mitigate this artifact. Note that this artifact typically wraps around in the PEG direction [28, 29].

Distorted bands of signal and void near the edges of the image (and occasionally toward the center as well) are called Moire artifacts. These typically arise due to a combination of wraparound and B0 inhomogeneities (Fig. 7.7). Re-shimming the magnet (trying to make the field more uniform) and attempting to better center the patient into the more uniform field in the center of the magnet may help [21].

Flow and Contrast Related

The periodic motion induced by pumping blood or CSF can give rise to a special type of motion artifact called pulsation artifact (Figs. 7.8 and 7.9). This still appears as a series of "ghosts" across the image, but these are typically more clearly demarcated. The circular structure of vessels in cross section mean ghosts can also be mistaken for lesions. Pulsation artifacts are of most concern in bright blood and contrast-enhanced sequences. Solutions are similar to those mentioned for regular motion artifact [20, 21].

Diffusion-weighted images are T2 weighted with diffusion additionally modifying the image contrast (Fig. 7.5). This means that bright structure on DW imaging could be due to restricted diffusion or could be because of bright signal on T2W (long T2 tissue). If the cause of the brightness is the latter, it is called T2 shine through arti-

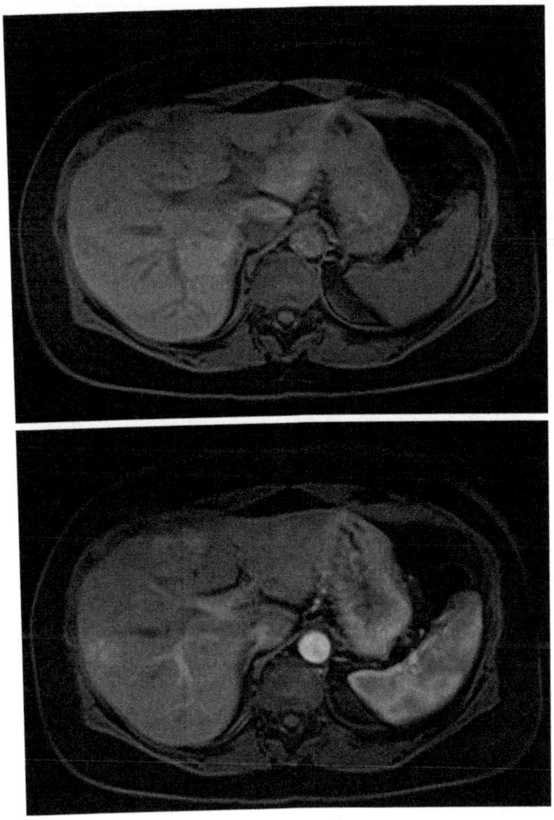

Fig. 7.9 Contrast enhancement. Top: unenhanced T1-weighted liver image. Bottom: post-contrast image clearly demonstrates hyperintense liver lesions where contrast agent was retained in the liver

fact [7, 8, 30]. Fat suppression can help, otherwise it is useful to refer to the T2W sequence and ADC map to determine if the cause of the brightness is T2W or DW. A similar shine through artifact occurs in contrast-enhanced angiography. Typically, background tissues are saturated, so they give little signal. However, if the suppression is weak, then short T1 tissues will demonstrate a bright signal due to the tissue T1, and not due to contrast uptake.

Timing in contrast-enhanced MR angiography is crucial to attain a proper image. If imaging is performed too early, then contrast-enhanced blood will not yet have reached the slice, and the lumen will appear dark. If contrast arrives after imaging of the slice has begun, then only the edges will appear bright. This artifact is typically known as Maki or ringing artifact. On the other side, if imaging begins too late, then contrast will have begun to fill the veins, and they will also be visualized on the MR image. This artifact is typically called venous contamination [31, 32].

Subtraction of a pre-contrast image from a post-contrast image is typically performed in breast MRI to evaluate the distribution of contrast media uptake and suppress signal from other tissues. If the patient moves between the pre- and post-contrast scans, then the subtraction will be incorrect, and not all non-contrast signal will be suppressed. Image processing (registration) can help reduce this artifact as can faster scanning to reduce the chance of patient motion ([33]; Table 7.4).

Table 7.4 Directionality of artifacts

Artifact	Motion/ pulsation ghosting	Chemical shift (first kind)	Wraparound	RF contamination
FEG		X		
PEG	X		X	X

Abbreviations: *FEG* frequency encoding gradient, *PEG* phase encoding direction, *RF* radiofrequency

Safety

Traditionally, concern for safety in MR imaging has lagged as issues of radiation dose have typically been at the forefront of safety concerns in medical imaging. As pulse sequences have become more complex, field strengths have increased, and utilization has expanded, MR safety incidents have also increased. In modern imaging, MR safety concerns are an important topic of discussion with many programs establishing a formal MR safety hierarchy similar to the radiation safety committee.

The MR area is explicitly broken into four zones [34, 35]. As the zone number increases, the risk increases. Zone I encompasses any area that can be freely accessed by the general public. This is outside the MR environment and may include hallways, offices, bathrooms, and other areas far enough from the magnet to be essentially minimal risk.

Table 7.5 MR safety zones

	Room examples	Risk from MR scanner	Comments
Zone I	Hallway, non-MR offices	None	Uncontrolled
Zone II	Reception and interview room	Small	Screening for ferromagnetic objects
Zone III	Scanner control room, hallway containing scanner room door	High	Contains 5 G line, requires MR training or level II personnel escort; all objects should be labeled based on MR safety
Zone IV	Scanner room	Highest	High static fields, MR safe or MR conditional objects only

Zone II is the transition between zone I, which is freely accessed by anyone (uncontrolled) and zones III and IV that are strictly controlled and monitored. Zone II typically includes reception, where patient interviews occur within the MR department, changing rooms, and the rooms where patients are screened for potentially hazardous materials (ferrous metals). Patients are not free to move through zone II unless supervised.

Zone III is the area where serious injury or death could occur for various reasons due to the fields of the MR scanner. There must be a physical barrier between zones II and III to block untrained personnel and non-personnel from entering unsupervised (locked door). Anyone who has not undergone sufficient MR safety, training must be directly supervised by sufficiently trained MR personnel (usually a technologist). Barring untrained personnel from unsupervised entry to zone III is a matter of safety and thus applies regardless of the person's standing (hospital administrator, physician, security, etc.). Zone III is generally made large enough to contain any static magnetic field 5 G or more in strength. It should be noted that such fields may extend to floors above and below the MR scanner as well.

Zone IV is the MR scanner room itself. The door to zone IV should be specifically marked as potentially hazardous due to the presence of very strong magnetic fields. Signage should have a red light and state that the magnetic field is always on. Further, a MR safety trained personnel working in zone III should have an unobstructed view of any access path into zone IV from their work area (typically this means technologists at the MR scanning console). If obstructions cannot be removed, then video monitors should be installed to allow for proper supervision of ingress sites by the properly trained staff. If an emergent situation occurs in zone IV, then only staff with proper MR safety training should enter the scanner room. They may initiate necessary life support (e.g., CPR) while moving the patient to a magnetically safe location outside of zone IV. Zone access restrictions must be maintained even in emergent situations to prevent potential injury to both patient and responders from untrained staff entering the area with MR unsafe equipment. Doors with access to zones II–IV should be clearly labeled with a sign to alert personnel and patients of the heightened safety risks (Table 7.5).

All people who will be in or near an MR scanner must have sufficient training to not be a danger to themselves and others or must be supervised by someone with such training [34, 35]. This includes patients, patient families, cleaning staff, security, physicians, technologists, scientists, etc. regardless of rank or position. The level of training for personnel generally has three levels. Non-MRI personnel are the lowest level and generally have no MR safety training. As such, they are required to be supervised at all times by level II personnel. The next level up is level I personnel. They have undergone training sufficient to ensure their own safety but lack specific training necessary to oversee the safety of others. They may enter zones III and IV, but not supervise others. Typically, security, cleaning staff, and transport personnel will be trained to level I. Level II personnel have training specific to ensuring the safety to others. Typically, MR technologists, MR scientists, qualified medical physicists, and radiologists will be level II.

A formal structure for MR safety, similar to radiation safety committee, has been suggested by the ACR [34, 35]. At the top of this structure is the MR medical director (MRMD). This is typically a radiologist who is responsible for all decision related to the safety of patients and personnel as related to the institution's MR scanners. Generally, the MRMD sets MR safety policy and procedures. They also have final say on scanning off-label for a given patient. Working under the MRMD is one or more MR safety officers (MRSOs). These are typically technologists that are delegated oversite and responsibility by the MR medical director and ensure that MR safety policies and procedures are applied in daily practice. They will make day-to-day safety decisions and consult with MRMD and other experts as needed. Finally, the MR safety expert (MRSE) is an advisor. The MRSE is typically an MR scientist or qualified medical physicist who acts as a resource for the MRMD and MRSO due to their depth of technical knowledge related to MRI and MR safety. The American Board of Magnetic Resonance Safety is a credentialing board that distributes Magnetic Resonance Safety Certified™ (MRSC™) credentials related to the MRMD, MRSO, and MRSE positions. While these credentials are not a requirement to work in these positions, they do convey that the person with these credentials has passed an examination related to relevant MR safety knowledge needed for that position.

The magnetic fields, gradients, and RF pulses all may interact with objects brought into the scanning room causing effects varying from image artifacts to thermal burns, to death. A standardized system is currently used to determine the safety of any object or implant that may potentially be brought into zone III or higher. All objects should be labeled with a sticker as MR safe (meaning they pose no danger due to the MR scanner), MR unsafe (meaning their presence due to the scanner is a serious danger and is contraindicated), or MR conditional (meaning that they are safe under tightly defined scanning parameters) [36]. Implants must be identified through patient interviews, screening, and the patient's medical record prior to scanning. A patient should generally not be scanned unless all implants are either MR safe or MR conditional. Generally, implant manufacturer Websites and manuals are the best resources to identify the safety of a given patient implant.

The Food and Drug Administration (FDA) and the International Electrotechnical Commission (IEC) require operating levels built into MR scanners based on the potential heating of the patient and time-varying magnetic field strength [37, 38]. There are three levels: normal mode, first-level controlled mode (sometimes called controlled mode), and second-level controlled mode (sometimes called experimental or research mode). Normal mode is set such that it is unlikely to cause stress to the body and thus is suitable for an average patient. First-level control mode is set such that the fields and/or heating may cause stress to the patient based on previous models and research. This mode requires medical supervision and a positive action (usually an acknowledgment on the machine by the operator) before scan initiation. Second-level control mode is set such that it may cause significant risk for patients. Explicit ethical approval (typically from an Institutional Review Board) is required before scanning.

Static Field (B0) and Static Gradient Field (AKA, Fringe Field)

The static magnetic field (B0) that is generated by the superconducting magnet is several orders of magnitude greater than the Earth's magnetic field. Due to its strength, B0 has the potential to cause biological effects. In addition, the field may interact with other electronic and mechanical devices causing serious injury or death to the patient. The magnetic field is always on for MR scanners although it is strongest at a volume in the center of the bore and is progressively weaker as one moves away from the scanner. The magnetic field that exists outside the scanner is called the fringe field or spatial gradient field.

In general, the biological effects that may be caused by B0 are temporary and dissipate once the person is removed from the field.

Magnetophosphenes are flashes of light sometime referred to as "starry eyes." They typically occur as the patient is pushed or walks through the static gradient field or moves their head while a gradient is applied inside the scanner. The changing B0 experienced in the eyes is translated into an electric field, which stimulates the retina causing the phenomena [39–41].

The magnetohydrodynamic effect is a name that has been used to describe two related phenomena. When a conductive fluid flows through a magnetic field a force and opposing current is created. The force acting on blood flow has been shown to increase blood pressure. This increase is negligible under 3 T and increases to only 4% in an 8 T magnet. Changes of greater than 10% are necessary to be deemed clinically significant, and such changes are unlikely to occur from fields less than 15 T [42].

The second phenomena attributed to the magnetohydrodynamic effect relates to cardiac monitoring. The deflection of blood and opposing current flowing from the effect cause a false amplitude increase in the T-wave of an electrocardiogram (ECG). This can result in incorrect cardiac gating and poor image quality. Using extra information such as pulse oximetry or vector ECG can eliminate the issue [43, 44].

Other temporary biological effects such as vertigo, dizziness, nausea, and a metallic taste in mouth are thought to be linked with the induction of currents in the respective anatomy of the body. Although potentially alarming or unpleasant to the patient, they pose no serious danger and dissipate once the patient is removed from the magnetic field. At 3 T or less, these biological effects along with magnetophosphenes typically require movement to generate sufficient induced current in the body. As a result, it is recommended that patients are moved into and out of the scanner slowly and counseled to remain as still as possible (even for parts of the body that are not actively being imaged).

Several studies have investigated and failed to demonstrate increased risk to an embryo or fetus from MR scanning without contrast in utero or from exposure of pregnant occupational workers. Rates of stillbirth, congenital anomalies, neoplasm, hearing loss, vision loss, spontaneous abortion, preterm delivery, and low birth weight were not significantly increased. However, it should be noted most studies relied on data that is acquired primarily at 1.5 T, and thus the exact effects at higher fields are not as clear [45–50].

While direct biological effects are typically mild and transient, the potential danger from mechanical effects of the static field is much more severe. The missile (projectile) effect refers to the magnetic field pulling a magnetic object into the scanner with such force that it causes injury or death. The missile effect has been responsible for several deaths in the past and is a serious concern. In general, the translational force an object feels is proportional to both the static field and the gradient felt across the object. Thus, the most dangerous place is not typically the center of the magnet where the gradient is zero, but the entrance to the magnet where the static field is strong and the gradient is also strong [51]. The force is also proportional to the amount of magnetic material and the type of material. Thus, large ferromagnetic objects such as typical oxygen canisters are very dangerous and can easily deliver a deadly blow if pulled by the magnet. Plastic and other nonmagnetic materials are generally MRI safe and feel no force. Typically, ferromagnetic materials should not be in the scanning room. Some weakly magnetic materials such as nitinol and titanium may be scanned under specific conditions (MR conditional). A note should be made about stainless steel. Unfortunately, stainless steel encompasses several different formulations some of which are ferromagnetic and others that are not. It is important that any stainless-steel object is tested for magnetic properties (typically with a strong hand magnet) before being brought into the scanning room.

In addition to the missile effect, other effects may attempt to push ferromagnetic or conducting objects. The static field may cause torque (twisting force) on magnetic objects to attempt to align it with the static field [52, 53]. The strength of the torque is determined by B0, material shape, and the material type. Torque is typically strongest in the center of the bore where field strength is highest. A second important consideration related to artificial heart valves relates to forces created by Lenz's Law. This law states that any conductor moving through a magnetic field will feel a force. This force increases with the velocity, and thus metal heart valves moving while placed in the static field of an MR scanner can be affected. This effect is negligible at 1.5 T; however, since this force increases with B0, it may become significant at 7 T [54].

The static field and static gradient field may cause stray electric currents in electronics near or moving through the field. It is important that all medical devices are cleared for their use in or near the MR scanner room. In general, the 5-Gauss line [36, 55] is contained inside zone III to prevent such a strong field from interacting with implanted devices such as a pacemaker and causing device failure. Very recently, this threshold has been increased to 9 Gauss. This is to reflect that more modern pacemakers are typically designed to be more resistant to magnetic field interactions. Importantly, other machines may have thresholds for malfunction much lower than 9 or 5 Gauss, and thus it is important to always reference manufacturer guidelines. Scanning of patients is always a risk-benefit analysis. Despite some articles claiming pacemakers (or other implants) are generally safe to scan, it is important to follow recommendations for each specific make and model of device.

Time-Varying Gradient Field

The fringe field discussed in the Static Field section is a gradient, that is, a change in the magnetic field with position. However, in MRI, the terms "gradient" and "gradient field" typically refer to time-varying gradients produced by the gradient coils of the MR scanner. As discussed above, these gradients are mainly used for localization purposes (SSG, FEG, and PEG) and to create gradient echoes. These gradient fields are not static, but instead change with time (gradient switching). The change in gradient strength with time is termed the slew rate. High slew rates are necessary for fast imaging (e.g., in EPI) but have implications in MR safety that will be discussed in this section.

A changing magnetic field can induce an electric field in an antenna and other conductive objects with suitable geometry. Resistance in the object can convert this electrical energy to heat causing burns. However, at current clinical strengths and speeds, thermal effects from gradient fields are typically not a concern. Currents induced in the body by gradient fields can, however, stimulate the body tissues and create stray electricity in implants. The most severe danger would be direct stimulation of the heart which has been caused in animal models [56, 57]. In current clinical practice, the induced currents do not reach the level of danger for inducing cardiac issues if scanners follow International Electrotechnical Commission (IEC) recommendations [37]. Further, typical clinical scans are designed to limit the stimulation of peripheral nerves, which occur at a much lower threshold than cardiac tissue [58].

Fast imaging (e.g., EPI) that uses strong gradients that switch quickly (high slew rate) can excite muscles and nerves by inducing electric fields in tissue. This stimulation is called peripheral nerve stimulation (PNS) [59]. PNS occurs at the patient periphery because this is where the rate of change in magnetic field is a maximum during scanning for the patient. PNS increases with large changes in magnetic field (dB) and fast changes in magnetic field (dt); thus the larger dB/dt, the larger the induced current, the more likely PNS is induced, and the more severe the stimulation effects will be. Similarly, the larger the slew rate, the more likely and intense is the PNS [40, 47]. Although older documents recommend a 20 T/s maximum, there is currently not an FDA-mandated quantitative slew rate or dB/dT limit in the United States, although guidance suggests that painful stimulation is to be avoided [38, 60]. The limit for PNS to be avoided may be determined by scanning volunteers or using previously derived models for whole-body gradients or electric field [61]. Most machines have operating modes set by the IEC that warn the user of potential PNS based on volunteer studies and mathematical modeling. Normal mode is limited such that it does not exceed 80% of the dB/dt limit for PNS. Level 1 controlled mode does not exceed 100% of that limit, and level II controlled mode does not have a limit.

The loud noises typically associated with MR scanning are due to forces on the MR scanner housing and components due to the time-varying gradients. Since the frequency of the gradient switching falls into the audible range, the scanner creates noise (just like an audio speaker playing music). Audible scanner noise increases with dB/dt and proximity of the patient's head to the scanner. If noise exceeds certain limits, then hearing loss may occur [62]. There is no significant risk of permanent hearing loss if peak unweighted sound pressure level is <140 dB and A-weighted root mean square sound pressure level < 99 dBA (with hearing protection). According to the FDA and IEC, hearing protection should be provided to patients where sound pressure exceeds these amounts [37, 60]. Newer machines may also offer "silent/soft gradients," which incorporate technology to reduce sound from gradient switching [63, 64]. It should be noted that studies of pediatric hearing failed to demonstrate any increase in hearing loss due to MR scanning in utero [50, 65].

Radiofrequency Pulse (RF or B1)

Diffuse thermal heating and focal burns are generally due to RF energy deposited into the patient by the MR scanner [66, 67]. Focal burns are the most-reported MR injury aside from contrast-related reactions according to the US Food and Drug Administration's Manufacturer and User Facility Device Experience. In general, RF energy is transmitted to the patient by either the body coil located in the scanner or the dedicated transmit/receive coils. Unlike the fringe field associated with the static field, RF generally does not extend beyond the scanner bore or transmitting coil volume and thus is not a substantial occupational risk.

Thermal heating of the patient is typically quantified by the specific absorption rate (SAR) [68–71]. SAR is calculated using proprietary methods that are typically vendor specific and may result in a spread of reported SAR values for the same patient undergoing the same or similar pulse sequences. Further, due to various methods used to calculate SAR, the machine reported value is not reliable for determining heating in implants [72]. The higher the SAR from a scan, the more heating the patient experiences. SAR increases with the square of the B0 and the square of the flip angle and depends on the specific shape of the RF pulse [1, 58]. Thus, the 180° pulse in a SE sequence delivers 4× the SAR of the 90° pulse to flip Mz into Mxy. In fast SE sequences, increasing ETL in fast SE imaging generally increases the number of 180° pulses per TR and thus substantially increases SAR. SE sequences will have larger SAR values than GRE sequences due to the 90° and 180° RF pulses that are not present in GRE imaging.

Recently, scanners have begun reporting B1 + rms as a more reliable metric of heating in the presence of implants. This metric is essentially a measure of the magnetic field component of the RF pulse sent to the patient. Since this can be indirectly measured by measuring the voltage needed to produce a given flip angle for the patient, it avoids vendor-specific assumptions about the absorption of RF energy in the body that hinders SAR. This is important as such factors are not necessarily applicable for local heating in the presence of an implant [73].

The ability of a patient to tolerate heating from the RF transmission is dependent on the air flow and temperature in the scanning room, patient clothing, body habitus, function of their thermoregulatory system, and other factors [74]. In general, larger patient will experience more heating due to the RF energy deposition because of smaller volume to surface areas, decreased airflow, and increased natural insulation. Special care should be taken with sedated individuals as they will be unable to voice heating concerns, and some drugs used for sedation can impact the thermoregulatory system. In most scanners, the patient weight is a component in determining the SAR value; thus it is important that patient weight is accurately recorded on the machine before scanning.

Focal burns are typically the result of some exterior object or implant focusing the RF energy and thus causing a substantial increase in local temperature [66, 75]. Proximity to the transmitting coil can cause near-field effects that result in burns to the patient. These are especially common in large patients that touch the bore walls. All coil wires should be checked for cracks, and at least 1 cm of insulation should be placed between the patient and coils. Conductive loops or U-shapes in the bore can resonate and convert RF energy into electricity and heat [66]. Care should be taken that wires are not directly in contact with the patient or do not form loop or U-shapes. The patient's body can also act as a current loop, and thus it is important that padding is placed between the patient's hands and thighs (assuming arms are down) and that hands, thighs, calves, and feet to not touch during scanning [76, 77].

Implants in the body may act as antennae, receiving the RF energy and establishing a standing wave that focuses the energy and quickly increases temperature at the tips of the antenna. An antenna resonates efficiently at half and quarter wavelengths of the incoming energy [78–80]. For a 1.5 T magnet, the transmit frequency is roughly 64 MHz and thus will have a quarter wavelength of 1 meter in air; however, when implanted into human tissue, the wavelength (and thus resonant wavelength) shortens to about 30 cm. At 3 T with a transmit frequency at roughly 128 MHz, the wavelength decreases to roughly 15 cm. Many implants, especially wires, may satisfy these resonant length requirements. Insulation of the wires may prevent resonant energy from focally dissipating into the body; thus, it is important that wires are intact when determining MR safety of implants. Further, it should be recognized that heating will generally occur at the tips of an antenna-like implant [78, 80]. At 7 T, the resonant length decreases to 7 cm and thus stents, and other currently "safe implants" may become heating risks. Finally, it should be noted that metallic drug delivery patches [81], tattoos [82], piercings [83], metallic makeup [84], and other metallic objects [85] may concentrate RF energy through one or more of the above mechanisms and cause serious injury in the form of skin burns.

The FDA and IEC have set several limits related to heating [37, 60]. These limits are listed both in terms of absolute temperature increases and SAR in Table 7.6.

Table 7.6 FDA and IEC heating limits

Anatomy	Dose	Exposure time (min)	SAR (W/kg)	Temperature (°C)
Normal mode				
Body	Whole body	6	2	< 0.5 increase
Head	Whole head	6	3.2	38
Trunk	Any 10 g	6	10	39
Extremities	Any 10 g	6	20	40
First-level control mode (controlled)				
Body	Whole body	15	4	< 1.0 increase
Head	Whole head	–	–	–
Trunk	Any 10 g	6	20	–
Extremities	Any 10 g	6	40	–
Second-level controlled mode (research/experimental mode)				
Body	Whole body	15 (FDA) 6 (IEC)	> 4	> 1.0 increase
Head	Whole head	10 (FDA) 6 (IEC)	> 3.2	> 38
Trunk	Any 10 g	6	> 20	> 39
Extremities	Any 10 g	6	> 40	> 40

Abbreviations: *SAR* specific uptake rate

Cryogen and Quenching

Modern MR systems utilize liquid helium, cooled to 4° Kelvin, to ensure that the scanner coils generating B0 stay superconducting. The system keeping the helium cool is called the cryogen. Under extraordinary circumstances, typically where elimination of B0 will save a human life, the magnet may be "quenched." This involves allowing the liquid helium to rise in temperature and thus boil off into a gas. This causes the coil to lose superconductivity and thus quickly eliminates B0 as electrical current in the coil dissipates.

Quenching is associated with long outages as service must be called in to ensure integrity of the system and re-initialize the currents in the superconductive coils. During the quench, gas should be vented to the outside through a specially designed venting system. The outflow should be positioned such that the supercooled gas cannot injure members of the public due to temperature or by displacing oxygen in the area. Quenching presents a hazard for those in zone IV if gas fails to properly vent and begins to fill the room. Each liter of liquid helium expands to more than 700 liters of helium gas [86]. This results in a pressure buildup that can rupture eardrums and may make it impossible to open doors that open into the magnet room. As the gas fills the room, the temperature puts those in zone IV at risk for frostbite and also for asphyxiation as the gas displaces oxygen in the room.

In general, it is reasonable to initiate a quench when the B0 field must be turned off immediately. This may occur due to a person being pinned to the magnet by an object or if a fire breaks out that cannot be easily contained and is likely to cause liquid helium to boil in the magnet. The boiling of liquid helium in the magnet without a quench is a significant explosive hazard as the pressure buildup can be so great as to breach the walls of the magnet with explosive force. In the event of a fire, fire personnel may insist on access to zone IV. If they need to bring in fire safety gear such as fire axes and other magnetic equipment, then the magnet must be quenched before they enter to avoid potentially deadly missile effects [34, 35].

Safety Oversight

Several organizations have taken on regulatory and advisory roles related to MR safety. The ACR was an early advocate of MR safety. It convened a blue ribbon paned to address MR safety issues and periodically issues a whitepaper that has come to be the standard for MR safety in the field [34, 35]. In addition to the MR safety whitepapers, the ACR publishes multiple practice parameters specific to modality and scan type. These parameters include guidance on protocols as well as safety considerations. The ACR periodically publishes The Contrast Manual [87], which is a summary of current literature related to MR and non-MR contrast agents, their safety, and recommended guidelines for use. The ACR also acts as an accreditation body and, as such, sets specific minimum requirements for image quality and safety in MRI. A component of accreditation are policies related to MR safety [34, 35].

The FDA is a regulatory body that has jurisdiction over the MR scanning machines and their marketing as medical devices. The FDA has previously issued guideline papers that set exposure limits for various quantities related to MR safety such as SAR, dB/dt, and acoustic noise as well as specifying minimum safety elements required in MR scanners sold in the United States [38, 60].

The IEC is a quasi-governmental agency that develops standards followed internationally. It performs a similar service internationally as the FDA in the United States and, as such, most MR scanners will adhere to both FDA and IEC standards. IEC standards for MRI are typically more prescriptive and quantitative [37].

The Joint Commission is a hospital accrediting body. It has routinely set minimum requirements related to quality and safety issues. It also routinely issues sentinel event alerts meant to bring attention and focus to areas of particular safety concern in medicine [88].

The Institute for Magnetic Resonance Safety, Education, and Research (IMRSER) [89] is an independent, multidisciplinary, professional organization that focuses on education and awareness. They have issued several guidelines related to safety issues such as patient screening, heating/

burn prevention, and MR scanning of those with implanted devices or other hardware. The popular site MRISafety.com is run by IMRSER and is often considered a source of information when determining MR safety of devices.

American Board of Magnetic Resonance Safety (ABMRS)

The American Board of Magnetic Resonance Safety (ABMRS) [90] is a not-for-profit corporation whose purpose is to improve the safety of medical and research magnetic resonance (MR) environments by certifying that MR personnel. Certification aims at ensuring MR personnel possess a baseline knowledge of underlying MR safety principles as well as practical knowledge that allows them to apply that knowledge in the clinical decision-making process as it relates to MR safety. The ABMRS develops and runs credentialing tests for MRMD, MRSO, and MRSE.

International Commission on Non-Ionizing Radiation Protection (ICNIRP)

The International Commission on Non-Ionizing Radiation Protection (ICNIRP) is a not-for-profit nongovernmental agency that provides scientific advice and guidance on the health and environmental effects of nonionizing radiation. They have published several papers related to the measurement, effects, and suggested limits of exposure for MR-related radiation [40–42, 46].

ASTM International (Formerly the American Society for Testing and Materials)

ASTM International is a voluntary standards developing organization [91]. MR relevant standards include MR safety labeling [36], force measurement [92], torque measurement [93], heating measurement [94], and evaluation of image artifacts [95].

Chapter Summary

1. MR technology is primarily based around using magnetic fields to induce a signal from the body.
2. Image contrast is determined by the specific parameters chosen and pulse sequence selected.
3. In addition to standard contrast weightings, specialized weightings may also be induced (e.g., flow, diffusion, contrast agent, etc.).
4. Scanning requires careful selection of several parameters each of which likely impacts several aspects of image quality and safety.
5. MR safety issues include forces on and induced electrical currents in implants and objects, heating/burns, acoustic noise, and contrast agents.
6. A formal MR safety hierarchy and site zone layout are recommended to ensure safety of patients and staff.

Glossary

Acquisition Time The time necessary to acquire an image or scan

Apparent Diffusion Coefficient An approximate measure of local water diffusion

Diffusion-Weighted Imaging Images with additional contrast dependent on the ability of water to spread

Echo Planar Imaging Rapid imaging sequences that acquire an entire image in a single flip of spins into the xy-plane

Echo Train Length The number of echoes produced per TR interval in fast spin echo imaging

Frequency Encode Gradient Magnetic field modulation that alters the Larmor frequency of protons to encode location

Gadolinium A chemical that has the ability to shorten T1 times of surrounding water and thus alter the contrast of the image

Gradient (Recalled) Echo Type of MR imaging that utilizes modulated magnetic fields to force protons to align and produce a signal

Image Contrast How different tissues are assigned different shades of gray in an MR image

Larmor Frequency Natural frequency that protons rotate at when placed in a static magnetic field

Magnetic Resonance Imaging Imaging utilizing magnetic fields to induce a signal from protons in the body

Proton Density Weighted An image where tissue contrast is mainly dependent on the density of mobile protons

Phase Encode Gradient Magnetic field modulation that changes the phase of proton magnetic fields in order to encode location

Quench Allowing the superconducting coils to heat up to stop the external static magnetic field

Radiofrequency Pulse In MRI, a pulse at a specific frequency used to rotate proton magnetic moments into a desired orientation

Receiver Bandwidth Range of frequencies collected by the receive coil during MR scanning

Resolution The ability to represent small detail and closely spaced objects as distinct

Specific Absorption Rate A metric that attempts to approximate the rate of absorbed heat energy from MR imaging

Spin Echo Type of MR imaging that utilizes a 180° RF pulse to force protons to align and produce a signal

Signal-to-Noise Ratio The magnitude of the desired object's intensity (signal) to the magnitude of the random pattern of gray levels that are inherent to all imaging (noise)

Slice-Select Gradient In 2D imaging, magnetic field modulation that alters the Larmor frequency of protons during the RF pulses to encode location

Static Field External magnetic field used to align the magnetic fields of protons in the body

T1 Weighted An image where tissue contrast is mainly dependent on the spin-lattice relaxation time characteristic of each tissue

T2 Weighted An image where tissue contrast is mainly dependent on the spin-spin relaxation time characteristic of each tissue

T2* Weighted An image where tissue contrast is mainly dependent on the spin-spin relaxation time characteristic of each tissue and inhomogeneities in the magnetic field

References

1. Sensakovic WF, Huda W. Review of radiologic physics. 5th ed. Philadelphia: Wolters Kluwer; 2024.
2. Hahn H. Spin echos. Phys Rev. 1950;80(4):580.
3. Bernstein MA, King KF, Zhou ZJ. Handbook of MRI pulse sequences. Burlington: Elsevier Academic Press; 2004.
4. Tsuruda J, Saloner D, Norman D. Artifacts associated with MR neuroangiography. AJNR Am J Neuroradiol. 1992;13(5):1411–22.
5. Weber J, Veith P, Jung B, Ihorst G, Moske-Eick O, Meckel S, et al. MR angiography at 3 tesla to assess proximal internal carotid artery stenoses: contrast-enhanced or 3D time-of-flight MR angiography? Clin Neuroradiol. 2015;25(1):41–8. https://doi.org/10.1007/s00062-013-0279-x.
6. Hagmann P, Jonasson L, Maeder P, Thiran JP, Wedeen VJ, Meuli R. Understanding diffusion MR imaging techniques: from scalar diffusion-weighted imaging to diffusion tensor imaging and beyond. Radiographics. 2006;26(Suppl 1):S205–23. https://doi.org/10.1148/rg.26si065510.
7. Mukherjee P, Berman JI, Chung SW, Hess CP, Henry RG. Diffusion tensor MR imaging and fiber tractography: theoretic underpinnings. AJNR Am J Neuroradiol. 2008a;29(4):632–41. https://doi.org/10.3174/ajnr.A1051.
8. Mukherjee P, Chung SW, Berman JI, Hess CP, Henry RG. Diffusion tensor MR imaging and fiber tractography: technical considerations. AJNR Am J Neuroradiol. 2008b;29(5):843–52. https://doi.org/10.3174/ajnr.A1052.
9. Hagberg GE, Scheffler K. Effect of r(1) and r(2) relaxivity of gadolinium-based contrast agents on the T(1)-weighted MR signal at increasing magnetic field strengths. Contrast Media Mol Imaging. 2013;8(6):456–65. https://doi.org/10.1002/cmmi.1565.
10. Ringe KI, Husarik DB, Sirlin CB, Merkle EM. Gadoxetate disodium-enhanced MRI of the liver: part 1, protocol optimization and lesion appearance in the noncirrhotic liver. AJR Am J Roentgenol. 2010;195(1):13–28. https://doi.org/10.2214/AJR.10.4392.
11. Sabach AS, Bruno M, Kim D, Mulholland T, Lee L, Kaura S, Lim RP. Gadofosveset trisodium: abdominal and peripheral vascular applications. AJR Am J Roentgenol. 2013;200(6):1378–86. https://doi.org/10.2214/AJR.12.8991.
12. Sensakovic WF. Regarding fat suppression in MRI, when are spectral techniques preferred over STIR, and vice versa? AJR Am J Roentgenol. 2015;205(3):W231–2. https://doi.org/10.2214/AJR.14.14174.
13. Ma J. Dixon techniques for water and fat imaging. J Magn Reson Imaging. 2008;28(3):543–58. https://doi.org/10.1002/jmri.21492.

14. Graessner J. Bandwidth in MRI. In Seimens (Ed.) MAGNETOM/Flash: Seimens; 2013. p. 3–8.
15. Hayes CE, Axel L. Noise performance of surface coils for magnetic resonance imaging at 1.5 T. Med Phys. 1985;12(5):604–7. https://doi.org/10.1118/1.595682.
16. Mohliger MA, Sodickson DK. An introduction to coil array design for parallel MRI. NMR Biomed. 2006;19(3):300–15. https://doi.org/10.1002/nbm.1046.
17. Dietrich O, Raya JG, Reeder SB, Reiser MF, Schoenberg SO. Measurement of signal-to-noise ratios in MR images: influence of multichannel coils, parallel imaging, and reconstruction filters. J Magn Reson Imaging. 2007;26(2):375–85. https://doi.org/10.1002/jmri.20969.
18. Pruessmann KP, Weiger M, Scheidegger MB, Boesiger P. SENSE: sensitivity encoding for fast MRI. Magn Reson Med. 1999;42(5):952–62.
19. Mansfield PF. Multi-planar image formation using NMR spin echoes. J Phys C. 1977;10:L55–8.
20. Morelli JN, Runge VM, Ai F, Attenberger U, Vu L, Schmeets SH, et al. An image-based approach to understanding the physics of MR artifacts. Radiographics. 2011;31(3):849–66. https://doi.org/10.1148/rg.313105115.
21. Zhuo J, Gullapalli RP. AAPM/RSNA physics tutorial for residents: MR artifacts, safety, and quality control. Radiographics. 2006;26(1):275–97. https://doi.org/10.1148/rg.261055134.
22. Ehman RL, Felmlee JP. Adaptive technique for high-definition MR imaging of moving structures. Radiology. 1989;173(1):255–63. https://doi.org/10.1148/radiology.173.1.2781017.
23. Feng C, Yang J, Zhao D, Liu J. CUDA accelerated method for motion correction in MR PROPELLER imaging. Magn Reson Imaging. 2013;31(8):1390–8. https://doi.org/10.1016/j.mri.2013.04.013.
24. Liu Z, Zhang Z, Ying K, Yuan C, Guo H. Improved motion correction in PROPELLER by using grouped blades as reference. J Magn Reson Imaging. 2014;39(3):700–7. https://doi.org/10.1002/jmri.24211.
25. Pipe JG. Motion correction with PROPELLER MRI: application to head motion and free-breathing cardiac imaging. Magn Reson Med. 1999;42(5):963–9.
26. Simmons A, Tofts PS, Barker GJ, Arridge SR. Sources of intensity nonuniformity in spin echo images at 1.5 T. Magn Reson Med. 1994;32(1):121–8.
27. Erickson SJ, Prost RW, Timins ME. The "magic angle" effect: background physics and clinical relevance. Radiology. 1993;188(1):23–5. https://doi.org/10.1148/radiology.188.1.7685531.
28. Axel L, Morton D. Correction of phase wrapping in magnetic resonance imaging. Med Phys. 1989;16(2):284–7. https://doi.org/10.1118/1.596378.
29. Heiland S. From a as in aliasing to Z as in zipper: artifacts in MRI. Clin Neuroradiol. 2008;1:25–36.
30. Lee SK, Kim DI, Kim J, Kim DJ, Kim HD, Kim DS, Mori S. Diffusion-tensor MR imaging and fiber tractography: a new method of describing aberrant fiber connections in developmental CNS anomalies. Radiographics. 2005;25(1):53–65. https://doi.org/10.1148/rg.251045085.
31. Lee VS, Martin DJ, Krinsky GA, Rofsky NM. Gadolinium-enhanced MR angiography: artifacts and pitfalls. AJR Am J Roentgenol. 2000;175(1):197–205. https://doi.org/10.2214/ajr.175.1.1750197.
32. Maki JH, Prince MR, Londy FJ, Chenevert TL. The effects of time varying intravascular signal intensity and k-space acquisition order on three-dimensional MR angiography image quality. J Magn Reson Imaging. 1996;6(4):642–51.
33. Harvey JA, Hendrick RE, Coll JM, Nicholson BT, Burkholder BT, Cohen MA. Breast MR imaging artifacts: how to recognize and fix them. Radiographics. 2007;27(Suppl 1):S131–45. https://doi.org/10.1148/rg.27si075514.
34. American College of Radiology. ACR manual on MR safety; 2024a. Retrieved from: https://www.acr.org/-/media/ACR/Files/Radiology-Safety/MR-Safety/Manual-on-MR-Safety.pdf. Accessed 10 Oct 2024.
35. American College of Radiology. MRI accreditation program requirements; 2024b. Retrieved from https://www.acraccreditation.org/modalities/mri. Accessed 10 Oct 2024.
36. ASTM International. F2503 – standard practice for marking medical devices and other items for safety in the magnetic resonance environment. West Conshohocken: ASTM International; 2005.
37. International Electrotechnical Commission. Medical electrical equipment – part 2–33: particular requirements for the basic safety and essential performance of magnetic resonance equipment for medical diagnosis. Geneva: International Electrotechnical Commission; 2015.
38. U.S. Department Of Health and Human Services, F. a. D. A., Center for Devices and Radiological Health. Guidance for industry: guidance for the submission of premarket notifications for magnetic resonance diagnostic devices. Rockville: U.S. Food and Drug Adminstration; 1998.
39. International Commission on Non-Ionizing Radiation Protection. ICNIRP statement on the "Guidelines for limiting exposure to time-varying electric, magnetic, and electromagnetic fields (up to 300 GHz)". Health Phys. 2009c;97(3):257–8. https://doi.org/10.1097/HP.0b013e3181aff9db.
40. International Commission on Non-Ionizing Radiation Protection. Guidelines for limiting exposure to time-varying electric and magnetic fields (1 Hz to 100 kHz). Health Phys. 2010;99(6):818–36. https://doi.org/10.1097/HP.0b013e3181f06c86.

41. International Commission on Non-Ionizing Radiation Protection. Guidelines for limiting exposure to electric fields induced by movement of the human body in a static magnetic field and by time-varying magnetic fields below 1 Hz. Health Phys. 2014;106(3):418–25. https://doi.org/10.1097/HP.0b013e31829e5580.
42. International Commission on Non-Ionizing Radiation Protection. Guidelines on limits of exposure to static magnetic fields. Health Phys. 2009b;96(4):504–14. https://doi.org/10.1097/01.HP.0000343164.27920.4a.
43. Chakeres DW, Kangarlu A, Boudoulas H, Young DC. Effect of static magnetic field exposure of up to 8 tesla on sequential human vital sign measurements. J Magn Reson Imaging. 2003;18(3):346–52. https://doi.org/10.1002/jmri.10367.
44. Gupta A, Weeks AR, Richie SM. Simulation of elevated T-waves of an ECG inside a static magnetic field (MRI). IEEE Trans Biomed Eng. 2008;55(7):1890–6. https://doi.org/10.1109/TBME.2008.919868.
45. Bulas D, Egloff A. Benefits and risks of MRI in pregnancy. Semin Perinatol. 2013;37(5):301–4. https://doi.org/10.1053/j.semperi.2013.06.005.
46. International Commission on Non-Ionizing Radiation Protection. Medical magnetic resonance (MR) procedures: protection of patients. Health Phys. 2004;87(2):197–216.
47. International Commission on Non-Ionizing Radiation Protection. Amendment to the ICNIRP "statement on medical magnetic resonance (MR) procedures: protection of patients". Health Phys. 2009a;97(3):259–61. https://doi.org/10.1097/HP.0b013e3181aff9eb.
48. Jaffe TA, Miller CM, Merkle EM. Practice patterns in imaging of the pregnant patient with abdominal pain: a survey of academic centers. AJR Am J Roentgenol. 2007;189(5):1128–34. https://doi.org/10.2214/AJR.07.2277.
49. Kanal E, Gillen J, Evans JA, Savitz DA, Shellock FG. Survey of reproductive health among female MR workers. Radiology. 1993;187(2):395–9. https://doi.org/10.1148/radiology.187.2.8475280.
50. Ray JG, Vermeulen MJ, Bharatha A, Montanera WJ, Park AL. Association between MRI exposure during pregnancy and fetal and childhood outcomes. JAMA. 2016;316(9):952–61. https://doi.org/10.1001/jama.2016.12126.
51. Schenck JF. Physical interactions of static magnetic fields with living tissues. Prog Biophys Mol Biol. 2005;87(2–3):185–204. https://doi.org/10.1016/j.pbiomolbio.2004.08.009.
52. ASTM International. F2213, standard test method for measurement of magnetically induced torque on medical devices in the magnetic resonance environment. West Conshohocken, PA: ASTM International; 2011b.
53. Teitelbaum GP, Bradley WG Jr, Klein BD. MR imaging artifacts, ferromagnetism, and magnetic torque of intravascular filters, stents, and coils. Radiology. 1988;166(3):657–64. https://doi.org/10.1148/radiology.166.3.3340759.
54. Robertson NM, Diaz-Gomez M, Condon B. Estimation of torque on mechanical heart valves due to magnetic resonance imaging including an estimation of the significance of the Lenz effect using a computational model. Phys Med Biol. 2000;45(12):3793–807.
55. Food and Drug Administration. A primer on medical device interactions with magnetic resonance imaging systems; 1997. Retrieved from https://www.federalregister.gov/documents/1997/05/22/97--13377/a-primer-on-medical-device-interactions-with-magnetic-resonance-imaging-systems-draft-guidance. Accessed 10 Oct 2024.
56. Bourland JD, Mouchawar GA, Nyenhuis JA, Geddes LA, Foster KS, Jones JT, Graber GP. Transchest magnetic (eddy-current) stimulation of the dog heart. Med Biol Eng Comput. 1990;28(2):196–8.
57. Yamaguchi M, Andoh T, Goto T, Hosono A, Kawakami T, Okumura F, et al. Effects of strong pulsed magnetic fields on the cardiac activity of an open chest dog. IEEE Trans Biomed Eng. 1994;41(12):1188–91. https://doi.org/10.1109/10.335868.
58. McRobbie DW. Occupational exposure in MRI. Br J Radiol. 2012;85(2012):293–312. https://doi.org/10.1259/bjr/30146162.
59. Ham CL, Engels JM, van de Wiel GT, Machielsen A. Peripheral nerve stimulation during MRI: effects of high gradient amplitudes and switching rates. J Magn Reson Imaging. 1997;7(5):933–7.
60. Food and Drug Administration. Criteria for significant risk investigations of magnetic resonance diagnostic devices; 2014. Retrieved from https://www.fda.gov/media/71385/download. Accessed 10 Oct 2024.
61. Zaremba L. FDA guidelines for magnetic resonance equipment safety. Paper presented at the annual meeting of the American association of physicists in medicine montreal, Canada; 2002. http://aapm.org/meetings/02AM/pdf/8356-48054.pdf
62. Price DL, De Wilde JP, Papadaki AM, Curran JS, Kitney RI. Investigation of acoustic noise on 15 MRI scanners from 0.2 T to 3 T. J Magn Reson Imaging. 2001;13(2):288–93.
63. Edelstein WA, Hedeen RA, Mallozzi RP, El-Hamamsy SA, Ackermann RA, Havens TJ. Making MRI quieter. Magn Reson Imaging. 2002;20(2):155–63.
64. Heismann B, Ott M, Grodzki D. Sequence-based acoustic noise reduction of clinical MRI scans. Magn Reson Med. 2015;73(3):1104–9. https://doi.org/10.1002/mrm.25229.

65. Reeves MJ, Brandreth M, Whitby EH, Hart AR, Paley MN, Griffiths PD, Stevens JC. Neonatal cochlear function: measurement after exposure to acoustic noise during in utero MR imaging. Radiology. 2010;257(3):802–9. https://doi.org/10.1148/radiol.10092366.
66. Dempsey MF, Condon B, Hadley DM. Investigation of the factors responsible for burns during MRI. J Magn Reson Imaging. 2001;13(4):627–31.
67. Shellock FG. Radiofrequency energy-induced heating during MR procedures: a review. J Magn Reson Imaging. 2000;12(1):30–6.
68. Bottomley PA, Edelstein WA. Power deposition in whole-body NMR imaging. Med Phys. 1981;8(4):510–2. https://doi.org/10.1118/1.595000.
69. Bottomley PA, Redington RW, Edelstein WA, Schenck JF. Estimating radiofrequency power deposition in body NMR imaging. Magn Reson Med. 1985;2(4):336–49.
70. Shellock FG. Thermal responses in human subjects exposed to magnetic resonance imaging. Ann N Y Acad Sci. 1992;649:260–72.
71. Shellock FGLC, Kanal E. MRI bioeffects, safety, and patient management: a review. Rev Magn Reson Imaging. 1992;4:21–63.
72. Bottomley PA. Turning up the heat on MRI. J Am Coll Radiol. 2008;5(7):853–5. https://doi.org/10.1016/j.jacr.2008.04.003.
73. Baker KB, Tkach JA, Nyenhuis JA, Phillips M, Shellock FG, Gonzalez-Martinez J, Rezai AR. Evaluation of specific absorption rate as a dosimeter of MRI-related implant heating. J Magn Reson Imaging. 2004;20(2):315–20. https://doi.org/10.1002/jmri.20103.
74. Allison J, Yanasak N. What MRI sequences produce the highest specific absorption rate (SAR), and is there something we should be doing to reduce the SAR during standard examinations? AJR Am J Roentgenol. 2015;205(2):W140. https://doi.org/10.2214/AJR.14.14173.
75. Kanal E, Shellock FG. Burns associated with clinical MR examinations. Radiology. 1990;175(2):585. https://doi.org/10.1148/radiology.175.2.2326485.
76. Friedstat JS, Moore ME, Goverman J, Fagan SP. An unusual burn during routine magnetic resonance imaging. J Burn Care Res. 2013;34(2):e110–1. https://doi.org/10.1097/BCR.0b013e3182642a40.
77. Knopp MV, Essig M, Debus J, Zabel HJ, van Kaick G. Unusual burns of the lower extremities caused by a closed conducting loop in a patient at MR imaging. Radiology. 1996;200(2):572–5. https://doi.org/10.1148/radiology.200.2.8685360.
78. Mattei E, Triventi M, Calcagnini G, Censi F, Kainz W, Mendoza G, Bartolini P. Complexity of MRI induced heating on metallic leads: experimental measurements of 374 configurations. Biomed Eng Online. 2008;7:11. https://doi.org/10.1186/1475-925X-7-11.
79. Yeung CJ, Susil RC, Atalar E. RF heating due to conductive wires during MRI depends on the phase distribution of the transmit field. Magn Reson Med. 2002a;48(6):1096–8. https://doi.org/10.1002/mrm.10310.
80. Yeung CJ, Susil RC, Atalar E. RF safety of wires in interventional MRI: using a safety index. Magn Reson Med. 2002b;47(1):187–93.
81. Kuehn BM. FDA warning: remove drug patches before MRI to prevent burns to skin. JAMA. 2009;301(13):1328. https://doi.org/10.1001/jama.2009.406.
82. Wagle WA, Smith M. Tattoo-induced skin burn during MR imaging. AJR Am J Roentgenol. 2000;174(6):1795. https://doi.org/10.2214/ajr.174.6.1741795.
83. DeBoer S, Fishman D, Chwals W, Straus C, Amundson T. Body piercing/tattooing and trauma diagnostic imaging: medical myths vs realities. J Trauma Nurs. 2007;14(1):35–8. https://doi.org/10.1097/01.JTN.0000264147.35051.ea.
84. Carr JJ. Danger in performing MR imaging on women who have tattooed eyeliner or similar types of permanent cosmetic injections. AJR Am J Roentgenol. 1995;165(6):1546–7. https://doi.org/10.2214/ajr.165.6.7484608.
85. De Wilde JP, Price DL, Renaud C. Magnetic resonance imaging safety issues including an analysis of recorded incidents within the UK. Prog Nucl Magn Reson Spectrosc. 2007;51(1):37–48.
86. Webb A. Magnetic resonance technology: hardware and system component design. Cambridge: Royal Society of Chemistry; 2016.
87. American College of Radiology. ACR Manual on Contrast Media; (2017). Retrieved from https://www.acr.org/clinical-resources/clinical-tools-and-reference/contrast-manual
88. Joint Commission. Preventing accidents and injuries in the MRI suite. Sentinel Event Alert. 2008;14(38):1–3.
89. IMRSER. Institute for Magnetic Resonance Safety, Education, and Research; 2001. Retrieved from http://www.imrser.org. Accessed 10 Oct 2024.
90. American Board of Magnetic Resonance Safety. ABRMS – American Board of Magnetic Resonance Safety; 2018. http://www.abmrs.org. Accessed 10 Oct 2024
91. ASTM. ASTM International; 2018. Retrieved from http://www.astm.org. Accessed 10 Oct 2024
92. ASTM International. F2052 – standard test method for measurement of magnetically induced displacement force on medical devices in the magnetic reso-

nance environment. West Conshohocken: ASTM International; 2006a.
93. ASTM International. F2213 – standard test method for measurement of magnetically induced torque on medical devices in the magnetic resonance environment. West Conshohocken: ASTM International; 2006b.
94. ASTM International. F2182 – standard test method for measurement of radio frequency induced heating on or near passive implants during magnetic resonance imaging. West Conshohocken: ASTM International; 2011a.
95. ASTM International. F2119 – standard test method for evaluation of MR image artifacts from passive implants. West Conshohocken: ASTM International; 2013.

8 Breast Imaging

Xiaoqin Wang, Jie Zhang, Nanditha George, and Margaret Szabunio

Introduction

Breast cancer is the second most common malignancy among women in the United States and the second leading cause of cancer deaths after lung cancer [1]. For nearly 50 years, mammography has been the cornerstone of breast cancer screening and diagnosis [2]. Breast ultrasound and magnetic resonance imaging (MRI) are important adjuncts to mammography, enhancing screening, diagnosis, and evaluation of breast disease—mainly breast cancer.

Breast imaging has been at the forefront of technological advancements, continually integrating innovations such as tomosynthesis, contrast-enhanced mammography, and artificial intelligence (AI). While these advancements offer significant benefits, they also introduce potential risks and new safety concerns. As emerging evidence informs evolving guidelines, radiology practices must remain current to uphold the highest standards of patient care and safety.

This chapter focuses on the quality and patient safety concerns associated with key imaging techniques dedicated to breast health. It reviews established quality assurance and control programs, recent updates to regulations and guidelines, and highlights ongoing efforts to improve imaging quality and patient safety.

Imaging Modalities

Mammography/Tomosynthesis

Mammography remains the benchmark for breast cancer detection, providing the high-spatial and high-contrast resolutions required to visualize small calcifications, distortions or masses which may indicate the presence of cancer in the breast. Mammography uses lower-energy x-rays, typically around 30 keV, compared to general-purpose radiography. Since the development of dedicated mammography units in the 1960s [3], continued improvements in technology have dramatically decreased breast radiation doses while improving its cancer detection ability.

Mammography can be performed with screen film or digital technique. Screen-film mammography (SFM) must be stored physically and viewed on a light box. Digital mammography, also called full-field digital mammography (FFDM), provides an electronic image which can be stored, viewed, and transmitted by computer. FFDM offers several advantages over SFM, including reduced radiation exposure, the ability

X. Wang (✉) · J. Zhang · N. George · M. Szabunio
Department of Radiology, University of Kentucky, Lexington, KY, USA
e-mail: xiaoqin.wang@uky.edu; jnzh222@uky.edu; nanditha.george@uky.edu; margaret.szabunio@uky.edu

J. Zhang (ed.), *Quality and Patient Safety in Medical Imaging*,
https://doi.org/10.1007/978-3-031-89007-9_8

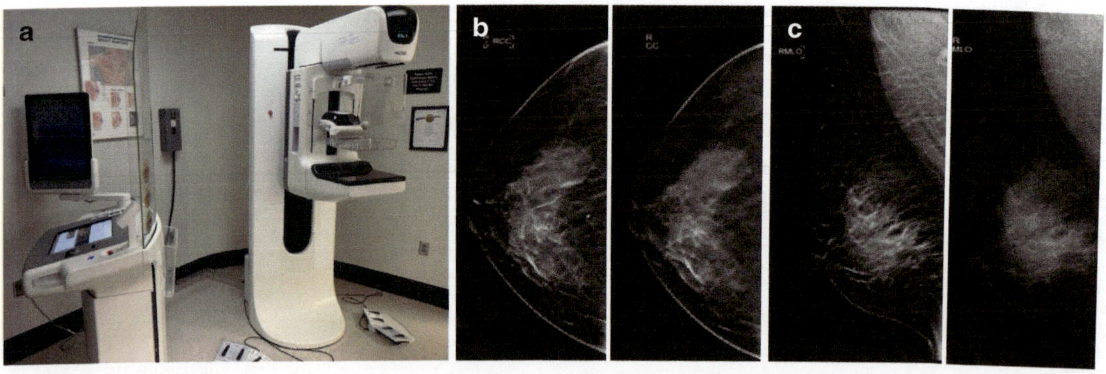

Fig. 8.1 (**a**) Digital mammography system capable of both 2D mammography and tomosynthesis. (**b**) Example of right breast mammograms in CC (2D mammography and tomosynthesis slice) views. (**c**) Tomosynthesis slice images in MLO (2D mammography and tomosynthesis slice)

to process images for better visualization, and easier storage and sharing. As a result, FFDM has completely replaced SFM in clinical practice despite the higher cost.

Digital breast tomosynthesis (DBT) is an advanced imaging technology that acquires x-ray projections from multiple angles to reconstruct a series of thin, planar images, providing a three-dimensional view of breast tissue. DBT was first approved by the FDA in 2011 as a supplement to FFDM and has been widely adopted in clinical practice. This technique mitigates the superimposition of overlapping structures, thereby improving the detection and localization of abnormalities within the breast. While DBT offers enhanced detection capabilities compared to 2D digital mammography [4–7], it also has drawbacks, such as higher radiation doses, longer interpretation times, increased image storage, and challenges in sharing images via picture archiving and communication system (PACS) among institutions.

DBT typically requires a 2D image for comparison with prior mammograms and accurate interpretation of calcifications; therefore, a 2D FFDM is performed after DBT. Synthetic mammography, a 2D reconstruction from the tomosynthesis dataset, was approved by the FDA in 2013 as an alternative to 2D FFDM. Synthetic mammography reduces acquisition time and radiation exposure while maintaining screening performance. However, studies have shown mixed results, with synthetic mammography being associated with higher false-positive rates for calcifications, reduced detection of asymmetries, and increased susceptibility to image artifacts (e.g., metallic artifacts, axillary blurring, and truncation) [8, 9].

Figure 8.1 shows a digital mammography system capable of both 2D mammography and 3D tomosynthesis.

Contrast-Enhanced Mammography

Contrast-enhanced mammography (CEM) is an emerging imaging technique that offers an alternative to contrast-enhanced breast MRI by combining functional and anatomical imaging at a lower cost. CEM uses intravenous iodinated contrast agents to highlight tumor neovascularity, utilizing dual-energy digital mammography to produce both standard low-energy images and iodine-enhanced images for improved lesion visualization.

Recent studies suggest that CEM improves diagnostic accuracy compared to digital mammography and ultrasound [10, 11]. It may also be valuable for screening women at increased risk of breast cancer, particularly women who are unable to undergo MRI. However, CEM involves increased radiation exposure and carries a minor risk of adverse reactions to iodinated contrast material.

Due to its recent introduction and limited data on long-term safety and quality, further discus-

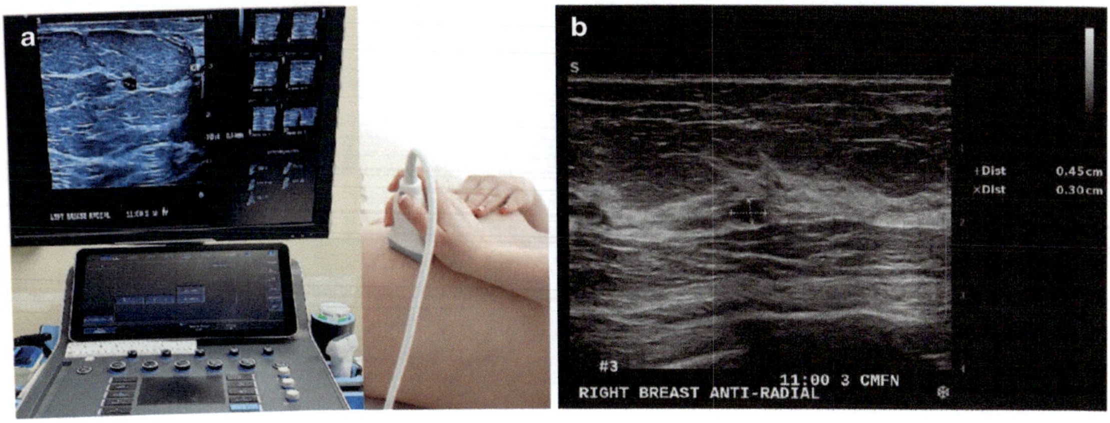

Fig. 8.2 (**a**) Ultrasound machine equipped with a high-frequency probe for breast imaging. (**b**) Ultrasound image displaying a small hypoechoic mass

sion on CEM is not included in this chapter until more robust evidence and established guidelines become available. For concerns related to radiation exposure, please refer to the mammography section in this chapter, and for iodine contrast safety concerns, please refer to the relevant chapter in this book discussing iodinated contrast agent safety.

Breast Ultrasound

Breast ultrasound is a nonionizing modality that is frequently used alongside mammography to improve screening and diagnosis [12–15]. It utilizes a frequency of 12 MHz or higher and is particularly useful for real-time characterization of lesion morphology and differentiating between cysts and solid masses with high specificity. Ultrasound is especially helpful in identifying small lesions that cannot be palpated.

Doppler ultrasound is commonly used for measuring blood flow in a tumor or lymph node, while breast elastography, a newer sonographic imaging technique, offers a noninvasive evaluation of lesion stiffness. Breast ultrasound is widely utilized for guiding breast biopsies and other interventional procedures. Technical advances such as compound imaging and harmonics have improved lesion characterization [16]. Figure 8.2 shows an ultrasound machine equipped with high-frequency probes for breast imaging.

Breast MRI

Breast MRI is a highly sensitive imaging technique that provides detailed anatomical and functional information about breast lesions. Unlike mammography and ultrasound, which primarily focus on structural aspects, MRI enables the evaluation of tissue composition, vascularization, and the dynamic changes of contrast agents within lesions. This capability makes breast MRI particularly valuable for detecting cancers that may be hidden by dense breast tissue or when other imaging modalities yield inconclusive results.

As a supplemental tool alongside mammography and ultrasound, breast MRI is particularly advantageous for screening patients at high risk, assessing the extent of a newly diagnosed breast cancer, evaluating residual disease in cases with positive surgical margins, and monitoring treatment response [17]. Studies have shown that MRI in combination with mammography significantly improves sensitivity in the detection of new cancer and quantification of disease extent [13, 18].

Figure 8.3 shows a breast MRI scanner with dedicated breast coil. Breast MRI is typically performed in an MRI scanner of 1.5 or 3 tesla. The imaging protocol generally includes T2-weighted image, pre-contrast T1-weighted image, and multiple post-contrast T1-weighted images. Despite its high sensitivity, breast MRI is not as widely used in clinical practice as mam-

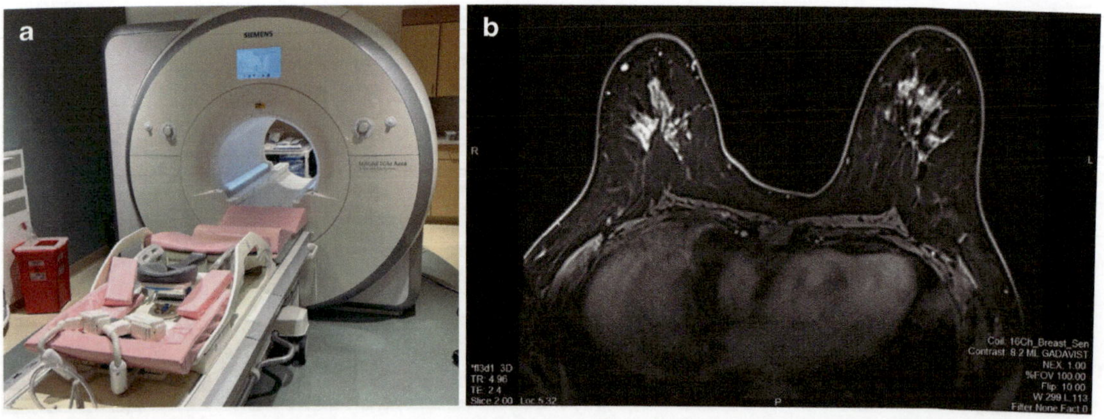

Fig. 8.3 (**a**) Breast MRI scanner with dedicated breast coil. (**b**) Axial T1-weighted breast MRI image with intravenous contrast and fat saturation

mography due to its limitations, including high cost, modest specificity, and the risk of false positives. As a result, it is primarily used as a supplemental tool to mammography [17].

Research to optimize MRI protocols is ongoing [19]. For example, one study showed that 3-min-abbreviated breast MRI protocols, consisting of only one pre- and one post-contrast sequence, could improve efficiency and accessibility by reducing scan time and increasing throughput [20].

Safety Concerns

Safety concerns in breast imaging primarily revolve around three key topics: radiation exposure from mammography, intense magnetic fields and intravenous gadolinium contrast agents in MRI, and, to a lesser extent, thermal effects and mechanical pressure from ultrasound.

Radiation Exposure from Mammography

Although mammography involves low levels of radiation, safety concerns remain, particularly for younger women, as breast tissue is highly sensitive to radiation. The mean glandular dose (MGD), which quantifies the radiation dose absorbed by breast tissue, serves as the standard metric for assessing the safety of mammography.

The average MGD for two-view FFDM exam is approximately 3.7 mGy, which is lower than the MGD for SFM, averaging around 4.7 mGy [21, 22]. DBT has an MGD comparable to a two-view digital mammogram [23]. The total radiation dose strongly depends on acquisition parameters and the number of views as well as breast composition [21]. In adults, the average effective doses for FFDM (0.44 mSv) and SFM (0.56 mSv) are relatively small compared to the annual effective dose from natural background radiation (excluding man-made and medical sources), which is approximately 3 mSv. For a single-view combined FFDM and DBT, the MGD for a 5 cm thick breast is around 2.5 mGy, which is lower than the Mammography Quality Standards Act (MQSA) limit of 3 mGy per view for a two-view screening mammography using an American College of Radiology (ACR) phantom [24, 25].

Although there is a theoretical risk of radiation-induced cancer, particularly in younger women, no confirmed cases have been directly linked to mammography [21]. The lifetime attributable risk (LAR) of developing breast cancer for a 40-year-old woman is estimated at five to seven cases per 100,000, with a mortality of 1.3–1.7 cases per 100,000 [21]. Given that approximately one in eight women will develop breast cancer in her lifetime, the benefits of regular mammography screening far outweigh the minimal risks.

In routine practice, mammograms are not recommended for women under 30 years old due to concerns about radiation exposure and the reduced sensitivity of the mammogram in younger women with dense breast tissue. Special care should be taken when imaging younger patients, and alternative modalities such as ultrasound may be considered according to the ACR's Appropriateness Criteria.

Although the radiation dose and associated risk from mammogram is very low for patients, medical professionals involved in breast imaging have a responsibility to ensure a safe working environment by keeping radiation exposure to staff and patient "as low as reasonably achievable." It is essential to assure that radiation doses to individual patients remain appropriate. To minimize unnecessary radiation exposure, nationally recognized guidelines, such as the ACR Appropriateness Criteria, should be followed when selecting the most appropriate imaging procedures. In addition, automated dose reduction technologies available on imaging equipment, as well as optimized manual techniques, should be implemented whenever appropriate to further reduce radiation exposure [26].

Breast MRI Safety

Breast MRI offers high sensitivity for detecting breast cancer but involves potential risks from the intense magnetic fields and intravenous gadolinium-based contrast agents.

Safety Concerns Related to Magnetic Fields

Magnetic Field Strength and Associated Risks Breast MRI uses powerful magnetic fields, typically ranging from 1.5 to 3 Tesla, which can pose risks if proper precautions are not taken. These risks include the potential for projectile accidents, where ferromagnetic objects (such as metallic implants, tools, or personal items) are drawn rapidly toward the MRI magnet, potentially causing injury to patients or staff. The ACR MRI Safe Practice Guidelines provide comprehensive safety protocols to minimize these risks, including strict screening procedures for all patients and personnel entering the MRI suite [27].

Adverse Incidents and Preventive Measures Incidents such as burns can occur from conductive materials, including wires, tattoos, or electrocardiogram (ECG) leads, that may heat up during the scan. Preventive measures include ensuring that all patients are screened for ferromagnetic objects, using nonconductive materials for monitoring equipment, and positioning patients properly to avoid skin-to-skin contact that could lead to burns.

Interference with Medical Devices MRI's electromagnetic fields can interfere with certain medical devices such as pacemakers, cochlear implants, neurostimulators, aneurysm clips, and breast tissue expanders, potentially leading to malfunction, device failure, or patient injury [28, 29]. Breast tissue expanders with magnetic ports can create artifacts that obscure imaging and pose risks of heating, displacement, or dysfunction of the port, making MRI nondiagnostic or unsafe.

Before undergoing MRI, all patients should be thoroughly screened for contraindications, including the presence of metallic implants, pacemakers, or other devices that may be affected by magnetic fields. Special attention is also needed for patients with tattoos, piercings, or nonremovable metallic objects. For those with medical devices, MRI safety and suitability should be determined through consultation with device manufacturers and clinical teams [30].

To ensure patient and staff safety, it is critical to adhere to the ACR MRI Safe Practice Guidelines. All staff working in MRI environments should receive comprehensive training on safety protocols and management of MRI-related emergencies.

Safety Concerns Related to Gadolinium-Based Contrast Agents

Most breast MRIs are performed with intravenous gadolinium-based contrast agents to enhance the visualization of tumor. While gadolinium is generally safe, it poses a risk of nephrogenic systemic fibrosis (NSF), a rare but severe condition characterized by fibrosis of the skin and other tissues, primarily in patients with severe renal insufficiency. To minimize this risk, it is recommended that gadolinium use be avoided in patients with an estimated glomerular filtration rate of less than 30 mL/min/1.73 m^2 [31]. Facilities should follow the latest guidelines in the ACR Manual on Contrast Media, which outlines protocols for screening and managing patients at risk for NSF [31].

Recent studies have raised concerns about the retention of gadolinium in the brain and other tissues following multiple contrast-enhanced MRI scans [32]. Although the clinical significance of these deposits is not yet fully understood, the FDA has issued warnings and is actively investigating the potential long-term risks. Patients with repeated exposure to gadolinium may need to be monitored, and the use of macrocyclic gadolinium agents, which are less likely to deposit gadolinium in the body, may be preferred over linear agents [33].

For patients who require gadolinium contrast but have underlying health conditions such as renal insufficiency, a risk-benefit assessment should be conducted, considering alternatives like non-contrast MRI or other imaging modalities. If gadolinium is necessary, macrocyclic agents are preferred, and kidney function should be closely monitored before and after the procedure.

Ultrasound Safety

Ultrasound is widely regarded as one of the safest imaging modalities for breast evaluation because it does not involve ionizing radiation. Breast ultrasound typically uses a high frequency linear transducer of at least 12 MHz [34]. While ultrasound operates through mechanical pressure from sound waves, which can theoretically cause thermal effects and mechanical cavitation, no adverse effects have been documented in breast ultrasound, making it extremely safe for routine use. Some patients may experience mild, temporary discomfort due to probe pressure, particularly in sensitive areas.

Although the risk is low, thermal and mechanical effects should still be considered in breast imaging. The thermal index (TI), which indicates the potential for tissue heating, becomes relevant when energy levels are high or scanning times are prolonged. The mechanical index (MI), which measures the likelihood of cavitation, poses a risk if ultrasound pressure waves are too intense. Ensuring TI and MI remain within safety limits is important to prevent potential tissue damage and maintain ultrasound as a safe imaging modality [35].

Safety Concerns Regarding Imaging-Guided Breast Interventional Procedures

Image-guided percutaneous breast biopsy performed with ultrasound, mammography, or MRI guidance is now widely accepted as a reliable alternative to open surgical biopsy [36, 37]. It offers several advantages including minimal scarring, better cosmetic effect, reduced morbidity, faster recovery, avoidance of general anesthesia, and shorter procedure times when compared to the excisional biopsy. In the United States, approximately 70–90% of the 1.6 million breast biopsies performed annually are image-guided percutaneous procedures [38]. Common types of imaging-guided breast procedures include core biopsy, wire or seed localization, and fine needle aspiration. These procedures may also serve therapeutic purposes such as abscess drainage or cyst aspiration.

Safety Considerations and Advantages of Different Modalities for Procedures

Ultrasound-guided procedures are the most commonly performed, especially for the non-palpable lesions visible on ultrasound. However, for lesions that are only detectable on mammogram or MRI, mammography-guided biopsy (stereotactic biopsy), or MRI-guided biopsy may be necessary. DBT-guided biopsy provides more positioning options and has shown positive clinical performance and feedback in practice [39].

Before performing any image-guided biopsy, it is essential to carefully assess the lesion images and determine patient suitability. This includes evaluating the risk of excessive bleeding due to underlying disorders or medications, identifying potential infection risks, and reviewing the patient's history for allergies or hypersensitivity to latex, lidocaine, or epinephrine. For stereotactic and MRI-guided procedures, additional considerations include ensuring the patient does not exceed the table's weight limit and can remain prone for the required duration. Breast thickness should also be assessed, as very small breasts may not be suitable for these techniques.

Complications Related to Image-Guided Breast Biopsy

Clinically significant complications from image-guided breast biopsy are rare [40]. The most common complication is hematoma, occurring in up to 27% of cases [41]. The risk of significant bleeding is higher for axillary lymph node biopsy due to the adjacent large vessels. Thus, fine needle aspiration instead of core biopsy can be performed with a cytologist present to ensure adequate sampling. Small hematomas usually resolve over time, but direct pressure should be applied to control bleeding. Large hematomas requiring surgery are exceedingly rare.

Infections are less common than bleeding with the use of sterile techniques. However, if an infection does occur, it should be promptly treated with antibiotics to prevent progression to abscess.

Pneumothorax is a possible complication of ultrasound-directed percutaneous biopsy. Pneumothorax can be avoided by using proper techniques to ensure the needle tip is always visualized to confirm correct placement and avoid penetration of the chest wall. Positioning the needle parallel to the chest wall is the key to avoiding this complication. Figure 8.4 shows proper needle positioning during an ultrasound-guided breast biopsy. Rare complications such as arterial–venous fistulae, pseudoaneurysm, and nerve injury can also occur but are largely preventable with appropriate planning and care [42].

Complications from local anesthesia are rare but can occur. For example, ischemia or skin sloughing is possible if lidocaine with epinephrine is injected in excessive volume to the skin. Proper training in the administration of local anesthetics and avoidance of epinephrine in the skin of certain patients can minimize these risks.

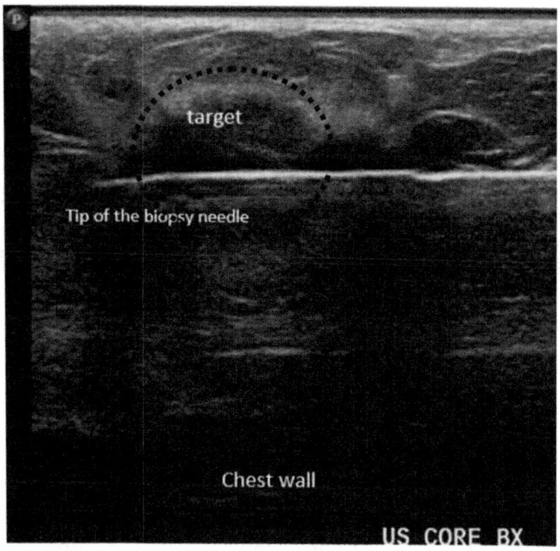

Fig. 8.4 Proper needle positioning during an ultrasound-guided breast biopsy. The needle is parallel to the chest wall and fully visualizable within the breast in relation to the target mass (dashed circle) and chest wall

To prevent tissue damage, such as necrosis, from accidental exposure to formalin, facilities should ensure that formalin is not placed on surgical trays and that specimens are only placed in formalin containers after the procedure is complete.

The Potential of Artificial Intelligence in Breast Imaging and Safety Considerations

AI offers transformative potential in breast imaging, including mammography, ultrasound, and MRI, by automating lesion detection, risk assessment, imaging quality improvement, and image triage [43]. It has demonstrated its ability to match or even exceed radiologists' diagnostic performance, improving breast cancer detection. In mammography, AI optimizes image contrast, reduces noise, and enhances resolution, particularly in dense breast tissue, which often poses diagnostic challenges. These advancements reduce the need for repeat imaging and contribute to more precise and safer diagnostic outcomes. In MRI, AI aids in segmentation and treatment response prediction, potentially reducing scan time and IV contrast usage.

While AI's potential is clear, its adoption is still evolving. Beyond computer-aided detection in mammography, most AI applications remain developmental and are not yet suitable for standalone clinical use. AI can assist radiologists but cannot replace them, especially in complex cases. Integration into clinical workflows also presents challenges [44].

AI adoption raises safety concerns, as its performance depends on training data quality, and biases or inaccuracies can lead to diagnostic errors [43, 45]. Without rigorous validation and ethical oversight, AI could introduce new risks into clinical practice. These risks are particularly concerning for underrepresented groups, where misdiagnoses could worsen healthcare inequalities. The "black box" nature of AI algorithms, where decision-making processes are opaque, further complicates their clinical use and increase the risk of overreliance on AI without human oversight [46]. Cautious implementation, strong safeguards, and continuous human supervision are essential to ensure patient safety.

Safety of Breast Imaging in Pregnant and Lactating Patients

The radiation dose to the fetus during a mammogram is minimal, and no lead apron is required, making mammography a safe option for pregnant women when necessary. Screening mammograms should not be delayed during pregnancy and should be determined based on the patient's age and risk status, as outlined by the ACR [47]. For women who do not meet the criteria for a screening mammogram but present with clinical concerns such as palpable masses or focal pain, ultrasound should be the first-line imaging modality. Ultrasound is more sensitive than mammography in pregnant women due to increased breast density during pregnancy. In cases when ultrasound findings are inconclusive or suspicious, a mammogram should be performed at the radiologist's discretion. However, MRI with gadolinium-based contrast should not be used in pregnant women, as the contrast crosses the placenta and the risks to the fetus are unknown [48, 49].

For lactating women younger than 40, ultrasound should also be the initial imaging choice because mammography is less sensitive during lactation due to increased breast density. If a mammogram is necessary, it is suggested that lactating women pump for 30 min prior to the procedure to reduce breast density and improve image quality. Other than that, lactating women can be imaged according to the same protocols as non-lactating women. Screening mammograms should not be delayed either. These guidelines ensure safe and effective imaging while minimizing risks to both pregnant and lactating patients [48].

Quality Concerns

High-quality breast imaging is critical for radiologists to detect and diagnose breast cancer with confidence and accuracy. Both false negatives (missed diagnoses) and false positives (overdiagnoses) can have serious consequences for patient care. False negatives may delay treatment, potentially increasing mortality, while false positives can lead to unnecessary imaging and invasive procedures and significant emotional distress for patients and their families. Ensuring optimal diagnostic accuracy requires both specialized imaging equipment and strict adherence to established protocols. This section explores key quality factors in mammography, breast ultrasound, and breast MRI.

Mammography

Mammography performed with the highest quality standards should accurately characterize the morphology of a mass, calcification, distortion of breast tissue, and the interval change from any prior studies. The critical elements to achieve and maintain high-quality imaging include well-trained and experienced personnel (radiologist, technologist, medical physicist), well-designed

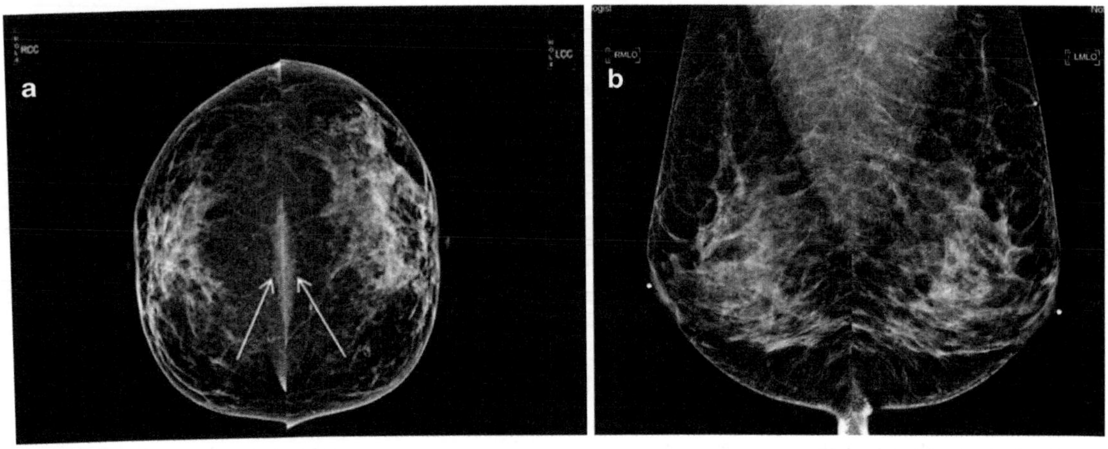

Fig. 8.5 (**a**) An ideal craniocaudal (CC) view showing retromammary space and pectoralis muscle (arrow). (**b**) An ideal mediolateral oblique (MLO) view showing the nipple in profile, well-visualized, convex pectoralis muscle margin, the edge of the pectoralis muscle extending below the level of the posterior nipple line (PNL), and an open inframammary fold

equipment for imaging acquisition and display, and systemic quality assurance (QA) and quality control (QC) programs for the assessment of the imaging quality. All mammography in the United States must be performed in concordance with the MQSA legislation and regulations published by the FDA [50].

Imaging Acquisition

High-quality mammographic imaging starts with appropriate imaging acquisition. Technical descriptions of acquisition using specific equipment can be requested from the manufacturers. Although each mammography manufacturer has specific device parameters and QC for mammographic imaging acquisition, the overall imaging quality is affected by tissue coverage, spatial resolution, contrast, latitude or dynamic range, noise, and artifacts [51].

Tissue Coverage

The goal of screening mammogram is to image the fibroglandular breast tissue as much as possible in the craniocaudal (CC) and mediolateral oblique (MLO) projections. Positioning is very important because only the breast tissue included on a mammogram can be evaluated for cancer. The X-ray beam and image receptor need to come as close to the chest wall edge of the breast support as possible. The image receptor should be large enough to image the breast for most women without loss of breast tissue. For imaging of large breasts, a large field of view can be used to reduce the radiation exposure from overlapped tiling. Both technologists and radiologist need to assess the positioning in digital mammograms to ensure the maximal amount of tissue visualization.

Figure 8.5 illustrates an ideal CC view and an ideal MLO view in mammography.

Ideal CC View

- Both the medial and lateral aspects of the breast should be clearly visualized.
- Ideally, a portion of the pectoral muscle should be seen.
- The posterior nipple line (PNL) should measure no more than 1 cm shorter than in the MLO view.

Ideal MLO View

- The nipple should be centered, but not at the expense of excluding breast tissue.
- The anterior edge of the pectoralis muscle should appear convex, ideally extending to the level of the nipple.
- The breast should be pulled up and out to include the maximal amount of posterior tis-

sue and an open inframammary fold, with a small portion of the upper abdomen visible.
- The PNL should be drawn perpendicular to the pectoralis muscle.
- The axillary tail should be visualized.

Spatial Resolution

Spatial resolution refers to the ability to distinctly display two adjacent structures in the image (i.e., sharpness). Mammography with low spatial resolution can affect the appearance of lesion characteristics, especially microcalcifications. Although geometric factors, receptor factors, and image processing can all affect the spatial resolution of mammography, motion blurring, often encountered in clinical practice, can have a particularly strong impact on image sharpness. Motion blurring can be minimized by using a short exposure time and appropriate breast compression. For dense breasts, higher tube voltage (kV) may be used to reduce the exposure time. Having the patient stop breathing instead of holding breath after deep inspiration may help limit breathing-related motion blurring. Magnification view using small focal spots and lower tube current (mA) requires longer exposure time and thus has higher potential for motion blurring.

Contrast Resolution

Contrast resolution refers to the signal difference between the structure of interest and its surroundings. High-contrast resolution is crucial for detecting subtle differences between cancer and normal glandular tissue. Contrast resolution is influenced by subject contrast and imaging contrast.

Subject contrast depends on the X-ray energy spectrum, which is determined by kV and filtration. Different target materials, such as molybdenum (Mo), rhodium (Rh), and tungsten (W), are used in mammography machines, and their X-ray spectra can be optimized with Mo, Rh, and silver (Ag) filters.

The selection of target and filter combinations plays a key role in achieving optimal contrast while maintaining a reasonably low radiation dose:

- Mo/Mo (target/filter): Provides high subject contrast while minimizing radiation dose, ideal for breasts 2–5 cm thick.
- Mo/Rh: Transmits 15–23 keV X-rays, making it suitable for dense breasts.
- Rh/Rh: Produces a spectrum effective for very dense, difficult-to-penetrate breasts.
- W target with an appropriate filter allows for higher effective energy and better tube heat management compared to the Mo/Mo combination.

Careful selection of target and filter materials ensures optimal contrast while maintaining an acceptable radiation dose for different breast densities.

Grids

Grids are used to reduce scatter radiation, which helps improve image contrast in contact imaging. However, grids are not used for geometric magnification views because the increased air gap between the breast and the detector naturally reduces scatter, making a grid unnecessary.

Compression

Breast compression is important for digital mammography quality. Proper compression can reduce motion blurring by immobilizing the breast; lower breast radiation dose by penetrating a more uniform, thinner tissue; and improve lesion detection by spreading out the overlapping tissue.

Noise

A high signal-to-noise ratio (SNR) is also important for mammography imaging quality as fine calcifications or subtle masses may not be visible in a noisy (underexposed) mammography, especially when noise is from software processing errors or digital detector deficiencies. To optimize SNR, a calibrated automatic exposure control (AEC) system is used to ensure appropriate exposure levels, improving image clarity while maintaining an optimal radiation dose.

Artifacts

Artifacts on mammogram can represent a serious quality concern because they can obscure true lesions. It is important for radiologists and technologists to recognize these artifacts and know how to mitigate them. While some artifacts are shared by SFM and FFDM, many are unique to FFDM, particularly artifacts related to detector or processing software. Artifact on FFDM can be vendor specific because the manufacturers use different detectors (direct or indirect) for digital imaging acquisition.

Common artifacts seen in digital mammography include patient-related artifacts (e.g., motion artifact), hardware-related artifacts (e.g., field inhomogeneity, grid lines, underexposure), and software-related artifacts (e.g., loss of edge, processing bars). The causes of these artifacts and methods for correction are discussed in detail in the reference [52].

Digital Breast Tomosynthesis

As discussed before, DBT generates thin (~1 mm) planar slices, minimizing tissue overlap and improving the detection and localization of masses, asymmetries, and architectural distortions compared to 2D mammography [53–56]. However, DBT has limitations in detecting and evaluating calcifications. The thin slices may capture only a fraction of the calcifications present, limiting their visibility. Additionally, increased noise from the lower radiation dose can negatively impact both the characterization and quantification of calcifications compared to FFDM [23, 24, 57]. Image blurring due to source and patient motion further reduces spatial resolution, diminishing DBT's sensitivity for calcifications [23, 24].

Imaging Display

The quality of the imaging display is a crucial factor in digital mammography. Digital mammograms can be displayed as either hardcopy (printed films) or softcopy (digital screens), but the advantages of digital mammography are best realized with softcopy display, which is now standard in most mammography units.

The ACR recommends that monitors used for FFDM interpretation be FDA approved for mammography. Display monitor QC should be performed weekly, and if a monitor fails to meet the manufacturer's criteria, corrective action must be taken immediately before interpreting images or imaging patients. QC guidelines should follow the American Association of Physicists in Medicine (AAPM) Task Group 18 recommendations for mammography-specific display standards [43]. MQSA regulations require a medical physicist to test a review workstation before its clinical use, and regular testing is necessary to ensure ongoing compliance [58, 59].

For optimal mammography interpretation, display monitors should have a maximum luminance of at least 400 cd/m^2, with 450 cd/m^2 or higher recommended, as increased luminance improves human eye sensitivity to contrast details. A minimum of 8-bit output luminance resolution is required, but 9-bit or higher is recommended if the "For Processing" image data exceeds 8 bits. Display specifications should closely match the acquisition matrix size, with a 5-megapixel (2048 × 2560 pixels) monitor recommended for diagnostic accuracy [60].

Ultrasound

Breast ultrasound is highly subjective and operator dependent, with significant variability in equipment and imaging techniques. The infrequent use of test phantoms further contributes to overlooked QC issues, leading to diagnostic inconsistencies. Unlike mammography, which is federally regulated, breast ultrasound lacks mandatory FDA quality assurance programs, resulting in wide disparities in image quality across clinical settings.

While there are no federal laws equivalent to the MQSA governing breast ultrasound, the ACR has established practice parameters to ensure high-quality breast ultrasound examinations.

These guidelines cover equipment specifications, technical settings, image annotation, and personnel qualifications, aiming to promote excellent radiological care [61].

Key imaging requirements outlined by the ACR include:

- Image Annotation: Each image must be annotated with key details, including clock face location, distance from the nipple, and orientation (radial and anti-radial views).
- Use of Doppler and Gray Scale Imaging: Doppler settings should be optimized for vascular assessments, while gray scale imaging must clearly distinguish between cystic and solid masses.
- Focal Zone Placement: The focal zone should be positioned at the depth of the lesion to ensure maximum resolution and precision.
- Depth Settings: The imaging depth must be adjusted to include the lesion and surrounding tissues within the field of view.
- Dynamic Range and Gain Settings: Dynamic range should prevent lesions from appearing anechoic or isoechoic, while gain settings should enhance visibility without introducing artifacts.
- Time–Gain Compensation Curve: This curve should gradually increase with depth to equalize echogenicity across all breast tissue layers.

Breast ultrasound, like other ultrasound modalities, exhibits various artifacts that can both hinder and aid diagnosis. For example, aliasing artifacts in ultrasound elastography can mimic solid masses when evaluating breast cystic lesions [62]. On the other hand, the twinkling artifact, used in real-time ultrasound, is valuable for detecting breast microcalcifications, improving diagnostic precision preoperative marking of calcification clusters [63, 64]. The blooming-like artifact in color Doppler ultrasound can help identify metallic biopsy markers in the breast and axilla, enhancing the accuracy of ultrasound-guided biopsies [65].

Breast MRI

Breast MRI requires a dedicated breast coil and a scanner with a field strength of at least 1.5 Tesla. The imaging protocol must include specific sequences, typically T2-weighted imaging, a pre-contrast T1-weighted image, and multiple post-contrast T1-weighted images, ensuring proper breast positioning and complete anatomical coverage of the entire breast and axillary tail. According to the Breast MRI Accreditation Program Clinical Image Guide, a high-quality breast MRI should have an adequate SNR to avoid graininess, good spatial resolution, and sufficient temporal resolution for dynamic series (60–90 s per phase). The image should also exhibit minimal or no artifacts, uniform signal and fat suppression, and good contrast enhancement. For pre-contrast and post-contrast T1-weighted series, accreditation standards require a slice thickness of ≤3 mm with no gap between slices, a maximum in-plane pixel dimension (phase and frequency) of ≤1 mm, and a total time from contrast injection completion to the end of the early phase of ≤4 min.

Artifacts in breast MRI are a common challenge that can significantly impact diagnostic accuracy if not properly managed. The most frequent artifacts include motion, poor or nonuniform fat saturation, susceptibility artifacts, aliasing (wrap-around), and signal nonuniformity [66–68].

Motion artifacts arise from blood flow, cardiac pulsation, respiratory motion, or patient movement, propagating in the phase-encoding direction and causing image blurring. Selecting the appropriate phase-encoding direction is crucial to minimize their impact: left-to-right for axial breast MRI and superior-to-inferior for sagittal imaging. Incorrect phase encoding, such as anterior-to-posterior, can obscure critical breast areas, potentially hiding lesions.

Chemical-shift fat suppression is essential in breast MRI protocols, improving contrast between tissues and enhancing lesion visibility. Subtracted series, where pre-contrast images are subtracted from post-contrast images slice by slice, are critical for both early and delayed phases of dynamic contrast-enhanced (DCE) imaging. However, artifacts affecting fat suppression, such as differential enhancement of fat and water, can degrade diagnostic accuracy. To mitigate these issues, a time-equivalent in-phase fat-suppressed 3D gradient–recalled echo sequence can be used to correct subtraction image errors [69].

Phase-wrap artifacts in bilateral axial DCE breast MRI can be minimized by positioning the intravenous line outside the field of view [70]. While multiparametric breast MRI protocols typically include DCE T1-weighted acquisitions, artifacts can still occur in different sequence and should be carefully identified to prevent misinterpretation [71].

Quality and Safety Improvement in Breast Imaging

Quality Assurance Program

An effective QA program ensures that all critical imaging elements remain consistently in place over time, covering everything from patient scheduling to final radiologic assessment. QC, a subset of QA, focuses on the technical aspects of imaging, including equipment maintenance, image acquisition, and ensuring adequate breast compression. Regular QC activities help maintain equipment integrity and imaging consistency, ensuring optimal diagnostic performance.

Mammography

Strict adherence to QA and QC measures is essential in all mammography facilities. Current QA and QC protocols align with guidelines from the United States FDA, MQSA, ACR Practice Guidelines, and select international standards [72].

FDA-approved FFDM QC includes various tests, such as phantom image quality assessment, collimation, exposure reproducibility, artifact evaluation, flat field uniformity, kV accuracy, beam quality (half-value layer), radiation output, and mammographic unit assembly evaluation. Monitor QC tests include monitor cleaning, viewing conditions assessment, monitor calibration checks, and image quality testing using the Society of Motion Picture and Television Engineers (SMPTE) test pattern [73].

Manufacturer-specific QC procedures, as mandated by the FDA, must be followed. Digital mammography system manufacturers define procedures and limits for corrective actions for daily, weekly, monthly, quarterly, and semiannual tests performed by a QC technologist, as well as annual tests conducted by a qualified medical physicist. These procedures are periodically updated.

Breast Ultrasound

There are four fundamental ultrasound QC tests used to assess clinical image quality: system sensitivity, uniformity, spatial accuracy, and contrast/spatial resolution.

- System sensitivity refers to the instrument's ability to detect small signals against background noise. High-frequency breast ultrasound provides better resolution but reduces sensitivity for deeper structures. A lower-frequency transducer is recommended for large breasts or deep axillary lymph nodes.
- Uniformity assesses image consistency in two planes: horizontal uniformity (parallel to the transducer face) and vertical uniformity (perpendicular to the transducer face). Horizontal uniformity is influenced by system-related factors, while vertical uniformity can be adjusted using time-gain compensation (TGC).
- Spatial accuracy has long been a standard component of QC tests, ensuring the correct positioning of structures in ultrasound images.
- Contrast and spatial resolution are crucial for image clarity, though evaluating these parameters in ultrasound can be challenging.

For ACR breast ultrasound accreditation, system sensitivity and uniformity are required, while spatial accuracy and contrast/spatial resolution are optional. The American Institute of Ultrasound in Medicine (AIUM) Quality Assurance Manual provides guidelines for grayscale imaging QC, detection of quality degradation, and routine quality assurance tests. The AIUM Medical Ultrasound Safety document offers recommendations for optimizing diagnostic ultrasound settings to obtain high-quality images with minimal patient risk.

While various ultrasound organizations recommend QC practices, the ACR is the only accrediting body that mandates ultrasound QC with specific requirements.

Breast MRI

All ACR-accredited MRI sites must comply with the minimum requirements outlined in the 2024 ACR MRI QC Manual. The ACR MRI Accreditation Program evaluates breast MRI facilities by reviewing personnel qualifications, equipment QC, MRI safety policies, and image quality.

The MRI Accreditation Program defines the roles and qualifications of key personnel:

- Qualified Medical Physicist/MRI Scientist: Responsible for establishing baseline equipment performance and overseeing all equipment-related QC activities.
- QC Technologist: Trained by the MRI scientist and responsible for conducting QC activities not assigned to the lead MRI radiologist or MRI scientist.
- Lead MRI Radiologist: Ensures that all QC requirements are met and that imaging quality and safety standards are maintained.

Ongoing Efforts to Improve Quality and Patient Safety

Federal/Organizational Efforts

Mammography Quality Standards Act, MQSA

The MQSA was enacted in 1992 to establish national standards for screening and diagnostic mammography, ensuring consistent image quality and patient safety across the United States. Implemented in 1994, MQSA mandates that all mammography facilities meet minimum quality standards for personnel, equipment, and record-keeping, with certification required by the FDA or an FDA-approved accrediting body [51]. The Department of Veterans Affairs (VA) has its own mammography quality program, exempt from FDA certification.

Since 1995, the FDA has conducted annual inspections to ensure compliance with MQSA. Over time, the regulations have evolved, incorporating updates based on inspection findings and advancements in imaging technology. Poor positioning has been identified as a leading cause of clinical image deficiencies. The Enhancing Quality Using the Inspection Program (EQUIP) initiative, introduced in 2016, emphasizes continuous quality review by requiring facilities to evaluate and correct clinical image quality beyond the standard annual MQSA inspection. Additional details on EQUIP and its three key inspection questions are available on the FDA Website [74].

Building on existing regulations, the FDA amended MQSA, with enforcement beginning September 10, 2024 [75]. Key updates include:

- Breast Density Notification Requirements: Facilities must classify breast density into one of four categories ("almost entirely fatty" to "extremely dense") and communicate clear, standardized information to patients about its impact on cancer detection.
- Revised Communication Timelines: Results categorized as "Suspicious" or "Highly Suggestive of Malignancy" must be delivered to both the healthcare provider and patient within 7 days.
- Annual Medical Outcomes Audits: Facilities must track key metrics, such as cancer detection rates, to ensure continuous quality improvement.
- Stricter Accreditation Standards: Facilities failing to meet accreditation requirements

after three consecutive attempts will face a one-year reapplication ban.

- Enhanced Recordkeeping Requirements: Improved documentation standards for mammogram storage and personnel qualifications to ensure compliance.

These updates reflect the FDA's ongoing commitment to improving mammography quality and patient safety, ensuring that facilities maintain high standards for imaging and effective patient communication.

ACR Accreditation and Quality Control

Through its accreditation programs and QC guidelines, the ACR continues to play a key role in ensuring high-quality breast imaging and patient safety.

The ACR is an FDA-approved accrediting body for both SFM and FFDM, ensuring compliance with FDA Final Rules [75]. Its accreditation process evaluates radiologist, medical physicist, and radiologic technologist qualifications, along with QC results, image quality, radiation dose, and recordkeeping. Phantoms used for accreditation must be ACR approved, and all mammography units within a facility must share the same accreditation expiration date, regardless of when each was accredited [76].

To support compliance with MQSA regulations (21 CFR 900.12), the ACR provides quality control guidance. The 1999 ACR Mammography Quality Control Manual established QC standards for screen-film mammography, while the 2018 Digital Mammography Quality Control Manual (revised in May 2020) introduced standardized QC testing protocols for digital mammography in collaboration with the FDA.

Since June 1, 2014, ACR Breast Ultrasound Accreditation has required acceptance testing and annual surveys by a qualified medical physicist or physician-approved designee, along with routine QC by trained sonographers or service engineers. Facilities must provide documentation of compliance with ACR QC requirements during accreditation, including reports from annual ultrasound surveys and records of corrective actions taken.

Unlike mammography, breast MRI is not regulated under MQSA, as the technology emerged after the act was passed. There is no federal regulatory program governing breast MRI quality; however, the ACR Breast MRI Accreditation Program provides quality standards and accreditation criteria. Facilities must have equipment for mammographic correlation, targeted breast ultrasound, and MRI-guided interventions or establish a referral agreement with a partnering facility for these services.

Although ACR accreditation is not mandatory, failure to achieve accreditation may impact Medicare reimbursement. Under the Medicare Improvement for Patients and Providers Act of 2008 (MIPPA), facilities performing advanced diagnostic imaging services, including breast MRI, must be accredited by a CMS-designated accrediting organization to qualify for Medicare reimbursement as of January 1, 2012. Compliance with these requirements is verified during ACR or CMS on-site surveys.

Clinical Efforts

While FDA and ACR regulations establish foundational quality and safety standards, additional clinical measures play a critical role in enhancing imaging quality and patient safety. Accreditation compliance is only the first step in a multistep process that requires continuous quality improvement (CQI) programs and well-defined performance standards across imaging facilities.

Achieving high-quality imaging and optimal patient care depends on effective communication and coordination among radiologists, medical physicists, technologists, support staff, and referring providers. Some key clinical efforts to improve quality and patient safety include:

- Optimizing imaging protocols to minimize radiation dose while maintaining diagnostic accuracy.
- Providing post-procedure follow-up calls within 24 h to address patient concerns and identify potential complications.
- Ensuring timely, comprehensive, and accessible diagnostic information to improve patient outcomes.
- Maintaining adequate capacity to offer convenient and timely access to mammography, breast ultrasound, and breast MRI.
- Conducting quarterly and biannual quality management meetings to review best practices and patient outcomes.

Radiologists play a central role in ensuring image quality and proper technique. Breast radiology teams must adhere to FDA and ACR guidelines, integrate QA programs into daily practice, and engage in continuous training and evaluation to improve diagnostic accuracy. The adoption of advanced imaging technologies and ongoing performance monitoring can further enhance clinical quality and patient safety in breast imaging.

Industry Efforts

Manufacturers continue to advance breast imaging technology with a focus on improving image quality, reducing radiation dose, and enhancing patient comfort. One major concern with DBT combined with 2D mammography is the increased radiation dose. To address this, Hologic (Marlborough, MA) developed synthetic software that reconstructs 2D images from 3D tomosynthesis data, eliminating the need for an additional 2D mammogram, thereby reducing radiation exposure and breast compression time [77, 78].

Several companies, including GE (Boston, MA), Sonocine (Reno, NV), and Philips (Amsterdam), have introduced automated breast ultrasound (ABUS) as a nonionizing alternative for dense breast screening. ABUS uses sound waves to create high-resolution breast images, offering a comfortable, fast, and effective supplemental screening method for women with dense breast tissue [79, 80]. The cUSBr-Patch, a wearable and conformable ultrasound device, has been developed to enable large-area, deep tissue scanning and multi-angle, repeatable breast imaging. It is capable of detecting lesions as small as 1 mm with high accuracy and reliability, as validated through in vivo comparisons with conventional ultrasound [81].

Automated image quality assessment software has been developed to analyze digital mammography images in real time. This technology provides immediate feedback to technologists, ensuring proper positioning and optimal image quality, which helps reduce repeat imaging and improves diagnostic accuracy [82].

Resources for Quality and Safety

Table 8.1 provides a summary of resources (e.g., QC recommendations, safety guidelines) for quality and safety specifically for breast imaging. The goal of this table is to provide readers with quick access to resources.

Table 8.1 Resources for quality and patient safety in breast imaging

Imaging modality	Organization or agency	Publication	Link
Mammography and stereotactic biopsy	ACR	Complete accreditation information: Mammography (revised 1-24-24)	https://accreditationsupport.acr.org/support/solutions/articles/11000063274-complete-accreditation-information-mammography-revised-1-24-24
	ACR	Technologist quality control forms	https://www.acraccreditation.org/modalities/mammography/tech-qc-forms
	ACR	Quality control: Mammography (revised 1-31-25)	https://accreditationsupport.acr.org/support/solutions/articles/11000056196-quality-control-mammography-revised-12-12-19
	ACR	Digital Mammography Quality Control Manual (2018—Revised May 2020)	https://edge.sitecorecloud.io/americancoldf5f-acrorgf92a-productioncb02-3650/media/ACR/Files/Clinical/Quality-Control-Manuals/Mammography-Quality-Control-Manual.pdf
	ACR-SPR	ACR-SPR Practice Parameter for Imaging Pregnant or Potentially Pregnant Patients with Ionizing Radiation (Revised 2023)	https://gravitas.acr.org/PPTS/DownloadPreviewDocument?ReleaseId=2&DocId=23
	ACR	ACR Practice Parameter for the Performance of Screening and Diagnostic Mammography (Revised 2023)	https://gravitas.acr.org/PPTS/GetDocumentView?docId=8+&releaseId=2
	ACR	ACR–AAPM–SIIM Practice Parameter for Determinants of Image Quality in Mammography (2022)	https://siim.org/resource/acr-aapm-siim-practice-parameter-for-determinants-of-image-quality-in-mammography-2022/
	ACR	ACR Practice Parameter for the Performance of Stereotactic/Tomosynthesis-Guided Breast Interventional Procedures (Revised 2024)	https://gravitas.acr.org/PPTS/GetDocumentView?docId=65+&releaseId=2
	US EPA	Federal Guidance Report no. 14: Radiation protection guidance for diagnostic and interventional X-ray procedures	https://www.epa.gov/radiation/federal-guidance-report-no-14-radiation-protection-guidance-diagnostic-and-interventional
	US FDA	Mammography quality standards act (MQSA) and MQSA program	https://www.fda.gov/radiation-emitting-products/mammography-quality-standards-act-mqsa-and-mqsa-program
	USPSTF	Final recommendation statement on breast cancer: Screening (April 30, 2024)	https://www.uspreventiveservicestaskforce.org/uspstf/recommendation/breast-cancer-screening#fullrecommendationstart
	NEMA	NEMA XR 22–2006 (R2020): Quality control manual template for manufacturers of displays and workstations labeled for final interpretation in full-field digital mammography (FFDM)	https://www.nema.org/standards/view/Quality-Control-Manual-Template-for-Manufacturers-of-Displays-and-Workstations-Labeled-for-Final-Interpretation-in-Full
	NEMA	NEMA XR 23–2006 (R2020): Quality control manual template for manufacturers of hardcopy output devices labeled for final interpretation in full-field digital mammography (FFDM)	https://www.nema.org/standards/view/Quality-Control-Manual-Template-for-Manufacturers-of-Hardcopy-Output-Devices-Labeled-for-Final-Interpretation-in-Full

(continued)

Table 8.1 (continued)

Imaging modality	Organization or agency	Publication	Link
Breast ultrasound	ACR	ACR practice parameter for the performance of a diagnostic breast ultrasound examination (Revised 2016)	https://flaus-us.org/arquivos/3-US-Breast.pdf
	ACR	Breast ultrasound accreditation program requirements	https://www.acr.org/accreditation/modalities/breast-ultrasound
	ACR	ACR Practice Parameter for the Performance of Ultrasound-Guided Percutaneous Breast Interventional Procedures (Revised 2021)	https://gravitas.acr.org/PPTS/GetDocumentView?docId=125+&releaseId=2
	AIUM	AIUM quality assurance manual for gray scale ultrasound scanners	http://aium.s3.amazonaws.com/resourceLibrary/14qa.pdf
	AIUM	AIUM: Standards and guidelines for the accreditation of ultrasound practices (June 16, 2020)	https://www.aium.org/resources/official-statements/view/standards-and-guidelines-for-the-accreditation-of-ultrasound-practices
	AIUM	AIUM practice guideline for the performance of a breast ultrasound examination	https://doi.org/10.7863/jum.2009.28.1.105
	AIUM	Medical ultrasound safety (MUS) manual	https://www.aium.org/resources/mus
	ASBS	The American Society of Breast Surgeons Performance and Practice Guidelines for breast ultrasound	https://www.breastsurgeons.org/docs/statements/Performance-and-Practice-Guidelines-for-Breast-Ultrasound.pdf
	NAPBC	National Accreditation Program for Breast Centers: Standards Manual (2018)	https://www.facs.org/media/pofgxojm/napbc_standards_manual_2018.pdf
Breast MRI	ACR	ACR MRI accreditation program	https://www.acraccreditation.org/modalities/mri
	ACR	Clinical image testing: MRI (revised 1-23-2025)	https://accreditationsupport.acr.org/support/solutions/articles/11000061017-clinical-image-testing-mri-revised-2-2-2024-
	ACR	ACR Practice Parameter for the Performance of Contrast-Enhanced Magnetic Resonance Imaging (MRI) of the Breast (Revised 2023)	https://gravitas.acr.org/PPTS/GetDocumentView?docId=6+&releaseId=2
	ACR	ACR Practice Parameter for the Performance of Magnetic Resonance Imaging-Guided Breast Interventional Procedures (Revised 2021)	https://gravitas.acr.org/PPTS/DownloadPreviewDocument?ReleaseId=2&DocId=123
	ACR	ACR Manual on Contrast Media (2024)	https://www.acr.org/Clinical-Resources/Clinical-Tools-and-Reference/Contrast-Manual
	ACR	ACR Manual on MR Safety (2024)	https://edge.sitecorecloud.io/americancoldf5f-acrorgf92a-productioncb02-3650/media/ACR/Files/Clinical/Radiology-Safety/Manual-on-MR-Safety.pdf
	ACR	ACS guidelines for breast screening with MRI as an adjunct to mammography	https://doi.org/10.3322/canjclin.57.2.75 https://acsjournals.onlinelibrary.wiley.com/doi/full/10.3322/canjclin.57.2.75
	IAC	IAC standards and guidelines for MRI accreditation	https://intersocietal.org/programs/mri/standards/

Abbreviations: *AAPM* American association of physicists in medicine, *ACR* American college of radiology, *ACS* American cancer society, *AIUM* American Institute of ultrasound in medicine, *ASBS* American society of breast surgeons, *IAC* intersocietal accreditation commission, *MR* magnetic resonance, *MRI* magnetic resonance imaging, *NAPBC* national accreditation program for breast centers, *NEMA* national electrical manufacturers association, *SIIM* society for imaging informatics in medicine, *SPR* society for pediatric radiology, *US EPA* United States environmental protection agency, *US FDA* US food and drug administration, *USPSTF* United States preventive services task force

Chapter Summary

This chapter provides an overview of breast imaging modalities and techniques, with a focus on quality, patient safety concerns, and strategies for improvement. It examines key imaging methods used in routine practice, including mammography, breast ultrasound, and breast MRI, outlining their roles, benefits, and limitations. The chapter also discusses risks associated with breast imaging, including radiation exposure, magnetic fields, contrast agents, and the safety of imaging-guided procedures, as well as special considerations for imaging pregnant patients. The emerging role of emerging techniques, like AI, in breast imaging is explored, along with its potential benefits and safety concerns. In addition, the chapter reviews QA and QC programs, regulatory guidelines, and industry efforts to improve imaging standards. A table summarizes key resources for quality and safety. While not exhaustive, this chapter provides essential insights into challenges and best practices for maintaining high-quality, safe breast imaging, with references for further reading.

Glossary

AAPM American Association of Physicists in Medicine
ACR American College of Radiology
ACS American Cancer Society
AI Artificial Intelligence
AIUM American Institute of Ultrasound in Medicine
ASBS American Society of Breast Surgeons
BEIR United States National Academy of Sciences Biologic Effects of Ionizing Radiation
CC Craniocaudal
CRCPD Conference of Radiation Control Program Directors
DEXA Dual-Energy X-ray Absorptiometry
EPA Environment Protection Agency
FDA US Food and Drug Administration
FFDM Full-Field Digital Mammography
IAC Intersocietal Accreditation Commission
ICRP International Commission on Radiological Protection
LAR Lifetime Attributable Risk
MGD Mean Glandular Dose
MLO Mediolateral Oblique
MQSA Mammography Quality Standards Act and Program
MRI Magnetic Resonance Imaging
NAPBC National Accreditation Program for Breast Centers
NEMA National Electrical Manufacturers Association
NHANES National Health and Nutrition Examination Survey
NRC Nuclear Regulatory Commission
NSF Nephrogenic systemic fibrosis
OSHA Occupational Safety and Health Administration
PEM Positron Emission Mammography
PNL Posterior Nipple Line
QA Quality Assurance
QC Quality Control
SFM Screen Film Mammography
SPR Society for Pediatric Radiology
SSR Society for Skeletal Radiology

References

1. Siegel RL, et al. Cancer statistics, 2023. CA Cancer J Clin. 2023;73(1):17–48.
2. US Preventive Services Task Force. Screening for breast cancer: US preventive services task force recommendation statement. JAMA. 2024;331(22):1918–30.
3. Van Steen A, Van Tiggelen R. Short history of mammography: a Belgian perspective. JBR-BTR. 2007;90:151–3.
4. Gennaro G, et al. Digital breast tomosynthesis versus digital mammography: a clinical performance study. Eur Radiol. 2010;20(7):1545–53.
5. Gennaro G, et al. Performance comparison of single-view digital breast tomosynthesis plus single-view digital mammography with two-view digital mammography. Eur Radiol. 2013;23(3):664–72.
6. Barton MK. Digital breast tomosynthesis may improve breast cancer detection rates. CA Cancer J Clin. 2013;63(5):291–2.
7. Brandt KR, et al. Can digital breast Tomosynthesis replace conventional diagnostic mammography views for screening recalls without calcifications? A comparison study in a simulated clinical setting. Am J Roentgenol. 2013;200(2):291–8.

8. Durand MA. Synthesized mammography: clinical evidence, appearance, and implementation. Diagnostics. 2018;8(2):22.
9. Hofvind S, et al. Digital breast tomosynthesis and synthetic 2D mammography versus digital mammography: evaluation in a population-based screening program. Radiology. 2018;287(3):787–94.
10. Suter MB, et al. Diagnostic accuracy of contrast-enhanced spectral mammography for breast lesions: a systematic review and meta-analysis. Breast. 2020;53:8–17.
11. Neeter L, et al. Comparing the diagnostic performance of contrast-enhanced mammography and breast MRI: a systematic review and meta-analysis. J Cancer. 2023;14(1):174–82.
12. Sehgal C, et al. A review of breast ultrasound. J Mammary Gland Biol Neoplasia. 2006;11(2):113–23.
13. Kuhl CK, et al. Mammography, breast ultrasound, and magnetic resonance imaging for surveillance of women at high familial risk for breast cancer. J Clin Oncol. 2005;23(33):8469–76.
14. Kelly K, et al. Breast cancer detection using automated whole breast ultrasound and mammography in radiographically dense breasts. Eur Radiol. 2010;20(3):734–42.
15. Nothacker M, et al. Early detection of breast cancer: benefits and risks of supplemental breast ultrasound in asymptomatic women with mammographically dense breast tissue. A systematic review. BMC Cancer. 2009;9(1):335.
16. Weinstein SP, Conant EF, Sehgal C. Technical advances in breast ultrasound imaging. Semin Ultrasound CT MRI. 2006;27(4):273–83.
17. DeMartini W, Lehman C, Partridge S. Breast MRI for cancer detection and characterization: a review of evidence-based clinical applications. Acad Radiol. 2008;15(4):408–16.
18. Eby PR, et al. Metabolic and vascular features of dynamic contrast-enhanced breast magnetic resonance imaging and 15O-water positron emission tomography blood flow in breast cancer. Acad Radiol. 2008;15(10):1246–54.
19. Sinha S, Sinha U. Recent advances in breast MRI and MRS. NMR Biomed. 2009;22(1):3–16.
20. Kuhl CK, et al. Abbreviated breast magnetic resonance imaging (MRI): first Postcontrast subtracted images and maximum-intensity projection – a novel approach to breast cancer screening with MRI. J Clin Oncol. 2014;32(22):2304–10.
21. Hendrick RE. Radiation doses and cancer risks from breast imaging studies. Radiology. 2010;257(1):246–53.
22. Hendrick RE, et al. Comparison of acquisition parameters and breast dose in digital mammography and screen-film mammography in the American College of Radiology Imaging Network digital mammographic imaging screening trial. AJR Am J Roentgenol. 2010;194(2):362–9.
23. Poplack SP, et al. Digital breast tomosynthesis: initial experience in 98 women with abnormal digital screening mammography. AJR Am J Roentgenol. 2007;189(3):616–23.
24. Uematsu T. The emerging role of breast tomosynthesis. Breast Cancer. 2013;20(3):204–12.
25. Feng SS, Sechopoulos I. Clinical digital breast tomosynthesis system: dosimetric characterization. Radiology. 2012;263(1):35–42.
26. American College of Radiology. ACR practice guideline for the performance of screening and diagnostic mammography; 2008.
27. American College of Radiology. ACR manual on MR safety; 2024.
28. Gimbel JR, et al. Safe scanning, but frequent artifacts mimicking bradycardia and tachycardia during magnetic resonance imaging (MRI) in patients with an implantable loop recorder (ILR). Ann Noninvasive Electrocardiol. 2005;10(4):404–8.
29. Wong JA, et al. Feasibility of magnetic resonance imaging in patients with an implantable loop recorder. Pacing Clin Electrophysiol. 2008;31(3):333–7.
30. van der Graaf AWM, Bhagirath P, Götte MJW. MRI and cardiac implantable electronic devices; current status and required safety conditions. Neth Hear J. 2014;22(6):269–76.
31. American College of Radiology Committee on Drugs and Contrast Media. ACR manual on contrast media. ACR; 2017.
32. Rogosnitzky M, Branch S. Gadolinium-based contrast agent toxicity: a review of known and proposed mechanisms. Biometals. 2016;29:365–76.
33. Fotenos A. FDA drug safety communication: FDA evaluating the risk of brain deposits with repeated use of gadolinium-based contrast agents for magnetic resonance imaging (MRI). Washington: FDA; 2017.
34. American College of Radiology. ACR practice parameter for the performance of a breast ultrasound examination. ACR; 2021.
35. Safety Group of the British Medical Ultrasound Society. Guidelines for the safe use of diagnostic ultrasound equipment. Ultrasound. 2010;18(2):52–9.
36. Brenner RJ, et al. Stereotactic core-needle breast biopsy: a multi-institutional prospective trial. Radiology. 2001;218(3):866–72.
37. Parker SH, et al. Percutaneous large-core breast biopsy: a multi-institutional study. Radiology. 1994;193(2):359–64.
38. Versaggi SL, De Leucio A. Stereotactic and needle breast biopsy; 2024. Available from: https://www.ncbi.nlm.nih.gov/books/NBK559147/
39. Schrading S, et al. Digital breast tomosynthesis–guided vacuum-assisted breast biopsy: initial experiences and comparison with prone stereotactic vacuum-assisted biopsy. Radiology. 2015;274(3):654–62.
40. Philpotts LE, Hooley RJ, Lee CH. Comparison of automated versus vacuum-assisted biopsy methods for sonographically guided core biopsy of the breast. Am J Roentgenol. 2003;180(2):347–51.
41. Jiang Y, et al. Mammotome(®) biopsy system for the resection of breast lesions: clinical experience in

two high-volume teaching hospitals. Exp Ther Med. 2013;6(3):759–64.
42. Gregg A, et al. Acquired arteriovenous fistula of the breast following ultrasound guided biopsy of invasive ductal carcinoma. J Clin Imaging Sci. 2013;3:38.
43. Mendelson EB. Artificial intelligence in breast imaging: potentials and limitations. Am J Roentgenol. 2019;212(2):293–9.
44. Hickman SE, Baxter GC, Gilbert FJ. Adoption of artificial intelligence in breast imaging: evaluation, ethical constraints and limitations. Br J Cancer. 2021;125(1):15–22.
45. Wang X, et al. Inconsistent performance of deep learning models on mammogram classification. J Am Coll Radiol. 2020;17(6):796–803.
46. Morgan MB, Mates JL. Ethics of artificial intelligence in breast imaging. J Breast Imaging. 2023;5(2):195–200.
47. diFlorio-Alexander RM, et al. ACR appropriateness criteria(®) breast imaging of pregnant and lactating women. J Am Coll Radiol. 2018;15(11s):S263–s275.
48. Peterson MS, et al. Breast imaging and intervention during pregnancy and lactation. Radiographics. 2023;43(10):e230014.
49. Aurela Clark M, Xiaoqin Wang, El Khouli R. Quality and safety in medical imaging during pregnancy and lactation –part I. Appl Radiol. 2024;5:4–14.
50. Monsees BS. The mammography quality standards act: an overview of THE regulations and guidance. Radiol Clin North Am. 2000;38(4):759–72.
51. American College of Radiology. ACR–AAPM–SIIM practice parameter for determinants of image quality in digital mammography; 2022.
52. Ayyala RS, et al. Digital mammographic artifacts on full-field systems: what are they and how do I fix them? Radiographics. 2008;28(7):1999–2008.
53. Caumo F, et al. Incremental effect from integrating 3D-mammography (tomosynthesis) with 2D-mammography: increased breast cancer detection evident for screening centres in a population-based trial. Breast. 2014;23(1):76–80.
54. Rose SL, et al. Implementation of breast tomosynthesis in a routine screening practice: an observational study. Am J Roentgenol. 2013;200(6):1401–8.
55. Haas BM, et al. Comparison of tomosynthesis plus digital mammography and digital mammography alone for breast cancer screening. Radiology. 2013;269(3):694–700.
56. Ciatto S, et al. Integration of 3D digital mammography with tomosynthesis for population breast-cancer screening (STORM): a prospective comparison study. Lancet Oncol. 2013;14(7):583–9.
57. Timberg P, et al. In-plane visibility of lesions using breast tomosynthesis and digital mammography. Med Phys. 2010;37(11):5618–26.
58. Siegel E, et al. Digital mammography image quality: image display. J Am Coll Radiol. 2006;3(8):615–27.
59. Norweck JT, et al. ACR–AAPM–SIIM technical standard for electronic practice of medical imaging. J Digit Imaging. 2013;26(1):38–52.
60. Kanal KM, et al. ACR-AAPM-SIIM practice guideline for determinants of image quality in digital mammography. J Digit Imaging. 2013;26(1):10–25.
61. Radiology, A.C.O. ACR Practice parameter for the performance of whole-breast ultrasound for screening and staging. Revised 2024 (Resolution 10).
62. Cho N, et al. Aliasing artifact depicted on ultrasound (US)-elastography for breast cystic lesions mimicking solid masses. Acta Radiol. 2011;52(1):3–7.
63. Kang J, et al. Real-time ultrasound detection of breast microcalcifications using multifocus twinkling artifact imaging. IEEE Trans Med Imaging. 2022;41(5):1300–8.
64. Relea A, et al. Usefulness of the twinkling artifact on Doppler ultrasound for the detection of breast microcalcifications. Radiologia (Engl Ed). 2018;60(5):413–23.
65. Asik M, Erdem G, Gezgin M. A novel color Doppler ultrasound artifact for identifying breast and axilla tumor markers: blooming-like artifact. Acad Radiol. 2024;
66. Harvey JA, et al. Breast MR imaging artifacts: how to recognize and fix them. Radiographics. 2007;27(suppl_1):S131–45.
67. Kapsner LA, et al. Prevalence and influencing factors for artifact development in breast MRI-derived maximum intensity projections. Acta Radiol. 2023;64(11):2881–90.
68. Bitencourt AGV, et al. Susceptibility artifact at breast MRI due to retained fragment of localization hookwire hiding breast cancer. Breast J. 2021;27(5):481–3.
69. Derakhshan JJ, et al. Characterizing and eliminating errors in enhancement and subtraction artifacts in dynamic contrast-enhanced breast MRI: chemical shift artifact of the third kind. Magn Reson Med. 2018;79(4):2277–89.
70. Slonimsky E, et al. Intravenous line phase-wrap artifact at bilateral axial 3-T breast MRI: identification, analysis, and solution. Radiol Imaging Cancer. 2020;2(6):e200004.
71. Bickelhaupt S, et al. Lesion-mimicking DIXON swap artifact in contrast-enhanced subtraction breast MRI. Radiol Case Rep. 2024;19(11):4921–4.
72. Farria DM, et al. Mammography quality assurance from a to Z. Radiographics. 1994;14(2):371–85.
73. American College of Radiology. ACR practice parameter for the performance of screening and diagnostic mammography; 2023.
74. U.S. Food and Drug Administration. Mammography quality standards act (MQSA) and MQSA program; 2024. Available from: https://www.fda.gov/radiation--emitting-products/mammography-quality-standards-act-mqsa-and-mqsa-program.
75. US Food and Drug Administration. Important information: final rule to amend the mammography quality standards act (MQSA); 2024. Available from: https://www.fda.gov/radiation-emitting-products/mammography-quality-standards-act-mqsa-and-mqsa-program/important-information-final-rule-amend-mammography-quality-standards-act-mqsa.

76. Destouet JM, et al. The ACR'S mammography accreditation program: ten years of experience since MQSA. J Am Coll Radiol. 2005;2(7):585–94.
77. Greer LRN. The benefits of using synthesized 2D (C-view™) images in breast tomosynthesis exams. Appl Radiol. 2014;11(5):1–4.
78. Nelson JS, et al. How does c-view image quality compare with conventional 2D FFDM? Med Phys. 2016;43(5):2538.
79. Kelly KM, et al. Breast cancer detection using automated whole breast ultrasound and mammography in radiographically dense breasts. Eur Radiol. 2010;20(3):734–42.
80. Boca Bene I, et al. Pros and cons for automated breast ultrasound (ABUS): a narrative review. J Pers Med. 2021;11(8)
81. Du W, et al. Conformable ultrasound breast patch for deep tissue scanning and imaging. Sci Adv. 2023;9(30):eadh5325.
82. Brahim M, et al. Automated assessment of breast positioning quality in screening mammography. Cancers (Basel). 2022;14(19)

Nuclear Medicine and Molecular Imaging

9

Jie Zhang, Blaine T. Mischen, and M. Elizabeth Oates

Abbreviations

AAPM	American Association of Physicists in Medicine
ACR	American College of Radiology
AIUM	American Institute of Ultrasound in Medicine
CR	Computed Radiography
CT	Computed Tomography
CTDI	Computed Tomography Dose Index
COR	Center of Rotation
CRCPD	Conference of Radiation Control Program Directors
DR	Digital Radiography
EPA	U.S. Environmental Protection Agency
FDA	U.S. Food and Drug Administration
HU	Hounsfield Unit
IAEA	International Atomic Energy Agency
ICRP	International Commission on Radiological Protection
IEC	International Electrotechnical Commission
IMRSER	The Institute for Magnetic Resonance Safety, Education, and Research
MIRD	Medical Internal Radiation Dose
NCRP	National Council on Radiation Protection and Measurements
NEMA	National Electrical Manufacturers Association
NM	Nuclear Medicine
NRC	U. S. Nuclear Regulatory Commission
MRI	Magnetic Resonance Imaging
OSHA	Occupational Safety and Health Administration
PET	Positron Emission Tomography
QA	Quality Assurance
QC	Quality Control
SID	Source-to-Image Receptor Distance
SPECT	Single-Photon Emission Computed Tomography
SNMMI	Society of Nuclear Medicine and Molecular Imaging
TOF	Time of Flight
US	Ultrasound

Introduction

Nuclear medicine (NM)/molecular imaging (MI) is a branch of medical imaging that uses small amounts of radioactive materials (radiopharmaceuticals) to diagnose and assess the severity of various diseases, including cancers, heart disease, and disorders of the gastrointestinal, genitourinary, endocrine, and neurological systems,

J. Zhang (✉) · B. T. Mischen · M. E. Oates
Department of Radiology, University of Kentucky, Lexington, KY, USA
e-mail: jnzh222@uky.edu; blaine.mischen@uky.edu; meoate2@uky.edu

J. Zhang (ed.), *Quality and Patient Safety in Medical Imaging*,
https://doi.org/10.1007/978-3-031-89007-9_9

among others. NM/MI provides insights into physiological processes by visualizing the biodistribution of radiopharmaceuticals in patients.

In NM/MI procedures, radioisotopes are combined with other elements or compounds to form radiopharmaceuticals. These radiopharmaceuticals are administered to patients orally, intravenously, Intraarterially, intradermally, intrathecally, or by inhalation. Once the radiopharmaceutical has distributed itself according to the physiological status of the patient (biodistribution), a radiation detector, such as a gamma camera or a PET scanner, is used to capture photons emitted from the radiopharmaceutical during its radioactive decay, thereby localizing the biodistribution to specific organs, organ systems, or cellular (molecular) receptors. NM/MI is a form of functional imaging with the ability to image the extent of a disease process in the human body, based on cellular and physiological functions, rather than relying solely on physical changes in the tissue anatomy.

The imaging modalities in NM/MI include planar imaging (using a scintillation gamma camera), single-photon emission computed tomography (SPECT), and positron emission tomography (PET). These methods use gamma rays, characteristic x-rays, or annihilation photons to generate images. The charged particles from radioactivity within a patient are mostly absorbed by the patient's tissues, minimizing external radiation exposure. Nowadays, these tomographic functional modalities are integrated with the anatomical modalities of computed tomography or magnetic resonance imaging (SPECT/CT, PET/CT, and PET/MRI).

This chapter aims to address key quality and safety issues across various NM/MI modalities, explaining each technology's fundamental principles and associated safety concerns. It highlights the importance of rigorous QC measures for the equipment to ensure high imaging standards and patient safety. The chapter also discusses ongoing efforts to enhance quality and safety, such as the Image Gently and Image Wisely campaigns, which promote responsible imaging practices and reduced radiation exposures. Overall, the chapter emphasizes the need for continual improvement in NM/MI.

Fundamental Principles of Nuclear Medicine/Molecular Imaging

NM/MI primarily involves administering radiopharmaceuticals (also known as radiotracers) orally or via intravascular injection, which then circulate and localize in specific organs or tissues. These radiotracers emit radiation, allowing external detection instruments to track and analyze their biodistribution. The resulting data, displayed as planar or tomographic images or cines, often with quantitative analysis (numbers, curves), reveal both the morphology and function of the organs.

The diagnostic mechanism in NM/MI hinges on how the body processes the diagnostic or therapeutic radiopharmaceuticals differently in various normal or pathological conditions. Radioisotopes, such as the commonly used ^{99m}Tc with its optimal imaging properties, are chemically bound to compounds that target specific body functions, forming radiopharmaceuticals (radiotracers). The presence of a disease usually alters the biodistribution or processing of these radiotracers. For example, methylene diphosphonate (MDP), which has a high affinity for bone, can be combined with ^{99m}Tc. This radiopharmaceutical, ^{99m}Tc-MDP, accumulates in the skeletal system, particularly in areas of heightened osteoblastic activity related to metastases, fractures, and metabolic bone disorders, appearing as "hot spots" of increased radiotracer concentration. Conversely, purely osteoclastic or lytic disease processes result in photopenic areas, or "cold spots."

The end product of this process is a "dataset" of one or more images. In dynamic datasets, the image array forms a time series showing a spatial sequence as the gamma camera captures the movement of the radiotracer within the body or organ system. In SPECT or SPECT/CT, rotating gamma camera images are reconstructed into image slices that provide a 3D view of the biodistribution within the patient's body.

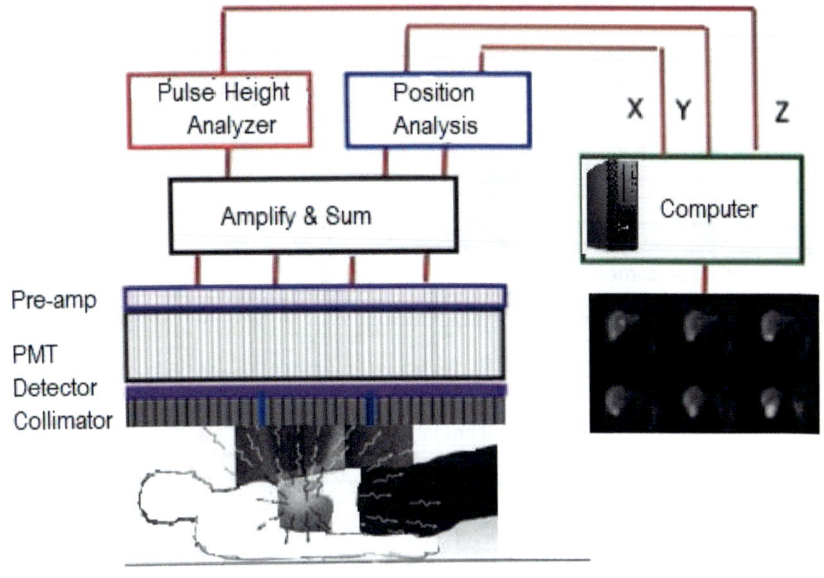

Fig. 9.1 Imaging chain of gamma camera

Gamma Camera

The gamma camera, also known as a scintillation or anger camera, is an essential device in NM/MI, designed to visualize gamma radiation from radiotracers administered to patients. It is widely used in drug development and medical diagnosis.

The imaging chain of a gamma camera (Fig. 9.1) begins with a key component, the sodium iodide crystal. This large, thin crystal is engineered to absorb gamma rays and convert them into visible light. The light is then detected by an array of photomultiplier tubes (PMTs), which transform the light into electronic pulses. These pulses undergo two primary processes: an energy pulse is created by summing the signals from the PMTs and the X and Y coordinates of the radiation event are calculated using position-dependent weighting factors.

The gamma rays from the radiopharmaceutical in each volume of a patient's body are emitted in all directions. To form a projection image, collimators have to be used to permit photons following certain trajectories to reach the detector and to absorb other scattered, off-axis photons. Most commonly, a parallel-hole collimator is used; it consists of numerous hexagonal holes separated by lead septa. The pinhole collimator allows for close proximity of the detector to a small region of interest, resulting in a magnified and inverted image, with increased spatial resolution. Collimation limits the performance of the scintillation camera since most emitted photons are wasted.

The crystal in the camera, generally 40–55 cm in diameter and 9.5 mm thick, must be hermetically sealed to prevent moisture absorption, as it is hygroscopic. The intensity of the scintillation produced in the crystal is directly proportional to the energy of the absorbed gamma ray. This scintillation is then converted into an electronic signal by the PMTs, where light induces electron emission, which is amplified through dynodes.

The pulse height analyzer plays a pivotal role in determining the energy of the detected event. It analyzes the signal, which is proportional to the gamma-ray energy, and sets an energy window to exclude scattered radiation, thereby enhancing image quality.

In modern systems, the imaging data from the gamma camera is digitally processed. The X and Y coordinates are stored in a computer matrix, with each detected event incrementally updating the matrix. This digital approach allows for the accumulation of detailed and precise data, leading to the formation of high-quality images that accurately represent the biodistribution of radiotracers within the patient's body.

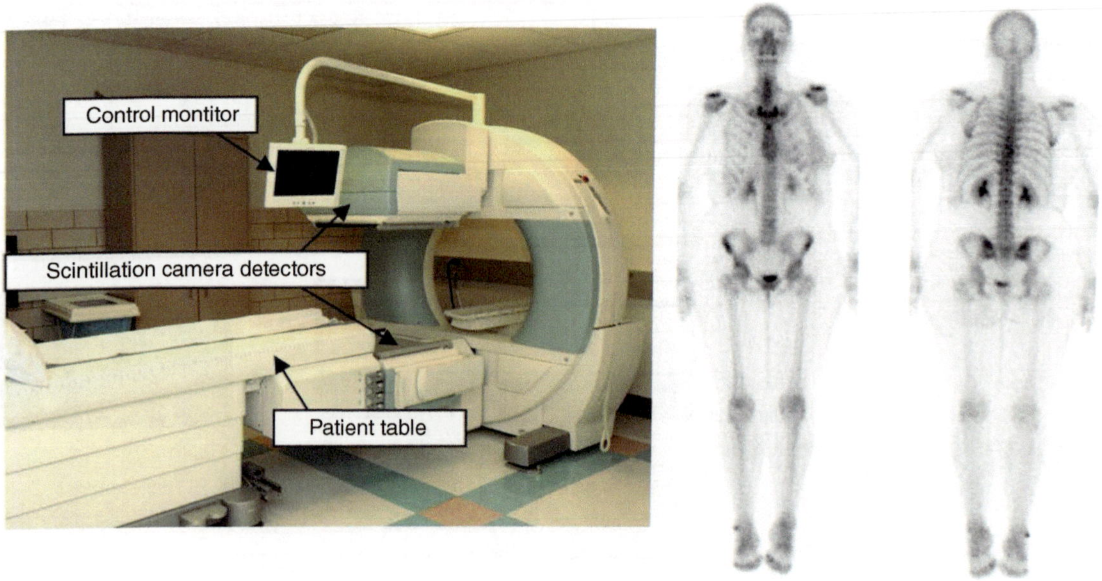

Fig. 9.2 A modern dual-detector scintillation camera and representative anterior and posterior whole-body bone images of a patient with left breast cancer. The patient was injected with 24.6 mCi of ^{99m}Tc- MDP intravenously and imaged approximately 3 h later

The scintillation camera can also be flexibly positioned to generate images from almost any angle. Figure 9.2 shows a modern dual rectangular head scintillation camera and representative anterior and posterior whole-body bone scan images. Planar imaging is still the standard for many NM/MI examinations such as whole-body bone scans, hepatobiliary, thyroid, renal, and pulmonary studies.

Single-Photon Emission Computed Tomography (SPECT) or SPECT/CT

Beyond the capabilities of traditional gamma cameras, which are limited to planar 2D imaging, SPECT produces enhanced resolution by accurately locating the radiotracer in 3D. This precision is critical when navigating complex anatomical structures.

The creation of 3D SPECT images involves intricate mathematical reconstruction of data from a gamma camera that revolves around the patient, capturing gamma rays emitted as the radiotracer decays. In SPECT, the systematic acquisition of data includes capturing a series of images, or projections, at multiple evenly spaced angles around the patient. These images are taken with the patient positioned so that the rotation axis aligns with their longitudinal body axis, creating a circular or semicircular arc as shown in Fig. 9.3. Typically, these projections encompass either a full 360-degree rotation or a 180-degree semicircle, with the number of projections varying from 50 to 150 based on the imaged area's size, the SPECT system's spatial resolution capabilities, and the number of detector heads.

SPECT requires capturing projection images from multiple angles around the patient. This is achieved by a gamma camera capable of rotating in a circular or elliptical path around the patient. A notable constraint of this rotating gamma camera system is its low sensitivity. The need for absorptive collimation to ascertain the trajectory of the interacting photons means that only a minimal share of the photons released by the patient are detected by the camera. Although using tighter collimation can enhance spatial resolution, it does so at the expense of sensitivity, resulting in increased noise in the image. One simple way to improve sensitivity is by increasing the number of detectors. Accordingly, dual-detector and multi-detector systems [1] have been introduced, which are more prevalent in modern practice.

The reconstruction process in SPECT is both complex and vital. Traditional methods like filtered backprojection (FBP) integrate projections into a comprehensive image. This method employs windowing functions to control the sharpness and noise levels. However, newer systems increasingly use iterative reconstruction (IR) methods, which begin with an initial estimate of the biodistribution and refine it through successive comparisons with actual projections. IR methods incorporate detailed models of data acquisition physics and noise, leading to more accurate image reconstructions.

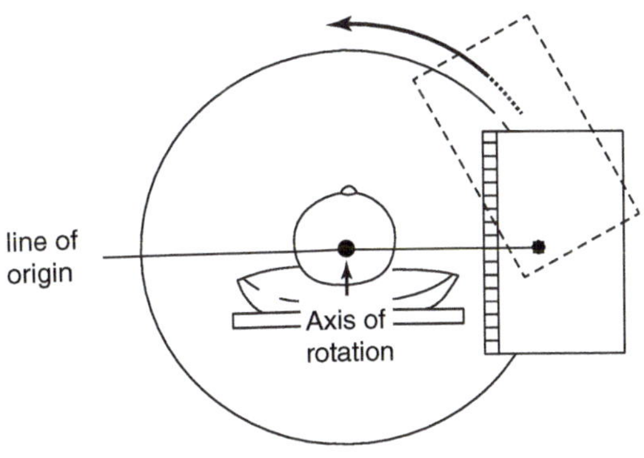

Fig. 9.3 A diagram demonstrating SPECT acquisition

Attenuation correction in SPECT imaging is essential for accurate quantification. It compensates for the variable absorption of photons by different tissues. Uniform attenuation correction is used for areas with constant tissue density, while nonuniform correction is necessary for heterogeneous areas like the thorax. Nonuniform correction requires detailed knowledge of internal tissue composition obtained through transmission images from an external photon source, enhancing the reliability of SPECT images.

Integrated (hybrid) SPECT/CT systems, which combine SPECT with helical CT scans, are increasingly common and are rapidly becoming the standard. They provide more precise attenuation correction and can generate diagnostic-quality CT images for a more comprehensive analysis. The CT component assists in characterizing internal materials for accurate nonuniform attenuation correction, although adjustments are needed due to the differing photon energies between CT and SPECT. These hybrid systems significantly improve diagnostic capabilities, offering a more integrated approach to imaging analysis. Figure 9.4 shows a typical SPECT/CT system and representative SPECT cardiac perfusion images.

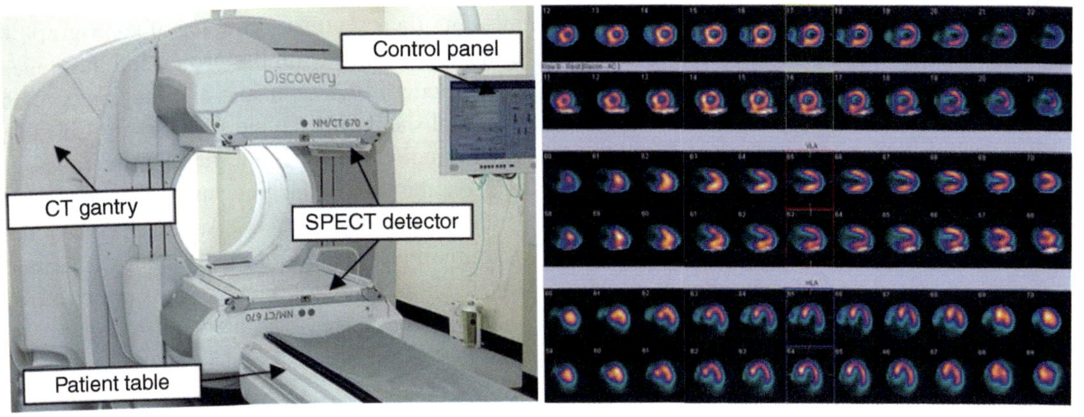

Fig. 9.4 A combined single-photon emission computed tomography/computed tomography (SPECT/CT) imaging system and representative stress-rest myocardial perfusion images of a patient. CT was used for attenuation correction. The patient was injected with 7.3 mCi of ^{99m}Tc sestamibi at rest and 22.3 mCi at peak stress. Attenuation correction was applied to mitigate the inferior wall attenuation artifact caused by the diaphragm

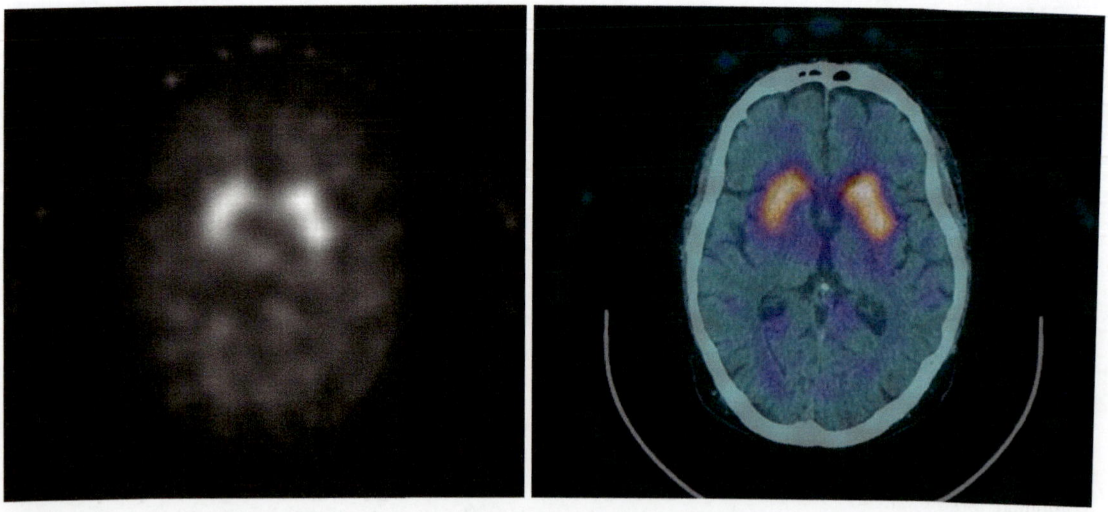

Fig. 9.5 SPECT/CT brain scan (5.9 mCi of ^{123}I ioflupane (DaTscan)). Normal uptake within the basal ganglia, not consistent with Parkinson's disease or other presynaptic Parkinsonian conditions

The ability of SPECT to accurately pinpoint locations within a 3D space renders it exceptionally useful for evaluating localized functions in internal organs. This attribute is particularly advantageous in detailed functional imaging of the heart and brain, where comprehending the spatial dynamics of organ function is vital. Figure 9.5 shows an NM/MI scan with SPECT/CT (^{123}I ioflupane, DaTscan) of a normal brain; the biodistribution pattern is not consistent with Parkinson's disease or other presynaptic Parkinsonian conditions.

Positron Emission Tomography (PET) or PET/CT

Positron emission tomography (PET) is an NM/MI technique that produces a 3D image of functional processes in the body. Positrons are positively charged particles emitted from some radioisotopes (e.g., ^{18}F). These radioisotopes can be combined with metabolically relevant compounds and administered to patients. The positron produced by the decay of the radioisotope combines with electrons from the surrounding tissues, and the mass of both is converted into two photons with directionality almost exactly 180 degrees from each other. This process is called annihilation and the emitted energy is called annihilation radiation. A PET scanner utilizes rings of detectors to detect the photon pairs produced during annihilation. Analogous to SPECT systems, PET systems then reconstruct a set of tomographic emission images from the projection data.

In modern PET scanners, 3D imaging is often accomplished with the aid of an x-ray CT scan performed on the patient during the same session and on the same machine, using an integrated (hybrid) PET/CT system. As for SPECT, the combination of PET with CT enables anatomic localization of abnormalities and correction of the emission images for attenuation. Figure 9.6

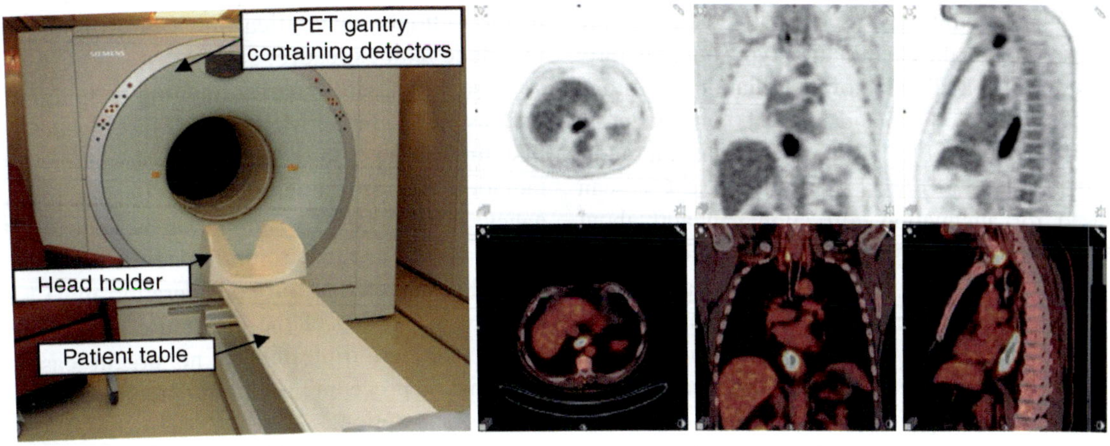

Fig. 9.6 A dual-modality positron emission tomography/computed tomography (PET/CT) imaging scanner with representative PET images (top row) and fused PET/CT images (bottom row) of the chest/upper abdomen. The patient was injected with 12.8 mCi ^{18}F FDG intravenously, followed by an incubation period of 58 minutes. A low-dose CT scan was performed for attenuation correction and anatomic localization

shows a PET/CT system and a set of PET and fused PET/CT images. PET has clinical advantages for certain diagnoses and the combined PET/CT systems have applications in cardiology, neurology, infection, inflammation, and oncology [2–5].

Safety Concerns in Nuclear Medicine/Molecular Imaging

Different from x-ray imaging, nuclear imaging depends on radioactive materials administered to the patient. Radioactivity may create a radiation hazard wherever it is used, stored, or discarded. Any radiation dose from radioactive materials inhaled, swallowed, or absorbed through the skin is called internal radiation dose. In NM/MI, internal radiation dose, as well as spill and disposal of radioactive materials, pose quality, patient, and personnel safety concerns.

Internal Radiation Dose and Administered Activity

A patient undergoing an NM/MI procedure will receive a radiation dose. The Medical Internal Radiation Dose (MIRD) committee develops standard methods, models, assumptions, and mathematical schema for assessing internal radiation doses from administered radiopharmaceuticals. Effective doses for adults for various NM/MI examinations vary significantly, from 0.2 mSv to 40.7 mSv, depending on the procedure and administered activity [6]. For a lung ventilation scan with ^{99m}Tc DTPA (diethylenetriaminepentaacetic acid), a very small radiation dose (0.2 mSv, similar to a chest x-ray) is delivered to the patient with an administered activity of 1300 MBq (megabecquerels, approximately 35 mCi) via nebulizer. The majority of the activity does not make it into the lungs, with the rest being swallowed by the patient, remaining in the nebulizer system, or dispersed into the room. For a cardiac stress-rest examination with ^{99m}Tc sestamibi or ^{99m}Tc tetrofosmin, a patient's effective dose is approximately **9–12 mSv** for an administered activity of **740–1110 MBq (20–30 mCi)**. While thallium-201 (^{201}Tl) chloride was historically used, the ^{99m}Tc radiopharmaceuticals have become more prevalent due to the lower radiation dose and better imaging characteristics. However, ^{201}Tl chloride may still be mentioned as it is occasionally used in specific clinical situations.

The dose for PET typically involves positron-emitting radiopharmaceuticals like ^{18}F FDG, with an effective dose usually around 8 mSv for adults, depending on the injected activity and imaging protocol. For SPECT, radiotracers labeled with

^{99m}Tc are commonly used, with doses varying depending on the examination type, but generally resulting in a slightly lower radiation dose than PET. On the other hand, the CT component of PET/CT and SPECT/CT contributes an additional radiation dose [7]. A low-dose CT scan used for attenuation correction can add about 1–7 mSv depending on the scan parameters [8]. However, a diagnostic-quality CT can deliver significantly higher doses, sometimes up to 30 mSv, especially when imaging larger body areas. For pediatric patients, it is particularly important to minimize the CT dose by using weight-based protocols and advanced dose reduction techniques to ensure diagnostic accuracy with minimal radiation exposure [9, 10].

The patient's effective dose is determined by the physical properties of the radiopharmaceutical, its route of administration (e.g., inhalation, ingestion, or vascular injection), the amount of administered activity, the rate of clearance from the body, and patient-specific factors. Details for the radiation dose for various NM/MI procedures and radioisotopes can be found in references [6, 11–14].

Imaging in Pregnancy

NM/MI in pregnancy presents significant safety concerns due to potential radiation exposure to both the mother and the fetus. Radiopharmaceuticals used in these procedures emit ionizing radiation, which can be harmful to fetal development, especially during early gestation when cells are rapidly dividing. One major concern is the possibility that radiopharmaceuticals can cross the placenta and deliver radiation to the fetus, which increases the risk of developmental defects, miscarriage, or long-term effects, such as a higher likelihood of cancer.

The choice of radiopharmaceutical is crucial. For example, iodine-131 (^{131}I) poses particular risks since it can cross the placenta and concentrate in the fetal thyroid, especially after 12 weeks of gestation, potentially leading to hypothyroidism or other developmental issues. To mitigate such risks, radiopharmaceuticals with lower fetal uptake and shorter half-lives should be used where possible, and the dosage of the radiopharmaceutical must be minimized to reduce fetal exposure.

In such cases, alternative imaging techniques, such as ultrasound or MRI, should be considered first line because they do not involve ionizing radiation and are generally safer during pregnancy. If an NM/MI examination is necessary, efforts should be made to minimize the administered dosage, and careful consideration must be given to the timing of the procedure, especially during the first trimester. In nonurgent cases, delaying the procedure until after pregnancy may be the safest option.

Pregnant patients should be thoroughly informed of the risks and benefits, and proper counseling must be provided to help them make informed decisions. Written and verbal guidance should be given on how to reduce radiation exposure if the procedure is unavoidable. Post-procedure fetal dose assessments may be required to ensure that exposure remains below the recommended safety limits, typically aiming for a fetal dose below 1 mSv according to current guidelines.

Recent guidelines by the International Commission on Radiological Protection (ICRP) and the National Council on Radiation Protection and Measurements (NCRP) provide specific recommendations for managing radiation exposure during pregnancy, emphasizing the need to keep fetal exposure as low as reasonably achievable (ALARA). These guidelines have been updated to reflect contemporary radiopharmaceutical use and safety standards in NM/MI [15, 16].

Pediatric Imaging

In pediatric NM/MI, special attention is given to optimizing the radiation dose. This is typically done through weight-based or age-based adjustments in the administered radiopharmaceutical dosage, ensuring the lowest possible dosage that still produces diagnostically useful images. Guidelines from organizations such as the Society of Nuclear Medicine and Molecular Imaging (SNMMI) provide specific dosage recommendations for pediatric patients to balance the need for diagnostic accuracy with radiation safety [17].

Techniques such as iterative reconstruction, which helps reduce image noise without increasing the radiation dose to the patient, play a critical role in pediatric NM/MI. Furthermore, hybrid imaging modalities like SPECT/CT and PET/CT enable practitioners to acquire functional and anatomical information in a single scan, reducing the need for multiple imaging procedures [18]. Protocols to optimize scan times and reduce motion artifacts, especially in younger children who may have difficulty remaining still during imaging, are also essential in ensuring high-quality images and accurate diagnoses [19, 20]. These tailored approaches help improve the safety and effectiveness of NM/MI procedures for pediatric patients.

Release of Individuals After the Administration of Radioisotopes

Patients who undergo imaging procedures involving radioactive materials may be released from medical supervision if certain conditions are met. The decision to release a patient is typically based on the estimated radiation dose that could be received by the public, particularly those in close contact with the patient, such as family members or caregivers. International bodies like the ICRP [21] and the NCRP [22] provide guidelines for this practice, but specific dose limits vary between countries. For example, limits in the United States differ from those in Europe and Canada.

Before releasing a patient, the licensee (medical facility or practitioner) must evaluate factors such as the amount of radioactive material administered, the patient's living situation, and possible exposure pathways to others. If the estimated radiation exposure is within regulatory limits, the patient can be released. In the United States, these practices are governed by 10 CFR 35.75 [23], which allows for patient release when it is determined that no member of the public will receive more than 5 mSv of radiation from the patient. If the estimated dose to the most exposed individual exceeds 1 mSv, the patient must receive written instructions on how to reduce radiation exposure to others. Special considerations are given to breastfeeding/lactating patients, who may be instructed to interrupt or stop breastfeeding/lactation to prevent exposing their child to radiation if the dose could exceed 1 mSv.

For NM/MI procedures which typically involve lower doses of radiation, patients are often not required to follow strict guidelines unless specific circumstances apply, such as breastfeeding/lactation. Diagnostic procedures generally do not require formal documentation of release instructions, though exceptions are made for particular cases, such as high-dose therapies or when radioactive materials remain in the body for an extended period.

The decision to release a patient is influenced by several factors, including the type of radiopharmaceutical used, the dosage administered, and the patient's ability to follow safety instructions. While the primary concern is the radiation dose to the most exposed individual, other factors such as the patient's living conditions and health status are also considered.

Although patients receive detailed instructions, it is important to note that they are not legally required to follow them, and no regulatory agency enforces patient compliance. The responsibility for following the recommendations rests with the patient, and the licensee cannot be held accountable if instructions are not followed.

For additional guidance, reference documents such as **NUREG-1556 Vol. 9, Rev. 3** [24] provide comprehensive protocols for the release of patients who have undergone imaging with radioactive materials, ensuring safety while allowing patients to return to their daily lives.

Radioactive Material Spill

During NM/MI procedures, spills of radioactive materials may occasionally occur. These spills are categorized as either major or minor, depending on the amount of material involved and the specific radioisotope. For example, a spill of ^{131}I involving less than 1 mCi is classified as a minor spill, while spills greater than 1 mCi are considered major spills. Similarly, for ^{99m}Tc, spills under 100 mCi are classified as minor, and those over 100 mCi as major. For isotopes such as ^{111}In and ^{67}Ga, spills greater than 10 mCi are considered major.

Every imaging facility must have a detailed safety protocol in place to handle radioactive material spills. These spills can lead to external contamination or accidental intake of radioactivity, such as inhalation. While minor spills generally pose a low radiation hazard, major spills can lead to significant contamination risks. Therefore, ensuring the safety of both patients and staff in the event of a spill within the NM/MI suite or during an NM/MI procedure is critical.

Quality Control Program

QC in Scintillation Gamma Camera

Routine monitoring of the quality and reproducibility of NM/MI instruments is an essential part of any clinical NM/MI program. There is no difference from other imaging modalities; the QC of an NM/MI instrument begins with its selection, site planning, and environmental constraints. Information concerning the QC of gamma cameras is summarized below. Detailed information can be found in references [25–27].

A scintillation camera requires frequent (daily, weekly, monthly, annual) QC. A QC manual should be available for each type of equipment, specifying the methods and frequency of testing. The recommended schedule for routine QC testing of a scintillation camera includes daily check of energy discrimination window, daily extrinsic or intrinsic low-count uniformity images of all camera detectors, and daily visual inspection of collimators for damage. These daily QC activities should be done before the first use each day. High count density extrinsic or intrinsic uniformity images of each camera detector, spatial resolution with bar or hole pattern, and efficiency of each camera detector should be tested weekly to monthly. Pixel size, head tilt angle, and extrinsic uniformity images should be checked quarterly. Each camera should have a complete evaluation at least annually, including all the listed items and multi-energy spatial registration and count-rate performance.

The uniformity of the scintillation camera can be assessed using a ^{99m}Tc point source, or a ^{57}Co planar source, or a fillable flood source. Sufficient counts have to be contained in the uniformity image in case quantum mottle masks uniformity defects. The spatial resolution is usually evaluated using a four-quadrant bar phantom placed on the camera (Fig. 9.7). The phantom should be imaged four times with a 90-degree rotation to evaluate all quadrants of the camera. Counting rate characterizes a scintillation camera's ability to function accurately at counting rates close to the maximum rate of camera operation. The test is usually performed with the source at the same distance. Then, the counting rate is calculated by recording the number of counts and counting time. Counting rate should be tested annually, or after any major repair, or any indicated significant change in dead time.

QC in SPECT or SPECT/CT

As presented above, SPECT is a rotating scintillation gamma camera system, performed with the same device as planar imaging. Therefore, the QC for the scintillation gamma camera applies to SPECT. Besides, there are several specific additional considerations for the QC in SPECT, including determination of field uniformity variations and their correction, the center of rotation, pixel size, camera-table alignment, and planar and transaxial resolution [25]. QC is critical to SPECT since malfunctions or maladjustments can markedly degrade image quality and, even worse, some artifacts may mimic pathology.

The test of field uniformity is to assure the uniformity of camera response. The camera uniformity should be controlled to within ±1%. Since the reconstruction algorithm tends to amplify the effects of nonuniformities, uniformity during rotation should also be performed. For example, a ring artifact caused by incomplete projections from a 360-degree arc may be inter-

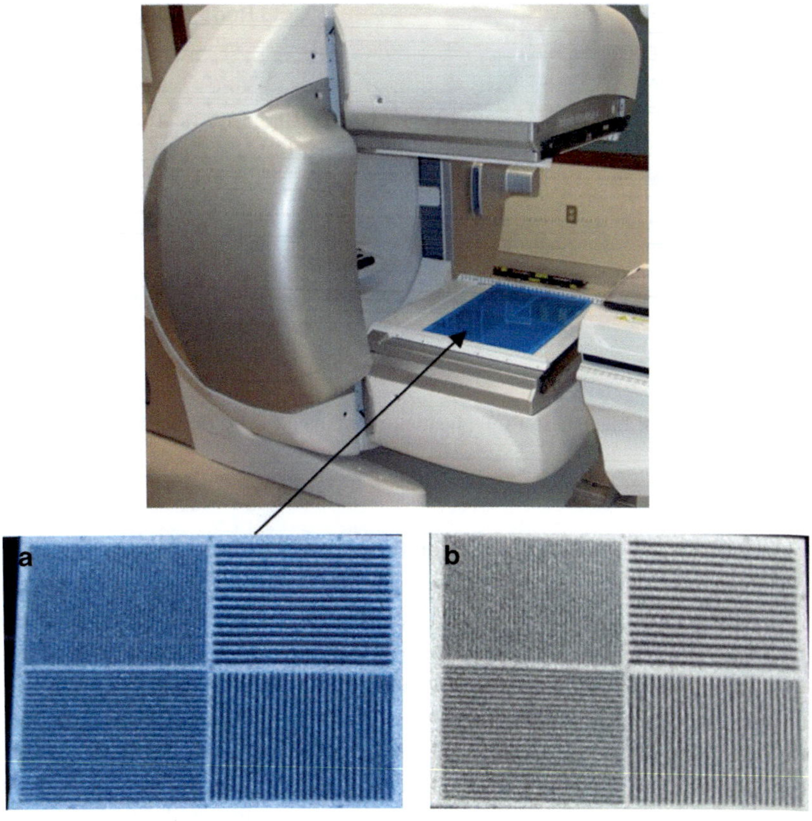

Fig. 9.7 Evaluation of spatial resolution of the scintillation camera using a four-quadrant bar phantom (**a**) and its associated image (**b**)

preted as high count density. It is very harmful, especially in examinations such as myocardial perfusion images with poor counting statistics and large variations in count density since the ring artifact may not be recognized at all.

The center of rotation (COR) is a critical factor in proper tomographic reconstruction, since the location of the COR is used to correctly calculate the 3D activity biodistribution from the projection images. In practice, the COR may vary from the mechanical axis due to variations in camera alignment and other effects. An uncorrected COR misalignment can cause a loss of spatial resolution and generate artifacts. Scintillation gamma camera vendors generally provide software to assess and correct COR misalignment and its effects.

Other tests are pixel sizing and spatial resolution. The effective size of the individual pixels must be known because most attenuation correction algorithms require projection path lengths through the body to function properly and because size and volume determination requires information of pixel size to scale image accurately.

QC in PET

The ACR accreditation program recommends that the QC testing for PET be performed in accordance with the ACR Technical Standard for Medical Nuclear Physics Performance Monitoring of PET Imaging Equipment [28]. The performance testing frequency recommended by the ACR is quarterly [29]. A semiannual performance test is a must.

The requirement on acceptance tests before clinical use is also applied to PET. Annual

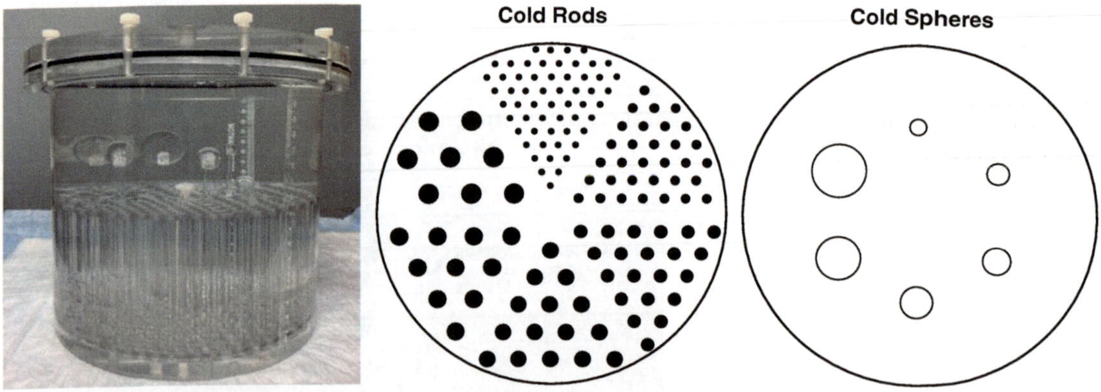

Fig. 9.8 Jaszczak Flangeless ECT phantom recommended by the ACR for the quality control of PET and SPECT systems

physics survey includes an ACR-approved phantom test and dose calibrators. The ACR-recommended Jaszczak Deluxe Flangeless ECT phantom (Fig. 9.8) can be used for both SPECT and PET to evaluate system performance, e.g., collimator, artifacts, calibration, and reconstruction parameters.

Dose Calibrator

The dose calibrator is a vital instrument in NM/MI because it ensures the accurate measurement of radiopharmaceutical activity before it is administered to patients. Proper quality control (QC) of the dose calibrator is critical to maintain the precision of dosage measurements, ensure patient safety, and comply with regulatory standards. Without accurate dosage measurements, patients could receive either too much radiation, increasing the risk of adverse effects, or too little, resulting in suboptimal imaging quality.

To ensure dose calibrators operate correctly, several key QC tests are required at various intervals, including tests for acceptance, constancy, accuracy, linearity, and geometry. Acceptance testing is performed when the dose calibrator is first installed. It verifies that the device meets the manufacturer's specifications and industry standards and establishes a baseline for future QC comparisons. This testing includes the evaluation of constancy, accuracy, linearity, and geometry.

Constancy testing is performed daily to confirm that the dose calibrator consistently measures the activity of a long-lived reference source. A radionuclide such as cesium-137 (^{137}Cs) is often used for this purpose, and its measured activity is compared to an established reference value. The acceptable range for constancy measurements is typically ±5%. This test ensures that the calibrator's performance remains stable over time and helps identify any drifts in measurement accuracy that could compromise patient safety.

Accuracy testing is conducted annually to verify that the dose calibrator provides correct activity readings across different radionuclides. It is essential to ensure that the calibrator measures a wide range of radionuclide energies accurately, as radiopharmaceuticals used in NM/MI have varying energy levels. Typically, two or more radionuclides, such as ^{131}I and ^{99m}Tc, are used to perform this test. The measured values should be within ±5% of the known activity to confirm that the dose calibrator remains accurate.

Linearity testing ensures that the dose calibrator measures both high and low activity levels accurately. This is particularly important because NM/MI procedures involve varying levels of radioactivity, depending on whether they are diagnostic or therapeutic. Linearity testing is typically conducted quarterly (recently changed to annually per the ACR) by measuring the decay of a high-activity radionuclide over time or by using a set of attenuators to simulate lower activity levels. The dose calibrator must maintain accuracy within ±5% across the full range of measured activities.

Geometry testing ensures that the dose calibrator provides consistent readings regardless of the size or shape of the container used to administer radiopharmaceuticals. Radiopharmaceuticals are delivered in vials and syringes of different sizes and volumes, and geometry testing verifies that these variations do not affect the activity measurements. The activity of a known volume of radioactive material is measured in containers of varying sizes, and the results are compared to ensure consistency, with deviations typically required to be within ±5%.

In addition, sensitivity tests may be performed to confirm that the dose calibrator can detect small amounts of radioactivity accurately. This is particularly relevant for diagnostic procedures where small dosages are administered and precise measurements are required.

Thyroid Uptake and Counting Systems

QC of thyroid uptake and counting systems is essential for ensuring accurate measurement of organ function and the assay of patient samples. These systems are primarily used to assess thyroid function by measuring the uptake of radionuclides like iodine-123 (^{123}I). Maintaining the system's accuracy and reliability through regular QC tests is critical for both diagnostic precision and patient safety. The key QC procedures include the following:

Energy calibration, linearity, and resolution: Energy calibration ensures that the system is correctly tuned to detect the specific energy peaks of radionuclides like ^{123}I. Regular checks using an ^{123}I capsule or a long-lived calibration source confirm that the system consistently identifies the correct energy peaks. Energy linearity verifies that the system responds correctly to a range of energies, ensuring accuracy across various radionuclides. Energy resolution measures the system's ability to distinguish between closely spaced energy peaks, ensuring that it can differentiate between radionuclides with similar energies. This combined testing ensures the system is precisely calibrated and capable of accurate radionuclide identification and measurement.

Minimum detectable activity (MDA) testing: MDA testing is crucial to verify the system's sensitivity to low levels of radioactivity. It determines the smallest activity level that the system can reliably detect, ensuring accurate measurement of low-level radionuclide uptake, which is especially important for assessing thyroid function. This test confirms the system's ability to detect trace amounts of radioactive material, ensuring clinical accuracy even in cases with minimal uptake.

Sensitivity testing: Sensitivity tests verify the system's capability to detect varying levels of radioactivity. This ensures that the system can measure both low and high activity levels accurately, which is essential for correct patient diagnosis. High sensitivity is critical for thyroid uptake studies, where the amount of radiopharmaceutical taken up by the thyroid gland may be very small.

Chi-square testing: The chi-square test is a statistical method used to assess the system's reliability and stability over time. By analyzing a series of counts from a constant source, the test checks whether the variations in the measured counts fall within the expected statistical range. Consistent chi-square results indicate stable and reliable performance, free from electronic instability or counting errors.

Background count: This test establishes a baseline radiation level by measuring environmental radiation in the absence of a radioactive source. Accurate background counting is essential for ensuring that patient sample measurements are not influenced by ambient radiation. By subtracting the background radiation from actual measurements, the system provides more accurate results.

High voltage/gain checks: High voltage or gain checks are critical to ensure the system's detector is operating at the correct voltage, which directly affects its sensitivity and energy calibration. Voltage fluctuations can lead to inaccurate results, so regular checks maintain stability and reliability in measurements.

Image Artifacts

Image artifacts in NM/MI, particularly in gamma camera, SPECT or SPECT/CT, and PET or PET/CT, can significantly affect diagnostic accuracy and patient safety. Artifacts arise from a variety of sources, including patient movement, equipment malfunction, and physical or technical limitations inherent to the imaging modality. In gamma camera imaging, one common artifact is related to nonuniformity in the detector response, often caused by improper calibration or issues with the photomultiplier tubes (PMTs). This can lead to areas of the image being falsely highlighted or diminished, potentially obscuring true pathological findings. Additionally, artifacts such as misalignment of the collimator or contamination on the detector surface can create false "hot spots" or "cold spots" in the image, which can be misinterpreted as abnormal findings [30, 31].

In SPECT imaging, artifacts frequently result from attenuation of the gamma rays by dense structures like bone or metal implants. This attenuation can cause errors in the reconstruction process, leading to distorted images. Attenuation correction techniques, such as those incorporating CT data in hybrid SPECT/CT systems, help mitigate these artifacts but can introduce new errors if the correction is not properly applied [32]. Motion artifacts are also a significant concern in SPECT, as patient movement during the scan can blur the image, especially in longer scans. Similarly, PET imaging is prone to artifacts from attenuation and motion. In addition, issues with time-of-flight (TOF) calibration, radiotracer biodistribution, or improper reconstruction algorithms can lead to false signals or distortions [31]. For both PET and SPECT, the presence of scatter from surrounding tissues also contributes to artifacts, which can degrade image quality and reduce the diagnostic utility of the scan [30].

Ongoing Efforts to Improve Quality and Safety

Efforts to improve quality and patient safety in NM/MI by organizations, clinical practice, and industry are discussed in the following:

Federal/Organizational Efforts

1. ACR accreditation

The ACR accreditation program is a continual effort to improve the quality of service to patients. The current NM/PET accreditation program includes general NM (planar imaging), body SPECT, nuclear cardiology imaging, and PET imaging. Besides applications for all modules performed at the site, the ACR also requires applications for all radioisotopes used on each unit. Similar to other imaging modalities, the ACR accreditation on NM has specific requirements for personnel (interpreting physicians, technologists, and medical physicists), performance testing, and QC program. In addition, the ACR accreditation program requires that the facilities monitoring cardiac stress studies have one individual who has current advanced cardiac life support (ACLS) certification present during the stress testing.

The ACR's efforts are also reflected in the optimization of radiopharmaceutical dosages through the establishment of diagnostic reference levels (DRLs) and achievable administered activities (AAAs). By adhering to these standards, imaging facilities can align their practices to ensure the use of the minimum effective radiopharmaceutical dosages while maintaining diagnostic image quality [33]. This strategy helps reduce patient radiation exposure, addressing safety concerns and enhancing the overall quality of diagnostic imaging.

2. Image Gently and Wisely Campaigns

Image Gently recently initiated the "Go-with-the-guideline" campaign dedicated to radiation protection for children undergoing NM/MI procedures. The campaign recommends following North American Consensus Guidelines for Administered Radiopharmaceutical Activities in Children and Adolescents by the Society of Nuclear Medicine and Molecular Imaging (SNMMI) [34]. The consensus includes dosages for 11 commonly used radiopharmaceuticals in terms of administered activity/kg and minimum administered radiopharmaceutical dosages for the smallest patients. The consensus guidelines differ significantly from the European Association for Nuclear Medicine (EANM) Pediatric Dose Card in several important respects:

- The administered activities in the consensus guidelines are slightly lower for infants and small children.
- Administered activities for ^{99m}Tc DMSA and ^{18}F NaF are considerably lower in the consensus guidelines.
- Administered activities for orally administered ^{99m}Tc-labeled radiopharmaceuticals and for radionuclide cystography provide a range of administered activities for each type of examination rather than an administered activity/kg.
- The consensus guidelines more closely represent clinical practice in North American pediatric centers.

The Image Wisely campaign [35] concerns radiation safety in adult medical imaging. The initiative aims to optimize radiation dose used in adult medical imaging and ensure that patients receive only necessary scans. It was a more recently launched campaign involving 3000 imaging providers at the time of access, including NM/MI.

The U. S. Nuclear Regulatory Commission (U. S. NRC) is considering requiring the reporting of NM/MI injection extravasations as medical events, a step aimed at enhancing quality and patient safety in NM/MI imaging. While the initiative seeks to improve transparency, reduce risks, and promote safer practices, it has generated some controversy. Critics argue that making extravasations reportable may impose additional regulatory burdens and question the clinical significance of some cases. Despite this debate, the proposal encourages the development of strategies to minimize extravasations and refine procedures, ultimately aiming to improve NM/MI imaging outcomes. For more details, visit the official NRC page [36].

Clinical Efforts

Clinical efforts to improve quality and patient safety include optimization of administered activity to reduce radiation dose, policies for the use and disposal of radioactive materials, radiation control by radiation safety committee, and continuous education program.

A number of NM/MI examinations deliver comparable patient effective doses as those by x-ray imaging, especially CT. However, there are no comparable effects to radiation dose reduction of NM/MI procedures as those in CT. This is partially due to the limited possibilities for the user. What the user can do is to control administered radioactivity with some options on the choice of equipment imaging parameters. The ability to detect and evaluate lesions depends largely on the concentration of the radiopharmaceutical in the organ/tissues, lesion itself, and biologic clearance rate. However, the relationship between NM/MI image quality and the amount of administered activity is controversial. It was reported that the image quality can be improved by increasing administered dosage [37]. This quality improvement is predicated on the increased radiation burden for the patient. The study on the relationship between administered radiopharmaceutical activity in myocardial perfusion scintigraphy and imaging outcomes showed that there was no evidence that higher activities improve imaging or clinical outcome [38]. The administered activity recommended by the SNMMI North American Consensus Guidelines for Administered Radiopharmaceutical Activities in Children and Adolescents is weight based. A recent study demonstrated that weight-based adjustment to the administered activity is suboptimal [39]. What we know so far implies that current administered activity for various NM/MI procedures may be far from optimized. Reduction in administered activity may still guarantee acceptable image quality [40]. Rigorous efforts are the key to balance the benefits of adequate image quality against the radiation risks.

Optimizing CT dose for attenuation correction in PET/CT and SPECT/CT imaging is essential to reduce radiation exposure, especially in pediatric patients. For low-dose CT attenuation correction, techniques such as lowering tube voltage, adjusting tube current, and utilizing automatic exposure control (AEC) are common [41]. Pediatric protocols are further optimized by tailoring radiation doses based on the child's size and weight, allowing sufficient image quality for attenuation correction without compromising patient safety. Iterative reconstruction methods like ASiR and SAFIRE further enhance image quality at reduced dosages [42].

The use of radioactive materials places another concern of patient safety. Every imaging facility has its own specific policies on the storage, delivery, and transfer of radioactive materials. Actions to radioactive spills and disposals are clearly addressed and strictly implemented. These policies are regularly reviewed and updated. Education lectures to staff are periodically provided.

Industry Efforts

PET (and PET/CT) and SPECT (and SPECT/CT) continue to evolve, with ongoing advancements in detector technology and image reconstruction algorithms. Industry efforts are focused on developing innovative detectors to improve detection efficiency, enabling more rapid image acquisition with higher quality and lower radiation doses for patients [43]. The increasing use of integrated (hybrid) modalities like SPECT/CT and PET/CT highlights the demand for continual improvements in detector systems to achieve better spatial resolution, sensitivity, and timing.

In parallel, newer reconstruction algorithms are being developed to integrate with improved hardware, particularly for handling time-of-flight (TOF) data. Novel approaches to attenuation and motion correction are also under active development, further enhancing image quality in PET and SPECT imaging. These innovations not only improve diagnostic accuracy but also reduce patient radiation exposure.

The integration of multi-modality techniques, such as SPECT/CT, PET/CT, and more recently, PET/MRI, is significantly advancing NM/MI. While NM/MI provides essential functional data, it is often complementary to CT or MRI, which offer superior anatomical details. SPECT/CT and PET/CT have become widely adopted in clinical practice due to their ability to combine both functional and anatomical information [2, 4, 44, 45], offering comprehensive insights into disease processes. Industry efforts to expand the clinical applications of PET/MRI, which reduces radiation by eliminating the need for CT, are rapidly growing, although the high cost and complexities of these systems limits widespread use [46–50].

The advent of modern digital detectors and whole-body PET/CT scanners has revolutionized NM/MI by improving detector efficiency. This allows for lower radiopharmaceutical dosages without compromising image quality, making frequent scans safer for patients, particularly in oncology, where repeated imaging is often required. TOF PET/CT scanners, for example, offer higher sensitivity, enabling reduced radiation doses and faster scanning times, while still detecting smaller lesions and improving diagnostic accuracy.

The integration of iterative reconstruction and AI-driven optimization in hybrid systems like SPECT/CT and PET/CT has significantly reduced radiation exposure while enhancing image quality. AI-based methods, such as deep learning algorithms, reduce noise, recover resolution, and leverage large datasets to produce clearer images, improving diagnostic accuracy and minimizing the need for repeat scans [51]. This not only reduces patient exposure to radiation but also allows for the use of lower dosages of radiotracers without compromising image quality. These advancements are especially crucial for vulnerable populations, such as children and patients requiring frequent imaging. By enhancing detector efficiency and enabling AI-assisted radiation dose management, these technologies push the boundaries of patient safety and ensure that lower radiation doses are used without sacrificing diagnostic precision.

Resources for Quality and Safety

Table 9.1 provides a summary of resources (e.g., QC recommendations, safety guidelines) for quality and safety in NM/MI. We include a selection of relevant references from the major organizations. The goal of this table is to facilitate readers' ability to readily access these resources.

It needs to be pointed out that most organizations do not function as enforcement agencies. Regulatory agencies that enforce the implementation of the recommendations/guidelines include the FDA, the Nuclear Regulatory Commission (NRC) and Agreement States, the Environment Protection Agency (EPA), and the Occupational Safety and Health Administration (OSHA).

Table 9.1 Resources for quality and safety in NM/MI

Nuclear medicine/molecular imaging (PET, SPECT)	
Planar imaging	**AAPM** Report No. 6: Scintillation Camera Acceptance Testing and Performance Evaluation **AAPM** Report No. 9: Computer-Aided Scintillation Camera Acceptance Testing **ACR** Nuclear Medicine/PET Accreditation Program **NCRP** Report No. 099: Quality Assurance for Diagnostic Imaging **ICRP** Publication 73: Radiological Protection and Safety in Medicine **ICRP** Report 80: Radiation Dose to Patients from Radiopharmaceuticals (Addendum to ICRP Publication 53) **ICRP** Report 53: Radiation Dose to Patients from Radiopharmaceuticals **NEMA** NU 1–2007: Performance Measurements of Gamma Cameras **NRC** 10 CFR 20.1201: Annual Dose Limits **NRC** 10 CFR: Part 35: Regulations on Medical Uses of Radioactive Material **NRC** 10 CFR 35.3045: Reporting Requirements for Medical Events **SNMMI**: North American Consensus Guidelines for Administered Radiopharmaceutical Activities in Children and Adolescents **IAEA** Quality Control Atlas for Scintillation Camera Systems
PET	**AAPM** Report No. 108: PET and PET/CT Shielding Requirements **ACR** Nuclear Medicine/PET Accreditation Program **ACR** Technical Standard for Medical Nuclear Physics Performance Monitoring of PET Imaging Equipment **NEMA** NU 2-2007: Performance Measurements of Positron Emission Tomography (PETs)
SPECT	**AAPM** Report No. 22: Rotating Scintillation Camera SPECT Acceptance Testing and Quality Control **AAPM** Report No. 52: Quantitation of SPECT Performance **ACR** Nuclear Medicine/PET Accreditation Program
General	**ICRP** Publication 84: Pregnancy and Medical Radiation **NCRP** Report No. 174: Preconception and Prenatal Radiation Exposure: Health Effects and Protective Guidance **IAEA** SPECT/CT Atlas of Quality Control and Image Artefacts, Human Health Series No. 36 **SNMMI**: 2024 Update of the North American Consensus Guidelines for Pediatric Administered Radiopharmaceutical Activities

AAPM: American Association of Physicists in Medicine
ACR: American College of Radiology
CRCPD: Conference of Radiation Control Program Directors
FDA: US Food and Drug Administration
IAEA: International Atomic Energy Agency
ICRP: International Commission on Radiological Protection
IEC: International Electrotechnical Commission
IMRSER: Institute for Magnetic Resonance Safety, Education, and Research
NCRP: National Council on Radiation Protection and Measurements
NEMA: National Electrical Manufacturers Association
NRC: Nuclear Regulatory Commission
SNMMI: Society of Nuclear Medicine and Molecular Imaging

Chapter Summary

This chapter presents both fundamental principles and associated intrinsic safety issues of the major NM/MI modalities: gamma camera, SPECT, and PET. While it is beyond this chapter's scope to comprehensively cover all details within these modalities, it is hoped that the major topics are addressed, and references within should provide more detailed explanations. We expect that this chapter provides essential information on quality and safety issues within the NM/MI modalities. Other quality and safety issues (e.g., informatics, communication issues) beyond imaging modalities are not covered in this chapter.

References

1. Johnson RD, et al. Introduction to the D-SPECT for technologists: workflow using a dedicated digital cardiac camera. J Nucl Med Technol. 2020;48(4):297–303.
2. Schöder H, Larson SM, Yeung HWD. PET/CT in oncology: integration into clinical management of lymphoma, melanoma, and gastrointestinal malignancies. J Nucl Med. 2004;45(1 suppl):72S–81S.
3. Andrade RS, et al. Posttreatment assessment of response using FDG-PET/CT for patients treated with definitive radiation therapy for head and neck cancers. Int J Radiat Oncol Biol Phys. 2006;65(5):1315–22.
4. Tian J, et al. Clinical application of PET/CT fusion imaging for three-dimensional myocardial scar and left ventricular anatomy during ventricular tachycardia ablation. J Cardiovasc Electrophysiol. 2009;20(6):597–604.
5. Lenze F, et al. Detection and differentiation of inflammatory versus fibromatous Crohn's disease strictures: prospective comparison of 18F-FDG-PET/CT, MR-enteroclysis, and transabdominal ultrasound versus endoscopic/histologic evaluation. Inflamm Bowel Dis. 2012;18(12):2252–60.
6. Mettler FA, et al. Effective doses in radiology and diagnostic nuclear medicine: a catalog1. Radiology. 2008;248(1):254–63.
7. Rinscheid A, et al. Radiation doses from low-dose CT scans in SPECT/CT and PET/CT examinations: a survey in Germany. Nuklearmedizin. 2022;61(4):294–300.
8. Li Y, et al. Effective radiation dose of 18F-FDG PET/CT: how much does diagnostic CT contribute? Radiat Prot Dosim. 2019;187(2):183–90.
9. Mohammadi N, Akhlaghi P. Evaluation of radiation dose to pediatric models from whole body PET/CT imaging. J Appl Clin Med Phys. 2022;23(4):e13545.
10. Saade C, Dib Nehme R, Zouain N. Weight-based protocols offer significant reduction in radiation dose without affecting PET-CT image quality. Radiol Technol. 2022;94(1):24–33.
11. ICRP. Radiation dose to patients from radiopharmaceuticals (Addendum to ICRP Publication 53). 1999, International commission on radiological protection.
12. ICRP. Report 53: radiation dose to patients from radiopharmaceuticals. International Commission on Radiological Protection; 1988.
13. NCRP. Report 124: sources and magnitude of occupational and public exposures from nuclear medicine procedures. National Council on Radiation Protection and Measurements; 1996.
14. Eckerman KF, Endo A. MIRD: radionuclide data and decay schemes. 2nd ed. Society for Nuclear Medicine; 2008.
15. Kappas C. Pregnancy and medical radiation. Radiat Phys Chem. 2022;201:110478.
16. 174, R.N., Preconception and prenatal radiation exposure: health effects and protective guidance. 2013.
17. SNMMI. 2024 Update of the North American Consensus Guidelines for Pediatric Administered Radiopharmaceutical Activities. [cited 2024 10/16]. Available from: https://snmmi.org/Web/Clinical-Practice/Procedure-Standards/Standards/2024-Update-of-the-North-American-Consensus-Guidelines-for-Pediatric-Administered-Radiopharmaceutica.Mobile.aspx
18. Giraudo C, et al. Pediatric imaging using PET/MR imaging. Magn Reson Imaging Clin N Am. 2023;31(4):625–36.
19. Chin J, et al. Update on pediatric nuclear medicine in acute care. Semin Nucl Med. 2023;53(6):820–39.
20. Poli GL, et al. Developing and implementing an imaging optimization study in pediatric nuclear medicine: experience and recommendations from an IAEA-coordinated research project. J Nucl Med. 2021;62(4):570–6.
21. Release of patients after therapy with unsealed radionuclides. Ann ICRP. 2004;34(2):v-vi, 1–79.
22. 155, N.R.N., Management of radionuclide therapy patients. 2006.
23. NRC, U.S., Guidance for the release of patients administered radioactive materials. 2019.
24. U.S. NRC NUREG-1556, V., Rev. 3:, Consolidated guidance about materials licenses: program-specific guidance about medical use licenses. 2019.
25. NCRP, Report No. 099: quality assurance for diagnostic imaging. 1998.
26. AAPM. Scintillation camera acceptance testing and performance evaluation. American Association of Physicists in Medicine; 1980.
27. AAPM. Computer-aided scintillation camera acceptance testing. American Association of Physicists in Medicine; 1981.
28. ACR. Technical standard for medical nuclear physics performance monitoring of PET imaging equipment. American College of Radiology; 2011.

29. ACR, PET module program requirements. American College of Radiology.
30. Pryma DA. Nuclear medicine: practical physics, artifacts, and pitfalls. Oxford University Press; 2014.
31. Rajai P, et al. Unusual artifacts encountered during routine studies on positron emission tomography-computed tomography and gamma camera. Indian J Nucl Med. 2024;39(1):43–6.
32. AGENCY, N.A.E., SPECT/CT Atlas of quality control and image artefacts. IAEA Human Health Series No. 36, IAEA, Vienna 2019.
33. Becker MD, et al. U.S. PET/CT and gamma camera diagnostic reference levels and achievable administered activities for noncardiac nuclear medicine studies. Radiology. 2019;293(1):203–11.
34. Image Gently's "Go with the guidelines" campaign 2024 [cited 2024 10/16]; Available from: https://www.imagegently.org/Procedures/Nuclear-Medicine
35. The Image Wiisely. [cited 2024 10/16]; Available from: https://www.imagewisely.org/Imaging-Modalities/Nuclear-Medicine
36. NRC. Reporting nuclear medicine injection extravasations as medical events. [cited 2014 10/17]; Available from: https://www.nrc.gov/materials/miau/med-use-toolkit/reporting-nuclear-medicine-injection-extravasations.html
37. Stefanoyiannis AP, Gerogiannis I, Geronikola-Trapali X, Armeniakos I, Prentakis A. Effect of administered radioactive dose level on image quality of brain perfusion imaging with 99mTc-HMPAO. J Eng Sci Technol Rev. 2008:66–9.
38. Robinson CN, et al. The relationship between administered radiopharmaceutical activity in myocardial perfusion scintigraphy and imaging outcome. Eur J Nucl Med Mol Imaging. 2008;35(2):329–35.
39. Sgouros G, et al. An approach for balancing diagnostic image quality with cancer risk: application to pediatric diagnostic imaging of 99mTc-dimercaptosuccinic acid. J Nucl Med. 2011;52(12):1923–9.
40. Díaz MP, et al. Administered activity optimization in 99mTc-MAG3 renography for adults. J Nucl Med Technol. 2003;31(4):216–21.
41. Bebbington NA, et al. Ultra-low-dose CT for attenuation correction: dose savings and effect on PET quantification for protocols with and without tin filter. EJNMMI Phys. 2023;10(1):66.
42. Gould S-M, et al. Optimisation of CT protocols in PET-CT across different scanner models using different automatic exposure control methods and iterative reconstruction algorithms. EJNMMI Phys. 2021;8(1):58.
43. Lewellen TK. Recent developments in PET detector technology. Phys Med Biol. 2008;53(17):R287.
44. Kim EE. Clinical PET-CT in radiology: integrated imaging in oncology. J Nucl Med. 2012;53(3):505.
45. Ell PJ. The contribution of PET/CT to improved patient management. Br J Radiol. 2006;79(937):32–6.
46. Judenhofer MS, et al. Simultaneous PET-MRI: a new approach for functional and morphological imaging. Nat Med. 2008;14(4):459–65.
47. Pichler BJ, et al. PET/MRI: paving the way for the next generation of clinical multimodality imaging applications. J Nucl Med. 2010;51(3):333–6.
48. Lee WW, et al. PET/MRI of inflammation in myocardial infarction. J Am Coll Cardiol. 2012;59(2):153–63.
49. Glaudemans A, Quintero A, Signore A. PET/MRI in infectious and inflammatory diseases: will it be a useful improvement? Eur J Nucl Med Mol Imaging. 2012;39(5):745–9.
50. Wang Y-R, et al. Low-count whole-body PET/MRI restoration: an evaluation of dose reduction spectrum and five state-of-the-art artificial intelligence models. Eur J Nucl Med Mol Imaging. 2023;50(5):1337–50.
51. Reader AJ, Pan B. AI for PET image reconstruction. Br J Radiol. 2023;96(1150):20230292.

Index

J. Zhang (ed.), *Quality and Patient Safety in Medical Imaging*,
https://doi.org/10.1007/978-3-031-89007-9

GPSR Compliance

The European Union's (EU) General Product Safety Regulation (GPSR) is a set of rules that requires consumer products to be safe and our obligations to ensure this.

If you have any concerns about our products, you can contact us on ProductSafety@springernature.com

In case Publisher is established outside the EU, the EU authorized representative is:

Springer Nature Customer Service Center GmbH
Europaplatz 3
69115 Heidelberg, Germany

Batch number: 10732809

Printed by Printforce, the Netherlands